Rethinking Sport and Exercise Psychology Research

Peter Hassmén • Richard Keegan • David Piggott

Rethinking Sport and Exercise Psychology Research

Past, Present and Future

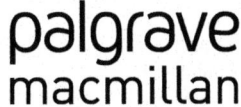

palgrave
macmillan

Peter Hassmén
School of Health and Human Sciences
Southern Cross University
Coffs Harbour
New South Wales
Australia

Richard Keegan
Research Institute for Sport and Exercise
University of Canberra
Canberra
Australian Capital Territory
Australia

David Piggott
Leeds Beckett University
Leeds
United Kingdom

ISBN 978-1-137-48337-9   ISBN 978-1-137-48338-6   (eBook)
DOI 10.1057/978-1-137-48338-6

Library of Congress Control Number: 2016957340

Cover illustration: © Daniel Rodríguez Quintana, iStock / Getty Images Plus

Printed on acid-free paper

This Palgrave Macmillan imprint is published by Springer Nature
The registered company is Macmillan Publishers Ltd. London
The registered company address is: The Campus, 4 Crinan Street, London, N1 9XW, United Kingdom

Contents

List of Figures

List of Tables

1

Why Rethink?

Introduction

The title of this book is ambitious; radical, even. It implies some fundamental change is needed in the way we do research in sport and exercise
psychology; and further, that we can diagnose the problems of the *past*
and *present* and prescribe the solutions for the *future*. It is important,
therefore, that we first qualify these bold claims—of past errors and for
better ways forward—and add the necessary caveats that all good fallibil-
ists must make. Foremost among these is the caveat that, since we have 'a
stake in the game', we aim to describe (Bourdieu, 1975: p. 40), we must
first acknowledge our own strategies and assumptions and the lenses
through which we will view the strategies of others. Since this is a book
partly about how sport and exercise psychologists *do* research, some of
our lenses are psychological and sociological (or historical) in nature. Yet
where we venture into questions of how research *should* be conducted
(and disseminated), theories from psychology and sociology have only
limited value. It is in these cases, then, that we draw more explicitly
on normative philosophical theory. In making our theoretical stance
more explicit, we hope to promote more open and transparent debate,

© The Author(s) 2016
P. Hassmén et al., *Rethinking Sport and Exercise Psychology Research*,
DOI 10.1057/978-1-137-48338-6_1

making it easier for our inevitable critics to engage with the arguments we intend to make.

An early example of the type of work we aim to undertake in this book is Rainer Martens' paper from the first issue of *The Sport Psychologist* characterising two sport psychologies: academic sport psychology and practicing sport psychology (Martens, 1987). Of these two approaches to research, the orthodox 'academic' approach tended to dominate the field up to the late 1980s, argues Martens, and continues to be highly influential (Keegan, 2015; Vealey, 2006). In this orthodox academic approach, research is conducted in laboratory settings by objective scientists, conducting controlled experiments, while seeking answers to questions that lack practical relevance. Martens criticises this approach to research, pointing out (rightly) that: (a) researchers are not and cannot be objective; (b) that psychological theories are insufficiently developed to allow for controlled lab-based research; and (c) that the findings of such studies lack relevance to practitioners. Martens' alternative 'practicing' sport psychology, based on a 'heuristic' view of science, is more appropriate, he argues, due to a close connection with practitioners and their real-world problems. The heuristic view involves a more realistic and flexible approach to research where prior knowledge and bias is acknowledged (and used), and where a range of alternative methodologies (e.g. more qualitative and idiographic approaches) are applied in problem solving situations.

Martens' paper raised some important questions for researchers in the late 1980s that remain relevant today. What kinds of research are people doing in sport and exercise psychology? What are the implications of taking different approaches? What can we claim (and not claim) for research findings derived from different 'paradigms'? What constitutes progress in sport and exercise psychology? Unfortunately, Martens' analysis was based on a personal and partial evaluation of research conduct of the time and his theoretical understanding of 'the scientific method' was narrow and occasionally misinformed. His ultimate conclusion—that the 'heuristic paradigm' is better and deserves much more attention to enrich the existing body of knowledge—is therefore difficult to accept. It is these two flaws—the lack of evidence of the existence of the two positions and the over-simplified conceptualisation of science—that we aim to address and correct in this book. By conducting more systematic surveys of research conduct in sport and exercise psychology on the one hand, and interpreting this conduct against more explicit psychological, sociological and philosophical theory on the other, we hope to bring up to date and develop the important discussion that Martens initiated back in the late 1980s.

Since Martens' analysis began with the flawed assumption that there is such a thing as an orthodox scientific method—a strange and incoherent hybrid of Baconian and Popperian ideas—it seems sensible and necessary to begin the book with an extended exploration of the different views on this subject, thereby allowing critics to examine our 'philosophical baggage' before it is taken on board, enabling a more constructive debate (Dennett, 1995: p. 21). Although this is a book about research in sport and exercise psychology, we argue throughout that in order to gain the necessary critical distance from the field, it is important to draw on ideas and theories from outside of the discipline. Hence, in this first chapter, we focus primarily on introducing the main sociological and philosophical ideas that underpin much of the analysis are arguments that follow in the more substantive chapters.

Philosophical Baggage

With the exponential growth of science in the last century, professional philosophers developed a parallel concern for explaining this progress. Starting with the so-called Vienna Circle in the 1930s, through the intellectual high-point of the 1960s and 1970s, and concluding with the so-called postmodern turn and the 'science wars' of the 1980s and 1990s, philosophy of science emerged as a fertile field of study in the twentieth century (Fuller, 2006). Of the many well-known names associated with the many and varied debates, we have chosen to focus on just four: Popper, Kuhn, Lakatos and Feyerabend. Aside from being perhaps the best-known philosophers of science of the last century (Agassi, 2014; Stove, 1982), our four protagonists also represent a broad range of contrasting positions, therefore enabling the widest possible debate. We begin this chapter proper with an outline of each position and the main points of agreement and disagreement between them. The order of presentation is chronological not hierarchical (i.e. Feyerabend does not necessarily represent an improvement on Popper), and it should be noted that, while we have tried to present a nuanced and critical narrative in each case, space demands a somewhat caricatured account.

Karl Popper and 'Critical Rationalism'

As the clock struck 7.30 p.m. on October 13, 1958, the audience looked on in anticipation as two men approached the lectern at the annual meeting of the Aristotelian Society in Bedford Square, London. The first man was a solid and self-confident figure; the second man was small and unimpressive with no presence at all. Yet to the surprise of the audience, still drying themselves after the downpour outside, it was the second man who was to give the presidential address. Over the following hour, the speaker proceeded to demolish hundreds of years of philosophising on scientific method, including the ideas of many members of the distinguished audience. According to one eyewitness report,[1] the ideas were too radical to be fully appreciated at the time, and the following debate focussed on particular historical interpretations of certain pre-Socratic philosophers. It would be another year before the president's landmark text, *The Logic of Scientific Discovery*, was published in English, and a further six years before 'Sir' Karl Popper would be considered the world authority on scientific method.

The summer of 1919 was instrumental in Popper's intellectual development (Popper, 1969). The ideas he would unleash on the unsuspecting audience at the Aristotelian Society almost 40 years later were forged in interwar Vienna. Many of Popper's core ideas were developed, characteristically, through a process of criticism, the most well known of which are probably *falsification* (or the *demarcation criterion*) and the *hypothetico-deductive* method. These related ideas first occurred to Popper as a 17-year-old as he noticed important differences in the popular scientific theories of the time. Specifically, he noticed that his socialist friends

---

[1] This 'creative non-fiction' is derived from Bryan Magee's account of his first face-to-face encounter with Popper (Magee, 1998). Magee's earlier book on Popper (Magee, 1973) is an excellent (and mercifully brief) introductory text.

and psychoanalysts were impressed by the seemingly infinite explanatory power of the theories of Marx and Freud, respectively. Everything could be explained by these theories, yet they ruled nothing out. Critics who raised contradictory evidence were summarily dismissed: the critics of Marx were under the spell of 'false consciousness'; those who denied Freud were suffering from un-analysed 'repressions' (Popper, 1969: pp. 46–47). In stark contrast, Einstein's theory, which had been tested that year by Eddington's observations, was:

> ...utterly different from the dogmatic attitude of Marx, Freud and Adler... Einstein was looking for crucial experiments whose agreement with his predictions would by no means establish his theory; while disagreement, as he would be the first to stress, would show his theory to be untenable. This, I felt, was the true scientific attitude... Thus I arrived... at the conclusion that the scientific attitude was the critical attitude, which did not look for verifications, but for crucial tests; tests which could refute the theory tested, though they could never establish it. (Popper, 1978: p. 38)

Popper began to see that these different types of theories were associated with very different methods. The theories of Freud and Marx were considered scientific because they had been arrived at through systematic and 'objective' observations; that is, they had an empirical basis. Einstein, by contrast, had proposed a bold and exciting conjecture and defined the conditions under which it should be tested. Later, in his *Logik der Forschung* (1934), Popper developed formal logical arguments against the theory of induction—the dominant explanation of scientific method since Bacon's *Novum Organum* inspired the Royal Society—and of the logical positivism of the Vienna Circle: the theories of science he felt had granted undeserved credibility to Freud and Marx.

With respect to induction, Popper argued that valid knowledge could not be the product of repeated observations for two main reasons: (1) all observation is preceded by theory; we cannot observe without a point of view—we are not 'white paper' as Locke supposed—so induction is mistaken; (2) since there might always be a falsifying instance, or 'black swan', around the corner, we have no reason (logically) to expect the future to follow the past. Induction, Popper argued, is neither logically or psychologically necessary as an explanation of the growth of knowledge. It is entirely dispensable; an optical illusion (Magee, 1973: p. 31). The only reasonable way to proceed, then, is to create bold and imaginative theories to solve problems and submit them to criticism by searching for falsifying instances. Theories that are formulated in such a way as to be easily testable, or *falsifiable*, are scientific (as was the case with Einstein); theories that avoid criticism, like those of Marx and Freud, are *pseudoscientific* and dogmatic (Popper, 1969). In this way, Popper developed his famous *demarcation criterion* between science and pseudoscience.

Popper's central argument here was to point out the logical asymmetry between verification and falsification: no amount of evidence can prove you right; yet any amount of evidence can prove you wrong. Much academic labour can be (and has been) wasted, warned Popper, searching for verifications of, or supporting evidence for, a theory. Building up huge piles of evidence in support of pet theories is, in Popper's view, anti-scientific; and the theories developed in this way *pseudoscientific*. So, if scientific theories are testable, in spite of being unprovable (Magee, 1973), we are left with knowledge that is *fallible*, but which can be improved (or made more 'truth-like') through rigorous theory testing and the elimination or errors. Popper was therefore both a realist and a fallibilist.

Truth, for Popper, was an important regulative concept. Progress in science 'involves increase in truth content' (Popper, 1974: p. 1102) which means that theories have to explain known facts (i.e. they have to be as good as rival theories in this respect) *and* predict new facts. Theories with greater empirical content have greater testability since they specify the conditions under which they would fail. Having been subjected to and survived a series of tests, a theory has a greater 'degree of corroboration' which is 'synonymous with the degree of severity of the tests it has passed' (Popper, 1959: p. 392). Scientists should therefore 'hold on, for the time being, to the most improbable of the surviving theories, or more precisely, to the one that can be most severely tested (i.e. that has greatest explanatory power, content, simplicity and is least *ad hoc*)' (Popper, 1959: p. 419). Saving a theory from criticism by inventing ad hoc hypotheses is a cardinal sin for the Popperian scientist, whose attitude is described succinctly by Magee (1973: p. 23):

Popper proposes, as an article of method [rather than logic], that we do not systematically evade refutation, whether by introducing *ad hoc* hypotheses, or *ad hoc* definitions, or by always refusing to accept the reliability of inconvenient experimental results, or by any other such device; and that we formulate our theories as unambiguously as we can, so as to expose them as clearly as possible to refutation.

Here we see, for the first time, another important element of Popperian thought: the distinction between logic and method. In much of his work, Popper used logical analyses as the basis for methodological *prescriptions*. He was prepared to accept, if only reluctantly, that scientists may act in illogical and irrational ways (e.g. by saving theories from criticism with ad hoc hypotheses), but remained optimistic in developing his normative theories for scientific method. Popper's so-called *hypothetico-deductive* method, therefore, is a prescription for developing theories to solve problems; deducing solutions (or making predictions); and then testing the predictions against experience. In later work, Popper came to express this method in a brief four-stage schema, represented below (Magee, 1973: p. 65):

$$P^1 \rightarrow TS \rightarrow EE \rightarrow P^2$$

P^1 stands for the initial problem, or *problem situation*, since all problems have a history, including previous unsuccessful attempted solutions. This problem must be formulated as clearly as possible by the researcher to enable others to understand, criticise and help solve the problem. **TS** is the *tentative solution* offered by the researcher, which is often the product of intuition or creative insight. Again, as we have seen, tentative theories must be formulated clearly; they must explain known facts and also predict new facts. As one of Popper's famous students put it: 'a theory must be made to stick its neck out' (Lakatos, 1970: p. 111). There then follows the all important **EE**, or *error elimination*, stage (sometimes written as CD for critical discussion). Here, the task is to design and execute the most severe test of the theory imaginable. The harsher the test, the greater the degree of corroboration of a theory. Again, this is a side of scientific activity which demands creativity, a quality that some Popperians have tried hard to promote (e.g. Medawar, 1969). By eliminating errors in theories, or discarding them altogether, we move towards more truth-like (or better corroborated) accounts of the phenomena under study. A by-product of this critical process is *new problems* (P^2), fundamentally different to the initial problem, which would have been temporarily solved or changed in light of the investigation.

To illustrate by example, consider how a Popperian researcher might engage with the popular psychological phenomenon of 'flow'. Csikszentmihalyi (2002) defines nine dimensions of flow, five of which describe broad characteristics of the experience (sense of control, action-awareness merging, loss of self-consciousness, time transformation, auto-telic experience), and four of which suggest conditions (challenge-skills balance, clear goals, unambiguous feedback, concentration). It is also argued that flow precedes optimal experience and, by association, optimal performance in sport (Jackson & Roberts, 1992). The Popperian may begin, therefore, by determining a problem to which flow presents a tentative solution (e.g. how can an athlete get into the optimal psychological state to perform at their best?). They would then proceed to articulate the theory in its simplest and strongest possible form and determine the conditions under which the theory would fail (i.e. they would need to specify what kinds of severe tests they could conduct).

This second step is problematic, as recent research has suggested that flow is undertheorised (Swann, Keegan, Piggott, Crust, & Smith, 2012). Specifically, the particular combination or sequence of conditions that cause flow are poorly understood. Moreover, there is not even agreement about how many of the 'dimensions' need to be present before a flow state can be classified (Cf. Jackson, 1996). In short, flow has a low level of corroboration because: (a) it has not been formulated in a testable form (though see Swann, Crust, Keegan, Piggott, & Hemmings, 2015) and (b) has therefore not been subjected to any serious criticism. Very few papers challenge Csikszentmihalyi's nine dimensions with much of the contemporary research employing psychometric instruments that continue to verify the theory (Jackson, Martin, & Eklund, 2008). One may argue that, from a Popperian perspective, flow researchers have been 'playing tennis with the net down' (Khalil, 1987: p. 123), and given that flow was first theorised 40 years ago, with applications to sport since 1992, this reflects very poor progress.

Popper was a perfectionist polymath genius and workaholic. He would frequently work through the night, all days of the week, for most of the year, only taking brief walking holidays in the Alps for recovery. He therefore made important advances in a range of fields, including logic, probability theory, epistemology, political science and metaphysics. We have only touched on a narrow segment of his work here—the philosophy of science that he came to call *critical rationalism*—yet the full force of Popper's thought is hard to appreciate without an understanding of the relationships between his ideas across these fields (Magee, 1973: p. 17; Fuller, 2006: p. 26). For the scientists, politicians and historians who have invested in this endeavour, Popper's 'philosophy of action' has had a 'highly practical effect' (Magee, 1973: p. 10). Nobel Prize winners in biology (Sir Peter Medawar, Jacques Monod), physiology (Sir John Eccles) and physics (Sir Hermann Bondi) and well-known economists (e.g. Taleb, 2007) have all expressed an explicit debt to Popper's very practical influence on their approach to science. However, Popper has had his fair share of criticism, too. The best known of his critics was the American historian, Thomas Kuhn, who opened up a critical debate where Popper's former students, much to his chagrin, would come to play a central role.

Thomas Kuhn and 'Normal Science'

At the age of 27, with a freshly minted PhD and a Junior Fellowship at Harvard, Thomas Kuhn strode confidently into the first of the 1950 William James Lectures, expecting a show. He was not disappointed. Having already decided to dedicate himself to the study of science, Kuhn was enraptured by the lecturer—one Karl Popper—and his narrative of bold and inventive scientists, liberally criticising one another's theories through crucial experiments. This story was very different from the prevailing positivist historical account, which characterised science as a plodding, objective and cumulative enterprise. Yet despite his attraction to Popper's revolutionary philosophy, Kuhn left the lecture theatre with a niggling sense of doubt about its accuracy as a historical account.[2] Fifteen years later, Kuhn and Popper would meet again, but on that occasion Kuhn, as author of the wildly successful text, *The Structure of Scientific Revolutions*, would have star billing.

The meeting in question took place on July 13, 1965, at the International Colloquium in the Philosophy of Science at Bedford College, London. Although Popper chaired the session that afternoon, Kuhn's work was very much the focus of attention in the subsequent publication (Lakatos & Musgrave, 1970). In their exchange, Kuhn initially took a highly deferential stance, possibly due to Popper's recent knighthood, pointing out all the points where he and 'Sir Karl' agreed. Like Popper, Kuhn argued that we approach everything in light of a preconceived theory and that science moves forward in leaps when scientists engage in criticism of theories (Rowbottom, 2011). Kuhn, however, fundamentally disagreed about the frequency with which such criticism might occur. Where Popper imagined criticism to be *the* crucial characteristic of science, Kuhn—through his historical studies of post-enlightenment astronomy, physics and chemistry—felt that this attitude occurred only very rarely, under special social conditions (Kuhn, 1970). In short, Kuhn felt that Popper had overemphasised the 'revolutionary' side of science, ignoring almost completely the actual practice of scientists, or what he called 'normal science'. Since Kuhn's book has become so popular, with over 80,000 academic citations to date, and thus subject to mass misinterpretation and widespread misunderstanding (not least by Martens, 1987), it is worth tracing his ideas closely, as they appear in *The Structure of Scientific Revolutions*, before engaging in a critical review.

In outline, Kuhn's (1962/1996) narrative has three main parts: (a) he begins with a description of the characteristics of 'paradigms', or social formations wherein scientists engage in 'normal science'; (b) he goes on to explain how 'scientific revolutions' occur, following the build-up of 'anomalies' which eventually lead to a 'crisis' in the community;

---

[2] This sketch is constructed from numerous sources, including Kuhn (1974: p. 817), Preston (2008: pp. 5–4) and a brief primary account from *The Harvard Crimson* (anonymous author, Feb 17 1950).

(c) finally, Kuhn describes 'conversion processes' and the ways in which young scientists are socialised into the new paradigm, before considering, in conclusion, how progress in science can be understood. We look at each of these three stages in more detail below.

In developing his concept of a paradigm, Kuhn drew explicitly on the work of Polanyi (tacit knowledge) and Wittgenstein (language games) (Kuhn, 1962/1996: pp. 44–45). Paradigms contain theories, exemplars and methods that are accepted without question by the community, binding members together through a common set of assumptions. He argues that scientific communities cohere around a paradigm, which, though often not understood explicitly, enables scientists to determine significant facts, suggest problems or puzzles to solve and offers exemplars for solving them (ibid: pp. 25–34). Paradigms are formed through a process of debate, where groups of scientists come to adopt similar views, eventually forming distinct 'schools' of thought. One school will eventually come to be perceived to be more successful—that is, its paradigm will be most effective in suggesting and solving new puzzles—at which point *all* scientists in the field will 'convert' to the dominant paradigm and engage in 'normal science' (see Fig. 1.1). To use Fuller's (2006: p. 37) colourful terms, the 'paradigm succeeds in monopolising the means of intellectual reproduction' much in the same way as did the Ministry of Truth in George Orwell's *Nineteen Eighty-Four*.

The paradigm, then, provides both the 'rules of the game' and the nature of the intended outcome in science (Rowbottom, 2011: p. 122). Kuhn was clear that, unlike Popper's notion of theory testing, activity in a paradigm was self-referential and inherently dogmatic. No scientist challenges the theory (or theories) at its centre, partly because of the way they have been trained, and partly because the paradigm has a real perceptual effect of closing down the scientist's awareness of alternative ways of looking at things. As Kuhn points out: 'work in the paradigm can be conducted in no other way, and to desert the paradigm is to cease practicing the science it defines' (Kuhn, 1962/1996: p. 34). This means that normal scientists develop a 'monomaniacal concern with a single point of view' (Feyerabend, 1970: p. 201), becoming 'intolerant of theories invented by others', with a literal 'inability to see phenomena that do not fit the paradigm' (Kuhn, 1962/1996: p. 24). Kuhn therefore characterised normal

Fractured Debate   Schools   Paradigm

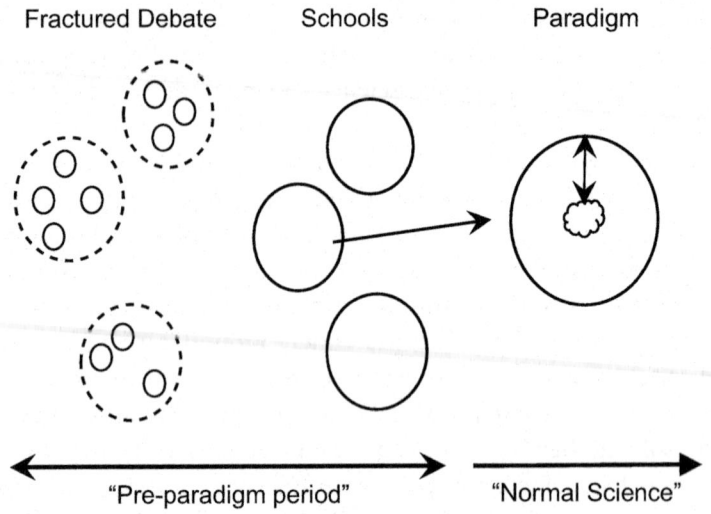

"Pre-paradigm period"   "Normal Science"

Fig. 1.1   The process of paradigm formation (Adapted from Kuhn, 1962/1996: p. 48)

science as a 'mopping-up operation' or puzzle-solving activity where the aim is to 'solve problems with known solutions (supplied by the paradigm) that test the skill of the scientist' (ibid: pp. 36–37).

Kuhn marshalled his historical examples—mainly from chemistry, astronomy and physics—to show that the paradigm (and associated professionalisation) has a twofold effect on science: first, it leads to 'immense restriction of the scientist's vision and to a considerable resistance to paradigm change' and, second, to an increase in the detail and precision of observation and information (e.g. the development of precision instruments and apparatus) (ibid: p. 65). For Kuhn, the first effect explains why periods of normal science may last for generations, while the second effect explains the great pace of 'progress' in science:

> So long as the tools a paradigm supplies continue to prove capable of solving the problems it defines, science moves fastest and penetrates most deeply through confident employment of these tools… retooling is an extravagance to be reserved for the occasion that demands it. (ibid: p. 76)

Kuhn drew on Bruner and Postman's psychological experiments on perception incongruity (ibid: pp. 62–64) to explain how these rare 'retooling' occasions, or revolutions, might occur. In short, he argued that the awareness of anomalies in the paradigm opens up a sort of window in which conceptual categories become adjusted. Since this is one of the most controversial parts of Kuhn's explanation (Cf. Fuller, 2006; Rowbottom, 2011), it is worth a closer look.

Under normal science, any scientist who discovers evidence that runs counter to the paradigm (i.e. an anomaly), which is at any rate highly unlikely, would assume a mistake on their part, rather than declare the paradigm 'refuted'. Like the poor carpenter who blames his tools, it is a poor normal scientist who blames his paradigm (Kuhn, 1962/1996: p. 80). Yet some anomalies are deemed worthy of scrutiny, and are identified by the scientist who 'can apply the precision instruments to locate anticipated phenomena, *but also* recognise that something has gone wrong' (ibid: p. 65). Kuhn offered some characteristic examples but admitted that he had 'no fully general answer' to the question of how such crises arise (ibid: p. 82). He conjectured that some anomalies that begin as puzzles eventually turn into Popperian counter instances and are likely to be noticed by younger scientists whose indoctrination is not yet total.

As anomalies accumulate and crisis sets in, so begins a brief but stormy period of extraordinary science. Here Kuhn draws on an extended analogy with political revolutions to explain the process of paradigm change. Revolutions are initiated by a growing sense that the existing institutions cannot solve important problems. And because there are no supra-institutional (or supra-paradigmatic) authorities to adjudicate between polarised 'camps', there is a 'resort to techniques of mass persuasion' (ibid: p. 93). Debates about the choice between paradigms are therefore necessarily circular since each group uses the paradigm to argue in the paradigm's defence (ibid: p. 94). In short, a paradigm shift is irrational.

Revolutions, for Kuhn, involve a Gestalt switch on the part of scientists who adopt new instruments and look in new places: 'what were ducks in the scientist's world before the revolution are rabbits afterwards' (ibid: p. 111). The conversion process to a new period of normal science, however, is a long, piecemeal process (see Fig. 1.1). Full conversion may occur over a generation, with conversions happening 'a few at a time until, after the last holdouts have died, the whole profession is practicing under a single, but now different, paradigm' (ibid: p. 152). Again, Kuhn's response to deeper and more detailed sociological question of 'how conversion is induced and resisted' is evasive: 'our question is a new one', he claims, 'so we shall have to settle for a very partial and impressionistic survey' (ibid: p. 152). One part of this process on which Kuhn had much to say, however, was the training of the next generation, once a new period of normal science has been established.

The process of socialisation into science was, for Kuhn, highly authoritarian. He believed that 'science students accept theory on the authority of the teacher and the text, not because of the evidence' (ibid: p. 80). Popper was disgusted, of course, countering that the normal scientist 'has been badly taught... a victim of indoctrination' (Popper, 1970: p. 53). Yet under Kuhn's system textbooks were a source of great importance and interest, representing critical 'pedagogical vehicles for the perpetuation of normal science' (Kuhn, 1962/1996: p. 136). Textbooks, thought Kuhn, are written in very deliberate ways to depict a version of history and an interpretation of the facts that fit the dominant paradigm. Indeed, the highly selective examples that 'entangle theory with exemplary explanation' often found in textbooks 'suggests applications *are* the evidence of the theory' (ibid: p. 80). Textbooks also play an important 'bonding' role in scientific communities through: (a) communicating the vocabulary and syntax of the scientific language; (b) actively obfuscating the ways in which normal science was established; and (c) through selection and distortion, depicting science as a cumulative (as opposed to a punctuated) activity (ibid: pp. 136–141).

Having explained the nature of a paradigm, the normal science that it entails, and the processes by which paradigms change and new generations are indoctrinated, Kuhn concludes by turning to the thorny issue of *progress*. As we have seen, Popper was a realist who used 'truth' as a regulative concept: a yardstick against which to measure progress. Kuhn, by contrast, was very much a relativist (although he argued otherwise). Since there can be no supra-paradigmatic standards for judging between theories, 'progress lies simply in the eyes of the beholder' (ibid: p. 163). Kuhn equated progress, rather, as a function of the *rate* of puzzle-solving.

Because of the absence of competing schools and the associated absence of peer scrutiny—since peers in a paradigm agree on fundamentals—scientists can 'get on with puzzle-solving largely uninhibited' (ibid: p. 163). Again, in complete contrast to Popper, progress is greatest, for Kuhn, when science is at its most dogmatic. The vision of the scientist as professional technician now appears, as Kuhn claim that 'unlike engineers and doctors… the scientist need not choose problems because they urgently need solution' (ibid: p. 164). For Kuhn, this fact also explains the different rates of progress in the natural and social sciences: where the latter choose difficult problems of social importance, the former, through their insulation from wider society, can simply busy themselves with puzzle-solving. Which group, asks Kuhn rhetorically, 'would one expect to solve problems at a more rapid rate?' (ibid: p. 164).

So what of Kuhn's influence in sport and exercise psychology? We take an example from one of the most popular fields of research at present: motivation and self-determination (Chap. 4 includes a more detailed investigation). In the preface to their *Handbook of Self-Determination Research*, Deci and Ryan (2002) describe the origins of their text, reporting on a 1999 conference, where:

> people came with a shared vocabulary, a shared set of concepts, a shared system of thought and a shared familiarity with the extensive research literature. This allowed everyone to begin immediately discussing important and penetrating issues. (p. x)

There follows a series of papers where Self-Determination Theory (SDT) is applied and extended in a host of disparate fields. Then, in the final chapter, where 'future directions' are suggested, Kuhn's influence is once again evident, with exhortations to 'test, extend and refine the tenets of SDT… apply the concepts to new domains… [and] integrate research findings from a multitude of studies' all under the metatheory which gives the concepts their 'true meaning' (Deci & Ryan, 2002: p. 432). In their final rallying call, Deci and Ryan (2002: p. 433) remind their reader that 'several major theoretical problems remain to be solved, new areas of application await careful consideration, and countless refinements would make the theory more exhaustive and precise'. In our own studies of the application of SDT in sport and exercise psychology (see Chap. 4), we have noted how studies over the last 5 years have drawn heavily on correlation methodology. There is a tendency to treat SDT as a paradigm—not a theory to be tested against experience—and when anomalies appear, they are explained away with reference to methodological errors or ad hoc hypotheses. Normal science, it seems, is alive a well in some corners of the field.

Returning to the start of the section, the substance of the debate that occurred at Bedford College in 1965 should now be clear. While academic etiquette required that Popper and Kuhn concede ground to one another, their basic visions of science and scientists could hardly have been more different. While reluctantly admitting that normal science exists, Popper (1970) saw it as 'a great danger to science and, indeed, to our civilisation' (p. 53). Moreover, he regarded the turn to psychology and sociology for enlightenment concerning the aims and possible progress of science as 'surprising and disappointing' (p. 57). Where logic has little to learn from psychology, argued Popper, 'the latter has much to learn from the former' (p. 58). Kuhn protested, of course, claiming that, as a historian, he had 'examined closely the facts of scientific life' which had consistently showed that much scientific behaviour had 'persistently violated accepted methodological [i.e. Popperian] canons' (Kuhn, 1970: p. 236). Where Popper saw ducks, Kuhn saw rabbits. Yet it should come as no real surprise that Kuhn the historian saw the world of science quite differently to Popper the logician. Indeed, their arguments were of fundamentally different kinds: Popper was making a *prescriptive* case for science, for the attitude and methodology scientists *ought* to adopt (i.e. that were logically sound); Kuhn on the other hand was concerned with *describing* science, attempting to lay bare the socio-psychological forces and factors that shaped behaviour. In many respects, they were arguing past one another.

Aside from some of the issues already mentioned—for example, that Kuhn 'leaves so vague' the conditions under which revolutions occur (Rowbottom, 2011: p. 119)—Kuhn's consistent ambiguity on the *description* versus *prescription* issue became a main source of criticism against him. Feyerabend (1970) accused Kuhn of deliberately avoiding the issue in trying to appeal to both camps: philosophers and historians. In his critical comparison, Fuller (2006) also notes that Popper's 'normative horizons were always more expansive than Kuhn's' (p. 26), and further that Popper and his followers seized upon a glaring weakness in Kuhn's theory: its lack of constitutional safeguards (p. 46). Scientists should always be *trying* to falsify their theories, just as people in democracies should always be *invited* to find faults with governments and consider alternatives (Fuller, 2006: p. 46). By contrast, Kuhn's authoritarian and irrational vision of science, governed by elite peers, where normal scientists lurch from one crisis to the next in 'contagious panics', is hardly appealing (Fuller, 2006; Lakatos, 1970). For his critics, then, Kuhn's normal scientist, disconnected from society, cuts a pitiful figure; with his explanation of revolutions fundamentally incomplete.

Despite these criticisms, there is no denying that it is Kuhn's vision that has become the dominant 'paradigm' of the day (Fuller, 2006). This is particularly so in the social sciences, where his descriptive account (not least misunderstandings of his concept of 'incommensurability') has been mistaken for an excuse to *avoid* criticism (Cf. Denzin and Lincoln, 2005). Or, as Feyerabend put it: 'by accepting Kuhn's account as a clear new *fact*... they [social scientists] started a new and most deplorable trend of loquacious illiteracy' (Feyerabend, 1978: p. 66). Whatever the consequences of Kuhn's success—an explanation for which is beyond the scope of this text—one of his early and unlikely champions was Popper's student and direct successor at the London School of Economics, Imre Lakatos. While some have intimated devious intentions on Lakatos' part (cf. Agassi, 2008), there is no doubt that, in bringing Popper and Kuhn together, Lakatos intended to create intellectual space for his own 'middle way' philosophy of science (Motterlini, 1999).

Imre Lakatos and Scientific 'Research Programmes'

Late in the evening on Friday, July 16, 1965, Imre Lakatos sat at his desk reflecting on a long and momentous day. Earlier that week, after years of effort, he had finally managed to engineer the meeting of his mentor, Karl Popper and the famous American historian, Thomas Kuhn.

A contented smile crept across his face as he reached for a paper and pen and dashed off a boastful note to his friend, Paul Feyerabend, who had been kept at home due to one of his regular bouts of illness. Lakatos had heard about the meeting second hand, so didn't comment on details, but he noted to his friend how the time was now right for his to own middle way philosophy of science to take centre stage. It took Lakatos a further 5 years to publish the papers from the 'International Colloquium in the Philosophy of Science' which, when it appeared under the title *Criticism and the Growth of Knowledge,* granted a measly 6 pages to Popper, 74 pages to Kuhn and 105 pages (one third of the text) to himself!

As a Popperian, Lakatos stood firmly against the irrational 'mob psychology' science he saw in Kuhn: 'submission to the collective will and wisdom of the community', thought Lakatos, was a poor recipe for normal science (Lakatos, 1970: p. 178). Moreover, since Kuhn identified no rational causes or standards in revolutions, he leaves us with only weak psychological or social psychological explanations which are useless as methodological prescriptions (ibid: p. 179). However, Lakatos also regarded Popper's logical standards as sociologically naive and historically untenable. His subsequent innovations on (or clarifications of) Popper were small but important; and his alternative historiographical methodology was arguably more sophisticated than Kuhn's (Feyerabend, in Motterlini, 1999: p. 16). His designs on winning the debate he staged in 1965, then, were at least partly successful. We will consider his Popperian methodological modifications and his historical methodology in turn.

In his co-edited volume of the 1965 conference (Lakatos & Musgrave, 1970), Lakatos begins his 105-page essay by arguing that Kuhn attacked a form of 'naive falsification'—a Popperian straw man—and further, that by strengthening the Popperian position, one can present the history of science 'as constituting rational progress rather than as religious conversions' (ibid: p. 93). Lakatos' distinction between 'naive' and 'sophisticated' falsification—a version he attributes jointly to himself and Popper (ibid: p. 181)—is summarised in Table 1.1.

Lakatos strengthened Popper's notion of falsification by making two important qualifications. First, we do not appraise single theories in isolation, but rather a series of theories: it is not possible to falsify a theory without the presence of a better alternative. A sport psychologist trying

Table 1.1 Naive versus sophisticated falsificationism

	Demarcation	Falsification
Naive	Any theory which is experimentally falsifiable is scientific	A theory is falsified by an observation statement that conflicts with it
Sophisticated	A theory is scientific only if it has corroborated excess empirical content over its predecessor (or rival)	A theory is only falsified if another theory has been proposed which: 1. has excess empirical content (predicts novel facts) 2. explains the previous success of its rivals 3. has some excess content that is corroborated (has passed tests)

Adapted from Lakatos (1970: pp. 117–122)

to understand the effects of arousal on the performance of a team of athletes, for example, does not *test* 'inverted-U theory' (Landers & Arent, 2010) without also having 'catastrophe theory' (Hardy, 1996) and 'reversal theory' (Kerr, 1997) in mind as possible alternatives. Hence, only a series of theories—or what Lakatos called a 'research programme'—can be considered scientific (ibid: pp. 118–120). Second, there can be no such thing as a crucial experiment; at least not if they are meant to be experiments that can instantly overthrow a research programme. (ibid: p. 173). Following Kuhn, Lakatos argued that the *defence* of a research programme (leading to greater stability) was just as important as its *attack*. In Lakatos' conception:

> criticism does not – and must not – kill as fast as Popper imagined. *Purely negative criticism... does not eliminate a programme. Criticism of a programme is a long and often frustrating process and one must treat the budding programme leniently...* It is only constructive criticism which, with the help of rival research programmes, can achieve real successes. (original emphasis) (ibid: p. 179)

What emerges, then, are a series of new methodological prescriptions, essentially based on Popper, but qualified by Kuhn-like socio-psychological insights. Or, as Lakatos put it in his final lectures: 'from a logical point of view, it is quite possible to play the game of science according to Popper's rules... the only problem is that it has never happened in this way' (Lakatos, in Motterlini, 1999: p. 98).

Lakatos' resulting 'sophisticated' methodological prescriptions can be summarised as follows (this list is a composite drawn from Lakatos, 1970; Motterlini, 1999 and Zahar, 1982):

1. Treat budding research programmes leniently (i.e. persist even in the face of criticism)
2. Nevertheless, try to look at things from different points of view
3. Put forward theories which anticipate novel facts (make theories 'stick their necks out')
4. Compare programmes on the basis of:

   (a) Their heuristic power (the extent to which they suggest fruitful new solutions);
   (b) Their degree of corroboration (assessment of the severity of tests theories have passed).

Research programmes, in general, are characterised by a *hard core* of accepted theories (rather like a paradigm), surrounded by a *protective belt* of auxiliary hypotheses. For example, social facilitation theory, as formulated by Zajonc (1965), contains a basic law concerning the relationship between performance and the presence of others: *well-learned skills remain robust under observation-induced stress, whereas poorly learned skills break down*. This general 'drive' or 'activation' theory could be said to be the hard core of the programme, and the multiple hypotheses that have been added more recently (e.g. evaluation apprehension; alertness and monitoring hypotheses; challenge-threat hypothesis; distraction-conflict hypothesis; self-presentation hypothesis), the protective belt (cf. Strauss, 2002). What remains, then, under the Lakatosian scheme, is to evaluate the extent to which such programmes are *progressive* or *degenerating*.

Progressive programmes are those in which scientists act in accordance with principles of sophisticated falsification, or where theories have excess empirical content over rivals which has also been corroborated (Blaug, 1991: p. 172). Put simply, they predict new facts and survive harsher tests. We may ask, for example, which of the three arousal theories already mentioned makes the most novel predictions, and which on balance has stood up to criticism? Such questions would be important for those conducting literature reviews prior to undertaking new empirical research in this field. Rather than simply selecting the most fashionable 'paradigm' (*a la* Kuhn), Lakatos would argue that researchers should identify the most progressive programme according to these criteria then work on corroboration.

Degenerating programmes, by contrast, make no novel predictions; they simply explain what is already known and 'save' theories from criticism by adding increasingly ad hoc auxiliary hypotheses (Motterlini, 1999: p. 2; Khalil, 1987: p. 124). Perceptive readers will notice a more than passing resemblance between degenerating programmes and Kuhn's normal science. But where Kuhn saw normal and revolutionary *periods*, occurring in a sequence, Lakatos saw progressive and degenerative programmes existing in a state of simultaneous and perpetual *interaction*, whose fluctuations were worthy of historical study (Feyerabend, 1970: p. 212; Zahar, 1982: p. 407).

Lakatos' new demarcation criterion, therefore, aimed to distinguish not between science and pseudoscience, but between *good* science and *bad* science (Motterlini, 1999: p. 3). To this end, Lakatos went so far as to recommended that scientists should identify and work on progressive research programmes and, moreover, that economic and intellectual resources be distributed in the same direction (Motterlini, 1999: p. 7). Some critics characterised such rationalist recommendations as pure propaganda, however, arguing that degenerating programmes are sometimes 'revived' by scientists and become progressive (Feyerabend, 1970). In such cases, deserting the degenerating programme may, in fact, be damaging to progress. Lakatos conceded that there was no purely rational case for following progressive programmes, but argued that a historiographical programme of research using 'progressive' and 'degenerating' as *ideal types* may at least help us identify how (and how often) such cases occur. Such a methodology of scientific research programmes (MSRP) would involve the 'rational reconstruction'[3] of individual cases in order to understand the 'reasons and strategies which have produced new ideas' (Motterlini, 1999: p. 16).

At the time of his death, nobody had applied MSRP to a historical appraisal of the social sciences (Lakatos, in Motterlini, 1999: p. 106), though the task has since been undertaken with some vigour in economics (Cf. Blaug, 1991; Hands, 1985; Khalil, 1987). Such examples have demonstrated the potential value of a Lakatosian historiography to other social sciences: identifying the hard core of programmes; describing their long-term growth; identifying ad hoc developments and patching-up procedures; and also debating where genuinely progressive shifts occur. We would argue that MSRP may be fruitfully applied in sport and exercise psychology, in systematic reviews and in justifying the selection of particular theories in, say, theses and dissertations. Taking the earlier example, based on Strauss' (2002) review, the hard core of social facilitation theory (SFT) was established in the 1960s following many years of 'anarchy'. It is worth asking, therefore, to what extent the auxiliary hypotheses added over the last 50 years represent progressive or degenerative shifts? Has SFT merely been 'patched-up', or have some of these hypotheses constituted bold new predictions that have been corroborated through experimental results? Without the conceptual toolbox of Lakatos, Strauss (2002) implies a series of degenerating shifts over the last 40 years in SFT yet is unable to reformulate the theory in a progressive way. The application of MSRP might therefore offer a valuable analytical tool for studying psychological research programmes in future.

To summarise, Lakatos felt that he had improved on Popper's methodological prescriptions, maintaining the rationalism of 'progressive' science, while salvaging from Kuhn the idea that some degree of tenacity is necessary in defending a programme against criticism, instilling some stability. In the final analysis, he was unable to offer clear reasons or criteria for moving from degenerating to progressive programmes (or vice-versa), or for when (and how vociferously) scientists should adopt a defensive or

---

[3] By 'rational reconstruction', Lakatos has in mind an explicitly theory-informed historical study, using his concepts as a particular lens through which to view historical cases. Feyerabend, though critical of Lakatos' prescriptions for science, considered this theory 'vastly superior to Kuhn's', and one that would 'definitely lead to more detailed research' (Feyerabend, in Motterlini, 1999: p. 16).

critical stance towards a research programme (Motterlini, 1999). Yet he remained resolute in the belief that 'in a game one has little hope in winning… it is better to play than to give up' (Lakatos, 1970: pp. 112–113). Here Lakatos was aiming a thinly veiled jab at his friend and most active critic: the anarchist—and master of 'giving up'—Paul Feyerabend.

Paul Feyerabend and 'Epistemological Anarchism'

On a cool wet day, sometime in late March 1973, Paul Feyerabend limped out of his perpetually dilapidated house, close to the campus of UC Berkeley, with his walking stick in one hand and a letter in the other. The letter was addressed to his close friend and critic, Imre Lakatos, and contained his infamous 'theses on anarchism' which he intended his friend, in the style of Martin Luther, to nail to the doors of the London School of Economics.[4] Less than a year later, Lakatos was dead. Their planned dialogue, *For and Against Method*, was never realised, leaving Feyerabend to publish his part the following year under the incomplete title: *Against Method* (Feyerabend, 1975).

Of the philosophers we have introduced so far, Feyerabend is by far the most elusive, and deliberately so, as we shall see. One of his favourite tactics was to pose as a rationalist—or 'undercover agent'—using rational arguments, in order to trick rationalists, such as Popper and Lakatos, into accepting irrational arguments (Feyerabend, 1975: p. 23). He would frequently and deliberately change his stance on issues, often arguing against positions he himself had once defended. He was, in short, an intellectual agitator of the highest order. Yet Feyerabend was more than a clever trickster: his methods were designed to disarm his opponents; to reveal to them the error of their rational ways. In the passages that follow, we will try to outline his methods and present Feyerabend's anarchist arguments insofar as they relate to, and help shed further light on, the ideas of Popper, Kuhn and Lakatos: three men he considered to be both personal friends and intellectual enemies.

---

[4] This conjectural sketch is based on Feyerabend's letters to Lakatos (from the Lakatos archive at the LSE) and brief biographical notes in Motterlini (1999).

Feyerabend's distinctive contributions to the debates we have featured—What makes scientific knowledge special? What method should scientists follow? How do scientists actually generate knowledge? How do we define progress in science? What criteria can we use to judge between theories?—are most clearly expressed in his two main texts: *Against Method* (1975) and *Science in a Free Society* (1978). He begins by establishing a central idea that he shared with Kuhn: *incommensurability*. To illustrate by example, consider two sport psychologists arguing over how best to motivate a group of disengaged basketball players. One is an ardent achievement goals theorist; the other a convert of self-determination theory. The first suggests a need to shift the goal orientations of the players by creating a more task-focussed environment: the coach should create games focussed on skill mastery, have players try to beat their own previous scores in skill-based games, offer process-based feedback (e.g. your feet are in a great position there—that's why you hit the shot!) and create systems for team selection based on effort or improvement. The second argues for greater autonomy supportive behaviours from the coach, such as allowing the players to set their own goals (within a team ethos); helping athletes generate their own feedback; work hard to help the athletes internalise the team's goals and performance model through regular discussions. How are we to decide who is 'right'? Which theory provides the best solution?

A Popperian/Lakatosian response would be to demand that both theories be formulated so as to make clear predictions about a possible intervention, conduct a test, then inspect the consequences. One of the two theories will survive the criticism of (or be better corroborated by) the evidence, and that is the more 'truth-like' theory (or more progressive programme), for the time being. However, since there is no such thing as 'theory-neutral' observation—a point on which all four of our protagonists agree—then there can be no recourse to 'the evidence' in judging between two theories since it, too, is entangled in theory (Feyerabend, 1975: pp. 22–23). What we are in fact doing in such cases is bringing a third theoretical view into the argument through which we interpret 'the evidence' and judge between the other two. This is Feyerabend's meaning of *incommensurability*.

If we accept the principle of incommensurability—that 'pure evidence' cannot be brought to bear on the decision to choose between different theories—it follows that a radically different approach to science is required. Feyerabend suggests the scientist:

> ...must compare ideas with other ideas rather than with 'experience' and he must try to improve rather than discard the views that have failed in the competition... Knowledge so conceived is not a series of self-consistent theories that converges towards an ideal view; it is not a gradual approach to the truth. It is rather an ever increasing *ocean of mutually incompatible alternatives*, each single theory, each fairy-tale, each myth that is part of the collection forcing the others into greater articulation and all of them contributing, via this process of competition, to the development of our consciousness. Nothing is ever settled. (Feyerabend, 1975: p. 21).

Feyerabend's method involved the articulation of historical counterexamples that were chosen to confound Popperian principles in two ways: first, he showed that some of the greatest advances in science occurred when scientists 'broke the rules' (Popperian rules); and second, he demonstrated that in some cases, theories that had been falsified (or 'degenerating' programmes) have, after centuries, been revived and led to great advances in science (e.g. the atomic theory of matter and the heliocentric theory of the solar system). For Feyerabend, rationalist principles such as 'take falsifications seriously' and 'avoid *ad hoc* hypotheses' not only give an inadequate historical account of science but 'are liable to hinder it in the future' (Feyerabend, 1975: p. 157). When it comes to method, then, if we base our judgements on existing standards, the only principle that does not inhibit progress is: 'anything goes' (Feyerabend, 1978: p. 39). Such disarming and initially unhelpful maxims often headline Feyerabend's work, yet he intended them to be read as a kind of 'medicine' for methodology; as a tonic to cure one of rationalist delusions (Feyerabend, 1975).

Having made such bold claims, Feyerabend immediately backtracks, agreeing with both Popper and Kuhn in that we initially approach enquiry through a 'medium of traditions' (Feyerabend, 1978: p. 34). Such traditions (or paradigms) prescribe methods and theories, which are necessary for progress in Kuhn's view, but represent modes of inhibition of freedom of thought for Feyerabend. Indeed, Kuhn's ideology, according to Feyerabend (1970: p. 197), 'could only give comfort to the most narrow-minded and most conceited kind of specialism… [and] would tend to inhibit the advancement of knowledge'. So, although he agrees with Kuhn that nature needs a point of view from which to be explored, he deplores Kuhn's 'specific twist' that involves the *exclusive choice* of one particular set of ideas (Feyerabend, 1970: p. 201).

Since he believed that all attempts to specify method inhibit progress—because they close down the invention of alternatives—Feyerabend's main methodological principle of 'anything goes' was intended to promote methodological pluralism. If there is no recourse to 'the evidence' to choose between theories (i.e. incommensurability), an 'essential part of the empirical method' lies in the invention of alternative theories (Feyerabend, 1975: p. 29). And the more the better, as each new theory forces others into fruitful competition. This approach is summarised by Feyerabend (1975) as follows:

> A scientist who is interested in maximum empirical content, and who wants to understand as many aspects of his theory as possible, will adopt a pluralistic methodology, he [*sic*] will compare theories with other theories rather than with 'experience', 'data' or 'facts', and he will try to improve rather than discard the views that appear to lose to the competition. For the alternatives, which he needs to keep the contest going, may be taken from the past as well. As a matter of fact, they may be taken from wherever one is able to find them – from ancient myths and modern prejudices; from the lucubrations of experts and from the fantasies of cranks. (p. 33)

Here we see a little more of Feyerabend's vision: the aim of science is increasing empirical content and enhancing understanding of theory; the way to do this is to compare theories with alternatives; and the alternatives may come from a very broad range of sources—much broader than his rationalist opponents (e.g. Popper and Lakatos) might allow.

Feyerabend's account of the history of science, then, involves both the reception of traditions and accepted methods *and* the simultaneous breaking of rules and invention of alternatives. To explain, he introduces an analogy of an adventurer who sets out into new territory with a rudimentary map. The map provides an image and a guide to reality which, like reason (i.e. methodology), contains idealisations. The adventurer uses the map to find his or her way, but also corrects the map as the adventure proceeds, removing old idealisations and introducing new ones. Using the map will soon get the explorer into trouble, but 'it is better to have maps than to proceed without them' (Feyerabend, 1978: p. 25). A graduate student employing grounded theory methodology for the first time, for example, may initially follow the directives of a well-known textbook (e.g. Strauss & Corbin, 1998) and the guidance of an experienced supervisor (Holt & Tamminen, 2010b). At some point, the student will get into difficulty—they will not understand how 'theoretical sampling' should work, or they will be unable to establish 'theoretical saturation'—and be forced to deviate from the book. In 'breaking the rules', they will create a slightly new and different approach to grounded theory, which they may eventually publish and force proponents of more traditional approaches into critical and fruitful discussion (see Chap. 4).

In other places, Feyerabend (1970, 1978) compares this view directly with Kuhn's, who he argued was wrong about the *successive* nature of the 'normal' and 'philosophical' components of science. In the normal component, scientists engage in a *practical* tradition of applying the paradigm; they follow a principle of *tenacity* (defending the paradigm, come what may); and demonstrate an attitude of *narrow-mindedness*. At the brief moments of extraordinary science, or the philosophical component, scientists engage in a *pluralistic* tradition of inventing alternative ideas; they follow a principle of *proliferation* of new theories that may compete; and demonstrate an attitude of *ignorance* towards the dominant traditions (see Table 1.2 for a summary). Contrary to Kuhn and like Lakatos, Feyerabend saw these two patterns in a relationship of 'simultaneity and interaction' (Feyerabend, 1970: p. 212). Where Kuhn had failed to

Table 1.2 Feyerabend's interactionist categories	Components	Normal	Philosophical
	Traditions	Practical	Pluralistic
	Principles	Tenacity	Proliferation
	Attitudes	Narrow-mindedness	Ignorance

explain how extraordinary science happens, Feyerabend noted that revolutions are mostly made by 'members of the philosophical component who, while aware of the normal practice, are also able to think in a different way' (e.g. Einstein's famous self-professed ability to escape from 'normal' training) (Feyerabend, 1970: p. 212).

At any given time, then, Feyerabend sees science as composed of two groups of people: (a) narrow-minded, practically focussed normal scientists who defend their views with great tenacity and (b) free-thinking, philosophically focussed pluralistic scientists whose goal is the proliferation of alternative ways of looking at things. While the second group are breaking rules, violating standards, inventing new theories and doing their own thing, the first group, 'whose highest aim is to solve puzzles', do not change their allegiance to a paradigm in a reasonable fashion. Rather, they may adopt new paradigms (invented by the second group) for a variety of capricious reasons (e.g. because the younger generation cannot be bothered to follow their elders, or because a public figure has changed his or her mind). Their tenacious work to deepen and extend knowledge in a paradigm, however, remains crucially important (Feyerabend, 1970: p. 214). So, while 'science was advanced by outsiders, or by scientists with an unusual background... science needs both *narrow-mindedness* and *ignorance*; the expert and the dilettante' (Feyerabend, 1978: p. 89).

Progress for Feyerabend was therefore characterised by proliferation, increasing pluralism, free debate and the challenging of standards (or conduct of research that violates standards). Only science that follows such a pattern will lead to growth in knowledge. However, by upholding anarchist principles such as preventing the elimination of old theories and advocating standard-violating research, Feyerabend had to invent new ideas concerning how it is possible to judge theories. His views on this matter are controversial but have begun to be operationalised to some degree in sport psychology in recent years (cf. Sparkes & Smith, 2009). Feyerabend (1970) has three main ideas, which are, of course, naturally limited and open to debate:

1. Claims for individual objectivity weaken rather than strengthen knowledge claims ("an enterprise whose human character can be seen by all is preferable to one that looks 'objective', and impervious to human actions and wishes") (p. 228)

2. Matters of taste are not completely beyond the reach of argument. In poetry, "every poet compares, improves, argues until he finds the correct formulation of what he wants to say. Would it not be marvellous if this process played a role in the sciences also?" (p. 228)
3. Better theories will have a smaller length of derivations (from theory to observation) and a smaller number of approximations (in derivations) (p. 229).

In summary, Feyerabend used his unorthodox arguments and 'propaganda' to strike terror into the hearts of confident rationalists by confronting them with an anarchist account of history. And despite his jovial and mischievous ways—jumping from one position to another; defending a point one day and attacking it the next—Feyerabend remained passionate about his central arguments and propositions. If one accepts incommensurability, pluralism and methodological rule-breaking appear to be sensible ways forward. As he notes in his conclusion to *Against Method*: 'I am convinced that science will profit from everyone doing his [*sic*] own thing… science needs people who are adaptable and inventive, not rigid imitators of "established behavioural patterns"' (Feyerabend, 1975: p. 159).

Having summarised Feyerabend's views and revealed his main differences with Kuhn, it is now possible to see how Feyerabend came to reject the views of his former teacher, Popper, and his friend, Lakatos. First, he felt that Popper's school of 'critical rationalism' was too narrowly prescriptive and full of simplistic rules, the following of which would inhibit (and had inhibited) progress (i.e. it will curb the creativity of the 'philosophical component'). He also pointed out that the high-minded standards of the Popperians (e.g. reject a theory following falsification; do not permit ad hoc hypotheses) were in themselves not open to criticism and therefore likely to stifle the invention of better alternatives. Indeed, Feyerabend claimed that it would be important for people to do research that violates existing standards, in order to engage in productive revisions (Feyerabend, 1978: p. 39).

Having considered Feyerabend's powerful critique of the other positions, it seems in the spirit of anarchism to turn that same critique on his own ideas. If Lakatos failed in the essential task of providing guidance for a scientist, for example, and Kuhn was accused of ambiguity on the, then what of Feyerabend's own positive prescriptive value? Guidance such as 'do your own thing', 'break the rules' or 'violate standards' might embolden a tenured professor but is likely to be of little consolation to a PhD student who may not have a 'thing' to do or know what 'standards' and 'rules' exist to be violated or broken. Yet Feyerabend's idea of simultaneous and interactive components or traditions seems to suggest that it is young scientists who have eschewed 'normal' training who are most likely to become the philosophical proliferators of new ideas. His ideas on theory evaluation also seem somewhat fanciful and wide open to debate (e.g. using principles from literary criticism to judge scientific theories). If Feyerabend's prescriptions appear logically robust but practically unrealistic (even untenable—certainly to a Kuhnian), he offers little more than did Popper. But Popper's methodology, as we have seen, has indeed had a powerful practical effect on a number of leading scientists, a fact for which Feyerabend offers a potentially illuminating explanation:

> Methodology, it is said, deals with what should be done and cannot be criticised by reference to what is. But we must make sure that the application of prescriptions leads to desirable results; and that we consider historical, sociological and psychological *tendencies* which tell us what is possible under given circumstances, thus separating feasible prescriptions from dead ends. (Feyerabend, 1975: p. 149)

Under what social conditions and with what psychological tendencies might anarchism—or critical rationalism for that matter—lead to desirable results? (Desirable results, in both cases, would presumably be the growth of knowledge and a reduction in preventable human suffering.) Are Popper's or Feyerabend's prescriptions likely to be feasible in certain circumstances, or will they lead to dead ends? To bring the question closer to home, what would happen if a young exercise psychologist, in the course of a PhD thesis, took an anarchist stance, both defending and attacking self-determination theory, violating standards in measurement and statistics and claiming, in defence, that 'anything goes'? Such an act would certainly demand the 'psychological tendencies' of confidence and bravery; not to mention favourable 'social conditions' of an amenable examiner and flexible institutional assessment guidelines. Although it is hard to imagine such a state of affairs, it is not impossible. So Feyerabend, if nothing else, invites us to invent alternative ways of thinking about and doing research, and he succeeds if we can, with effort, bring about the conditions under which epistemological anarchism might thrive.

Applying Philosophy to the Past, Present and Future

We began this chapter with a critical inspection of Marten's (1987) influential paper identifying two approaches to research in sport psychology. We noted that his formulation of 'orthodox' science was too simplistic and mistaken in some important ways. In the rest of the chapter we explored four different approaches to understanding science and research and attempted to differentiate between descriptive and normative theories (i.e. theories that attempt to describe the past and present state of science; and theories that attempt to prescribe logical ways forward). We began with Popper's critical rationalism and his vision of the scientist testing bold and imaginative theories through the process of conjecture and refutation. We compared Popper's so-called naive view first with Kuhn's notion of the puzzle-solving normal scientist and then with Lakatos' sophisticated falsification and theory of scientific research programmes. We concluded by considering Feyerabend's penetrating critique of all three positions and his unlikely and enigmatic prescription of anarchism. In this final section, we turn these analytical tools back on the present situation in sport and exercise psychology in an attempt to establish their value. We do so by taking a critical look at the field's most influential textbook: Weinberg and Gould's *Foundations of Sport and Exercise Psychology* (FSEP), partly because of its enduring popularity and partly because of the influence of Marten's (1987) paper on the view of science established therein.

As we have seen, Kuhn regarded textbooks as authoritative 'vehicles for the perpetuation of normal science' (Kuhn, 1962/1996: p. 136). Often authored by the academic elite—those with sufficient symbolic capital to dictate the accepted dogmas and paradigmatic boundaries (Bourdieu, 1991)—textbooks establish scientific norms with respect to the problems, theories and methods valued (or even permitted) within an academic community. Over the six editions of FSEP, there has been very little change in the first two chapters which establish a historical and methodological consensus (they are conflated into a single chapter in the later editions). Our first conclusion, then, is that between 1995 and 2015, according to Weinberg and Gould, there has been no significant shift in the paradigm. But what is the nature of the science practiced in this 'paradigm'? FSEP actually contains three distinct views on research, which we summarise in Table 1.3 and then critique.

First, the goal of research in general, we are told, is to 'describe, explain, predict and allow control of behaviour' (Weinberg & Gould, 1995: p. 24). In 'studies' this entails the discovery of theory that organises a large number of facts in a pattern that helps others understand them. The main exemplar here is Zajonc's development of social facilitation theory. According to the authors, 'Zajonc saw a pattern in seemingly random results [in performance in the presence of different kinds of audience] and formulated a theory' (ibid: p. 24). Consolidating facts in a simple theory that practitioners can apply in practice, is thus established as a central

Table 1.3 Three approaches to research in FSEP

Approach	Description	Suggested weaknesses
'Studies'	Involve objective observation of a series of facts and marshalling of facts into an explanatory theory	Unable to establish cause and effect relationships
'Experiments'	Involve the manipulation and control of variables; objective measurement and the collection of unbiased data	Variables cannot be controlled in social science; the researcher influences the object of study
'Professional practice'	Based on real-world problems and folk theories of practitioners; high on external or ecological validity (theories are useful to athletes, coaches etc.)	Theories lack internal validity and reliability

Adapted from Weinberg and Gould (1995: pp. 24–30)

objective of sport psychology studies. In other words, studies should follow the inductive, empiricist principles of science that Popper attacked (successfully) back in the 1930s. As we have seen, the twin ideas—(a) starting research with observations and (b) discovering valid and reliable theory (i.e. true facts)—have been comprehensively defeated by all four of our philosophical protagonists. As followers of Lakatos (and Popper) have noted, research programmes that 'merely rationalise known facts deserve little applause; such ingenuity has merit but involves no progress' (Blaug, 1991: p. 172).

'Experiments', by contrast, though not always distinguished from 'studies', are where 'scientists are trained to be as objective as possible' in the systematic control and manipulation of variables and where the 'goal is to collect unbiased data' (Weinberg & Gould, 1995: pp. 24–25). It is interesting to note that FSEP later goes on to undermine this approach, arguing that 'psychology is a social science' and that 'human beings change over time; they think about and manipulate their environment, making behaviour more difficult to predict' (ibid: p. 30). This then sets up the alternative of 'professional practice' knowledge, which is premised on the acceptance of very different assumptions about the social world and how it can be studied. This final approach is also criticised in FSEP for lacking objectivity and reliability. What is more problematic, however, is the fact that FSEP does not take a stance. Based on the rather obvious starting point that psychological research happens in the social world and involves humans, only one of these two sets of assumptions can be right. It is not a choice; it is a matter of understanding the arguments and drawing conclusions for research methodology.

So what, in summary, do we make of this picture of research painted in FSEP? After jettisoning the notion of 'studies', it is important to note that the remaining two approaches ('experiments' and 'professional practice') are underpinned by fundamentally conflicting assumptions about the nature of the social world, only one of which can be accepted. We would side broadly with the 'open system' view of social science which denies the possibility of experimental control of variables (Cf. Sayer, 2010) and with the widely accepted view, detailed in this chapter, that all observation, or data collection, is theory-laden (i.e. individual objectivity is impossible). But this still leaves a number of unanswered questions about the possible nature of research. We therefore conclude the chapter by posing the salient methodological questions from the perspective of the four philosophical approaches we have outlined (Table 1.4). These questions, and the answers supplied by our protagonists, inform our approach (implicitly and explicitly) to the rest of the book.

Table 1.4 Historical and normative questions raised by the four philosophers

<< Backward looking	Present Forward Looking >>
Kuhn	**Popper**
What theory, methods and exemplars are embedded in the paradigm (i.e. what does normal science look like)?	How do we increase the content of our theories so as to make them more 'testable'? (How do we make our theories 'stick their necks out'?)
What puzzles, as defined by the paradigm, were deemed worthy of solving?	How do we better corroborate theories (i.e. increase the severity of our tests)?
When did anomalies turn into counterinstances? (And who decided this?)	Under what conditions should we give up our theories and admit to being wrong?
How were the new generation of scientists socialised into the new paradigm?	
Lakatos	**Feyerabend**
What constitutes the 'hard core' of the research programme?	What kinds of alternatives could we invent (or revive) in order to force greater competition between theories?
What novel facts has the programme predicted (over its rivals)?	Who constitutes the 'philosophical component' in science and how might they fruitfully interact with the 'normal' component to achieve growth in knowledge?
What ad hoc moves have been made to protect the programme from criticism? (degenerative)	How could principles from art and literary criticism be brought to bear on the judgement of scientific theories?
What has been done in the spirit of sophisticated falsificationism? (progressive)	What social conditions and psychological tendencies are necessary for scientists to adopt anarchism to achieve desirable
Have scientists moved in progressive directions? (i.e. left degenerating programmes in favour of progressive programmes)?	ends (growth of knowledge; elimination of preventable suffering)?

Moving Forward

In the next chapter, we draw explicitly on Kuhn and Popper to raise and answer crucial questions about the history of psychology in general and of sport and exercise psychology in particular. We ask if certain paradigms (or research programmes) have become dominant, and consider the consequences for knowledge in our subject. We draw on Popperian thinking in Chap. 3, where the focus is on the role of criticism and the cultivation of the critical attitude. Chapter 4, by contrast, applies Kuhnian and Lakatosian theories directly to a critical analysis on the current state of affairs in the application of theory (specifically self-determination theory) and theory generation (grounded theory) in sport and exercise psychology. We then turn back to Kuhn and Popper in Chap. 5 as we explore the so-called paradigm wars and the influence of economic and political forces on the selection (or deselection) of dominant methodological approaches in the field. Kuhn's sociological ideas also support our analysis in Chap. 6, which focuses on cultural norms and the subtle yet systematic ways in which dominant groups maintain an 'intellectual monopoly' in sport and exercise. In Chap. 7 we raise critical questions about dominant approaches to measurement, specifically in achievement goal theory, and draw on Popperian ideas to suggest alternatives. Similarly, in Chap. 8, we begin with an analysis of the well-documented research-practice gap in sport and exercise psychology and once again draw on normative philosophical theory to chart a more positive path. Chapter 9 aims to establish a clear argument for the application of an explicitly Popperian approach to research practice, publishing and education in sport and exercise psychology. This provides an intellectual platform for the final chapter, where we look forward to a possible future in which sport and exercise psychology research is more explicitly informed by positive philosophical theories and standards, while remaining cognisant of the sociological and psychological reality in which we must operate.

2

The Emerging Field of Sport and Exercise Psychology

When trying to critically discuss the future, it is difficult to ignore the present and forget the past. The field of sport and exercise psychology is no exception, especially as it relates to research and its scientific foundation. Chapter 1 therefore aimed to describe—after having answered the question 'Why rethink?'—the reasoning of some of the more influential twentieth-century thinkers, not least Popper and Kuhn. We focused on their philosophy of science, because it continues to shape what is considered acceptable research. Their writings also constantly encourage us to rethink what we do and how we do it: because what and how research is performed now and in the future is very much influenced by how science was defined, and research performed, in the past.

The link between Chaps. 1 and 2 is thereby clearly visible; if for nothing else than the fact that many of the earlier empiricists stemmed from the ranks of philosophers, although they may later have ventured into medicine or general psychology, or even sport and exercise psychology. While the main aim of Chap. 2 is to describe the past, the historical perspective is but one facet. Another aim is to point to historical developments that have shaped the research process. Why, for example, is sport and exercise psychology still dominated by quantitative methods? The

© The Author(s) 2016
P. Hassmén et al., *Rethinking Sport and Exercise Psychology Research*,
DOI 10.1057/978-1-137-48338-6_2

answer is not surprising given the strong historical roots planted by the early psychophysicists; psychometrics is an area that remains strong and standardised instruments continue to be the preferred choice for many researchers with a sport and exercise psychology focus. In contrast, those favouring qualitative methods in sport and exercise psychology still seem to be forced to defend their approach to a much higher degree than quantitatively inclined researchers (cf. Sparkes, 2013, 2015). To understand this unequal balance, a historical perspective is enlightening.

It is instructive, therefore, to look more closely at the work of some of the earlier researchers in psychology that lay the foundation for modern day sport and exercise psychology research. As Nicholls (1989) points out below, this is neither about being right or wrong, nor is it about highlighting historical mistakes; it is always easier in hindsight to determine who ultimately had stronger or weaker arguments in any academic debate. But by considering the origin of science, psychology and ultimately the emergence of sport and exercise psychology, we seek to better understand where we stand today. This, in turn, may assist us in going forward to create some new answers, but most likely also create some new questions—and this, in Nicholls' words, is the ultimate form of respect.

> To take someone's ideas seriously enough to question them is a significant form of respect. It builds communities where controversy stimulates thought instead of enmity; where the clash of ideas leads not to victory for one party but to new questions and new answers for everyone (Nicholls, 1989, p. 1).

Early Psychophysics

Psychophysics contains many prime examples of when one researcher respectfully disagreed with another. In a paper published by Stevens in 1961, entitled 'To honor Fechner and repeal his law' (with the subtitle 'A power function, not a log function, describes the operating characteristic of a sensory system'), Stevens acknowledges the immense importance of Fechner's work, performed a century earlier, but also reveals some flaws in it. Fechner himself was probably aware of much of the criticism that Stevens voiced long after Fechner's departure into history. Because contemporaries such as Plateau (1872) and Brentano (1874) had already raised many of the issues that Stevens 100 years later reiterated. In fact, Fechner spent much effort to prove his peers wrong, but as stated by Stevens (1961), 'It was asking too much, perhaps, to expect a professor to change his mind after two decades of devotion to an ingenious theory' (p. 80). We will return to this issue in Chap. 7, when considering the impact of some other theories and theorists in sport and exercise psychology that have prevailed over time.

The ingenious theory—using Stevens' words—dawned on Fechner while he rested in bed early in the morning of the 22 October 1850. This day is still celebrated as 'Fechner Day' (http://www.ispsychophysics.org). His magnum opus was published 10 years later: 'Elemente der Psychophysik' (Elements of Psychophysics; Fechner, 1860/1966). When published, it was controversial. Nowadays, however, many see Fechner's book as the birth of psychophysics as an independent discipline, a discipline that immensely influenced how psychology and subsequently sport and exercise psychology developed.

Fechner's main contribution was that the relationship between the objective and the subjective could finally be described and expressed as a mathematical function—albeit incorrectly, according to Stevens. But merely stating that Fechner, a well-known and respected professor, was inclined to tenaciously defend his theory solely because of his stature did not satisfy Stevens. Stevens wrote:

> I have puzzled so often about the ability of this fancy [i.e., Fechner's law] to persist and grow famous that I have accumulated a list of possible reasons for it (1961, p. 80).

These reasons that Stevens accumulated may also explain why the research process in general is conservative, and that normal science (Kuhn) prevails until some major shift occurs (Popper). Stevens raised the following: no competition, the universality of variability, wide applicability, easy on the observer, model-maker's delight and pseudo differential equations (pp. 80–83). Whereas some of these may be more specific to measurements per se, others such as 'no competition', 'wide applicability' and 'model-makers delight' merit further consideration.

That a theory can survive longer when no competing theories are around seems logical (a Kuhnian monopoly); we will later in the book consider achievement-goal theory, and the defenders and proponents of this theory that was originally suggested by Nicholls (1984, 1989). This is indeed the same Nicholls who is cited at the beginning of this chapter. So by choosing Nicholls' theory as an example, we in his own words show him 'a significant form of respect' (1989, p. 1). However, it is not because of a lack of competing theories that achievement-goal theory has survived—even thrived some may say. Its survival is more a combination of a basically sound theory, together with prolific researchers that also vigorously defend it against any criticism, and who do not hesitate to launch counter-criticism whenever and wherever deemed necessary (see Chap. 7 for an extensive discussion).

As for wide applicability, the search for a theory or method that supersedes all other theories or methods is universal, at least as a dream. Stevens (1961, p. 82) himself made a strong argument for direct ratio scaling methods, reasoning that:

> Is there any substantive problem relating to the assessment of a subjective variable whose solution cannot be reached by direct ratio scaling procedures?

Chapter 7 in this book is devoted to measurement issues, and we will then see that there are alternatives to direct ratio scaling. Despite Stevens' belief, ratio scaling procedures did not, in fact, render all other scaling methods obsolete. Maybe 'model-makers delight' was the crucial component that led Fechner to vigorously defend his thinking about the relationship and the law that later came to bear his name? The concept of pet theories comes to mind. At the same time, even Popper—who almost considered 'normal science' and 'bad science' as synonyms—stated that

> I believe that science is essentially critical… But I have always stressed the need for some dogmatism: the dogmatic scientist has an important role to play. If we give in to criticism too easily, we shall never find out where the real power of our theories lies (Popper, 1970, p. 55).

When Stevens published his article 10 years before Popper, he could, of course, not refer to dogmatism as an explanation for Fechner's attacks on anyone criticising his way of thinking. Nor did Stevens mention Thomas Kuhn, who stated that 'The scientist who pauses to examine every anomaly he notes will seldom get significant work done' (1962/1996, p. 82). Suffice to say, there are many reasonable explanations why a theory, model or method remains in fashion long after its expiration date.

It may be appropriate at this point to ask ourselves, as authors of this book: Are we disciples of Popper or Kuhn? The obvious answer is of course 'both', at least in our everyday scientific work. This includes what Kuhn (1962/1996, Chap. 3) labelled the puzzle solving facets of science, and the importance of classification and prediction, theory-experiment alignment and articulation for 'normal science' to also be good science. Popper (1963) on the other hand was convinced that a critical attitude was essential, and 'the tradition of free discussion of theories with the aim of discovering their weak spots so that they may be improved upon, is the attitude of reasonableness, of rationality' (p. 67). By writing a book entitled *Rethinking Sport and Exercise Psychology Research*, we have clearly decided to look at the past, present and future through the eyes of Feyerabend, Lakatos and Popper, acknowledging that much of what we will see results from what Kuhn labelled normal science. Of course, much of our own research from years past has humbly aimed to help solve a tiny piece of the sport and exercise psychology puzzle; consequently we willingly admit that no one stands above criticism. As long as it is constructive, it can only help move the field forward. That said, we are, of course, not naïve enough to believe that what we present herein will be accepted without criticism from our peers (though, following Nicholls, we treat criticism as a form of respect).

Having made our viewpoint somewhat clearer (though more of this in Chap. 9), we are ready to proceed, by revisiting Fechner, because what we so far have touched upon is his so-called outer psychophysics. But Fechner also described 'inner psychophysics', which over the years has received considerably less interest from other researchers including psychophysicists. At first, this seems strange, because Fechner in the 'Foreword to Volume 2' (1889) explained the need for both an outer and inner psychophysics:

...the stimulus does not immediately arouse a sensation, but in addition, an inner physical activity takes place between it and the sensation. In short, according to one particular view, which we will decide about in the following chapter, we call that which is aroused by the stimulus, and which now carries directly along with it a sensation, the psychophysical activity. The lawful relation between the outer and inner end-links of this chain – namely, stimulus and sensation – necessarily translates itself into what occurs between the stimulus and this middle link, on the one hand, and between the middle link and the sensation, on the other hand. In outer psychophysics, we have skipped this middle link, so to speak, inasmuch as, subsequent to immediate experience, we were able directly to establish only the lawful relation between the end-links of this chain, of which the stimulus is the outer and the sensation is the inner experience. To enter into inner psychophysics we have to make a transition from the outer end-links to the middle link, in order further to consider this relationship, instead of the relation of the outer to the inner. Thus, after it has served its purpose in bringing us to the middle link, we shall drop consideration of the stimulus.

Much of what Fechner longed to study is nowadays topics within neuropsychology and techniques such as fMRI (functional magnetic resonance imaging) enable also sport and exercise psychology researchers to study what happens in the brain between a sensation and the following perception (e.g. Smith, 2016; Nauman et al., 2015). In Fechner's time, this was not possible, which he expresses in the following lines:

Our information about the anatomy and physiology in the inner physical mechanisms that serves as a basis for our mental activity is presently far too imperfect to allow for reliable inference about the general nature of psychophysical processes. Are they electrical, chemical, or mechanical? Are they in some way made of a perceptible or an imperceptible medium? Do we simply say we do not know? (Fechner, 1889, pp. 377–378).

If Fechner had stopped at this point, by merely expressing the need for better apparatus and techniques to make it possible to study what happens in the 'black box', then few contemporary researchers would have objected to his idea of an inner psychophysics.

But, like any scientist, Fechner was not independent from the times he was living in, where religion played an important role; nor could he shed his background as a physicist. And to simply admit that he did not know and stop was probably not an attractive alternative. He therefore presents an intriguing theory of waves:

> Our principal waves, on which our principal consciousness depends, pro-duce waves on which our special conscious phenomena depend; but can our principal waves for their part also be considered as overwaves of some larger principal wave? If physical waves can work like this, why not also psychophysical? The total activity of the earthly system can thus be repre-sented under our schema as a larger wave, and the systems of activity of the individual organic creatures are part of it as mere overwaves. The systems of activity of the heavenly bodies are likewise only overwaves of the general system of the totality of the processes of nature. The stepwise construction that goes on inside us also carries on outside of us (Chapter 45, p. 541).

Fechner published the above in 1889; in 1905 Einstein, a fellow physicist, published his Special Theory of Relativity, which he followed up with his General Theory of Relativity in 1915. Einstein also discussed among other things the possible existence of gravitational waves: ripples in spacetime. In 2015, gravitational waves from colliding black holes were for the first time detected by scientists working at the Laser Interferometer Gravitational-Wave Observatory in Louisiana and Washington, respec-tively. Fechner probably did not refer to ripples in spacetime when he wrote: 'activity of the heavenly bodies are likewise only overwaves of the general system of the totality of the processes of nature.' Fechner did continue (p. 542), however, by drawing the following conclusion:

> The consequence of this conception leads to the view of an omnipresent, conscious God in nature, in whom all spirits live, move, and have their being, as He also lives in them. The heavenly bodies and the individual spirits intermediate beings dwell in between Him and us, and these creature-spirits carry our sensory experiences just as undivided and united in themselves, as for their part they are carried in the divine God; like us, these creature-spirits carry their own sensory circles that carry within them their own special perceptions.

Fechner's later writings may have been more a reflection of his upbringing, because his father was a pastor, than of him being a scientist. Fechner nevertheless combined his background as a physicist (being a Professor of Physics between 1834 and 1839, when he contracted an eye-disorder while studying colour and vision) with a streak of philosophy and religion to become the first psychophysicist. Maybe the explanation for his outer and inner psychophysics is simple, at least in hindsight. As a physicist, Fechner studied phenomena that he could observe, that is in the outer world. This was not, however, enough so he pondered questions that today are studied in cognitive psychology and neuropsychology, processes that are not easily observed—at that time, it was impossible—hence the term 'inner'. As suggested earlier, Fechner was probably not satisfied with admitting that he did not know. So he instead attributed what he did not know to what for him was logical and in line with his upbringing: a divine spirit or God. Had Fechner been alive today, he would probably have been excited about signal-detection theory and new techniques such as fMRI that could offer him alternative explanations to answer some of the questions that he struggled with during a long and productive career.

Fechner's career, to some extent, formed how Stevens approached research, as director of the Psycho-Acoustic Laboratory at Harvard University, which was later renamed the Psychological Laboratories. Stevens, however, did much more than repeal Fechner's law. Maybe his most noteworthy contribution was his description of different scales of measurement.

Scales of Measurement and Modern Psychophysics

Any basic textbook dealing with research methods and statistics include a description of the four levels of measurement that Stevens presented in 1946. Measurement being defined as assigning numerals to objects, or events, according to rules. In this historically influential paper, Stevens presented four levels: nominal, ordinal, interval and ratio; the latter is common in the natural sciences such as weights and lengths. In psychology, ratio scales have been around for a considerable time, with the Sone scale by Stevens and Davis (1938) as one of the earliest efforts to compare loudness ratios by comparing pairs of tones, thereby focusing on the subjective perception of something, in this case perceived loudness.

This method is known as indirect scaling because a person is comparing pairs and judging whether one stimulus is, for example, louder, stronger, heavier or brighter than the other stimulus; not *how much* louder, stronger, heavier or brighter one stimulus is compared to the other. Stevens and his colleagues at Harvard (1937) therefore devised methods such as bisection (determining when the intensity of a stimulus falls midway between two others) and fractionation (adjusting the intensity of one stimulus to make its sensory magnitude appear to be some fraction of that of a fixed stimulus).

Scaling became much more user friendly when magnitude estimation was introduced (Stevens, 1975). A person is asked to estimate the magnitude (by assigning a number) of a stimulus. This number can be chosen arbitrarily, for example 10 or 100, and is referred to as free magnitude estimation; if a subsequent stimulus is perceived to be double the intensity the person is expected to say 20 (or 200), if it is perceived as half the intensity, 5 (or 50) would be expected. This creates numbers that conform to the standards of ratio scaling (having a true zero, equal intervals and order between stimulus).

The work by Fechner and Stevens, and the journey from the older to the newer psychophysics, was taken into the world of physical activity and sport by, among others, Gunnar Borg (1962). Devising a scale for ratings of perceived exertion (RPE)---or as it is now widely known, Borg's RPE scale—made it possible not only to measure and compare individuals physiologically but also psychologically. However, the RPE scale is not a ratio scale as it lacks a true 0 (the numerical range goes from 6 to 20), and some question whether the intervals between the verbal anchors (ranging from 'No exertion at all' to 'Maximal Exertion') are equal. Most statisticians will concede that the RPE scale allows ordinal measurements. In reality, however, researchers most often treat it as an interval scale, which allows the calculation of means and standard deviations and the use of parametric statistical analyses.

A further development was made in the 1980s when the first category-ratio scales were created, often used for pain but in contrast to the RPE scale that is used solely for perceived exertion, CR scales have more general verbal anchors (typically ranging between 'Nothing at all' constituting a zero to 'Maximal', sometimes with an open end-point to avoid ceiling-effects). This makes it possible to rate many modalities apart from perceived exertion and pain, for example, taste, smell, noise and vibration (Borg, 1998). Today, the Borg scales are frequently used in sport and exercise studies as a complement to heart rate, oxygen consumption, respiration rate, blood/muscle lactate and other physiological correlates.

Experimental Psychology

The history of psychology—indeed of any science—becomes known through its scribes. One such influential person was Edwin G. Boring, who in 1929 published *A History of Experimental Psychology*. He stated,

> Fechner, because of what he did and the time at which he did it, set experimental quantitative psychology off upon the course which it has followed. One may call him the 'founder' of experimental psychology, or one may assign that title to Wundt. It does not matter. Fechner had a fertile idea which grew and brought forth fruit most abundantly – and the end of that growth is not yet (p. 286).

Historians of psychology are—of course—not in total agreement, and some remain faithful to the belief that the lab devoted to experimental psychology and led by Wilhelm Wundt from its conception in 1879 constitutes the real starting point. Suffice to say, the foundation of experimental psychology was laid from 1850 onwards in Germany—why Germany?

One explanation favoured in books on the history of experimental psychology is that experimental physiology was already well accepted and established in Germany. Further, scholars such as Ernst Weber (1795–1878), Hermann von Helmholtz (1821–1894) and Gustav Theodor Fechner (1801–1887) all started out by studying medicine, physics and/or physiology before entering psychophysiology (Weber and Helmholtz) and psychophysics (Fechner). They were all interested in the interface between body and mind, a trend that prevailed, as we shall see when we consider the earlier efforts within the field of sport and exercise psychology. Another explanation for the early dominance by German researchers is that science was viewed more broadly than in England and France where it basically was limited to chemistry and physics. A third explanation relates to the context. Germany before 1870 was not a unified nation but a loose confederation with many well-financed universities. In contrast, England had two: Cambridge and Oxford. The former even vetoed a request to add experimental psychology to the curriculum in 1877, because it would 'insult religion by putting the human soul on a pair of scales' (Hearnshaw, 1987, p. 125) —again showing the time when Fechner were presenting his ideas about an inner and outer psychophysics. Cambridge changed their mind 20 years later, but it took Oxford nearly 60 years before experimental psychology was taught there.

Suffice to say, Wilhelm Wundt (1832–1920) had many advantages over his contemporaries in England and France. Wundt's early academic career is very similar to the ones described above: He started out by studying medicine with the explicit goal of becoming a physician. Apart from anatomy and medicine, his agenda included chemistry and physics; he was even appointed as laboratory assistant to Helmholtz. Wundt successively became more interested in psychological questions, manifested in a course on physiological psychology held at the University of Heidelberg; allegedly the first offering of such a course in the world. The publication of *Grundzüge der Physiologischen Psychhologie* (Principles of Physiological Psychology, in two parts, 1873 and 1874) paved the way for the establishment of the first laboratory of experimental psychology (several already existed devoted to experimental physiology). In Wundt's own words:

> The present work shows by its very title that it seeks to establish an alliance between two sciences that, although they both deal with almost the same subject, that is, pre-eminently with human life, nevertheless have long followed different paths. Physiology informs us about those life phenomena that we perceive by our external senses. In psychology, the person looks upon himself as from within and tries to explain the interrelations of those processes that this internal observation discloses (pp. 1–2).

It is hardly surprising that the methods used by Wundt were developed within the natural sciences and, of course, particularly by physiologists. Neither is it surprising that psychophysical methods—linking Fechner to Wundt—were used to study everything from auditory to visual perceptions including colour, colour blindness, visual contrast and visual size. Time perception and particularly reaction time was also a hot topic in Wundt's laboratory, and—as we shall see later—a topic that also arose the interest from early sport psychology researchers on the other side of the Atlantic Ocean.

The description above is far too short to include such names as Hermann Ebbinghaus (1850–1909), Franz Brentano (1838–1917) and Edward Bradford Titchener (1867–1927). But without them, sport and exercise psychology may not have developed along the path it has. The same applies to Francis Galton (1822–1911), who devoted considerable effort to the concept of individual differences. Not to say that many scientists before him—such as Weber, Fechner and Helmholtz—had been unaware of the fact that people differed psychologically in a great number of ways. Galton, however, explored this further when he turned his attention to mental ability, and specifically intelligence, and how to measure it by using mental tests.

But maybe Galton's most important contribution to science was the correlation that is the statistical method that makes it possible to calculate the strength of association between two variables (r_{xy}). From its humble origin, correlations remain at the base of all factor analytic methods including structural equation modelling that has become increasingly popular also in sport and exercise psychology research. Methods that benefitted from the development of the computer, which make advanced calculations easy to an extent that would have amazed Galton. Quantitative researchers within sport and exercise psychology thereby benefit from work performed well over 100 years ago not only by Galton, but indeed also by Fechner and Wundt.

To make this brief historical account of experimental psychology somewhat complete, we need to also mention James McKeen Cattell (1860–1944) and Alfred Binet (1857–1911). In the tradition of Galton, both Cattell and Binet were fascinated with the potential of the emerging statistical methods. This set Cattell apart from the man who had employed him as his laboratory assistant: Wilhelm Wundt in Leipzig. Cattell returned to the United States after receiving his doctorate, and shortly thereafter to Cambridge University in England where he met Galton. Whereas Wundt in his laboratory in Leipzig had favoured experiments with few participants, Cattell instead enlisted significantly larger groups of participants, thereby making the raw data suitable for testing out statistical techniques. Galton's work on measuring mental ability was further developed by Cattell who in 1890 published a formative article in *Mind* entitled 'Mental tests and measurements'.

This, in turn, inspired Binet, because he did not agree with Galton and Cattell that mental ability could be measured by testing sensory-motor processes. Binet instead tried to measure cognitive functions, such as memory and comprehension, as he believed this to be closer to intelligence—the intelligence quotient and the Binet–Simon Measuring Scale for Intelligence was the precursor to what still exists: the Stanford–Binet Intelligence Scales.

So why is this worth mentioning in a book dealing with sport and exercise psychology? One reason is that the research and researchers described lay a very important foundation for sport and exercise psychology research; Wundt's experimental paradigm and his laboratory in Leipzig where measurements were at the centre had paramount influence on how Lawrence Scientific School at Harvard University and the Yale Psychology Laboratory conducted research. It also explains why quantitative research methods got a head start over qualitative approaches, and why groups of participants were favoured over case studies as they allowed statistical analyses to be performed.

The Dawn of Sport and Exercise Psychology Research

Given the historical account above and the emergence of experimental psychology, who were the equivalents of Wundt, Fechner and all those other early researchers that became instrumental for developing sport and exercise psychology? One such important person—in fact a former student of Wilhelm Wundt in Leipzig—was Edward Wheeler Scripture, who came to be leading the Yale Psychology Laboratory. Scripture's work involved athletes and with a clear psychological focus; here, we see the beginnings of American sport psychology. In 1894 (p. 721), he wrote:

> A proper knowledge of the laws of rhythmic action might make a change in the winning of a boat-race. I respectfully suggest to the oft-defeated Harvard crew that they take a course in experimental psychology with special attention to reaction-time and time-memory. Indeed it might not be a bad thing to give all our college boys a little more mental training! If psychology is practically applied in this way, the bulletins of the twentieth century may read in this fashion: "Yale at this time was half a length ahead, but gradually fell behind for some reason. After the race an examination of the automatic record made by each oar revealed that the rhythmic movements of No. 2's oar had dropped below the required regularity. The mean error from the average was great enough to cause a decided loss of power." We may also read: "Mr. B., of the Chicago eleven has lately made several bad plays in passing the ball. Tests at the psychology laboratory revealed a large increase in discrimination time."

The influence from Wundt's laboratory is unmistakable, as timing issues and reaction time were often at the forefront in Leipzig. Scripture consequently used the techniques he was taught by Wundt, but applied them to sport, most notably fencers and the relationship between reaction time and time of muscle movement, linking in with Wundt's 'physiologischen psychologie'. Scripture's contemporary, George Wells Fitz of Harvard University, also devoted some of his career to study reaction time in athletes. Also noteworthy in the citation above is Scripture's suggestion: 'it might not be a bad thing to give all our college boys a little more mental training!' This is probably one of the earliest suggestions made by a sport psychology researcher to use the research results to inform practice, with the intent to enhance sport performance.

Both Fitz and Scripture are frequently mentioned in historical accounts of psychology. It is therefore somewhat ironic that Norman Triplett, as a result of his 1898 Master thesis in which he analysed official records of bicycle racing performance and also assessed the impact of audiences on sport performance, is honoured as being the first real sport psychology researcher (with a social psychology focus). Triplett's main result presented in his Master Thesis was that cyclists riding against a competitor performed better than when riding alone; he later shifted to study 'The psychology of conjuring deceptions', which became the title of his doctoral dissertation, published in 1900.

Another notable American who collected empirical data on topics related to sport and exercise psychology was Coleman Roberts Griffith. The time between 1920 and 1940 has even been called 'The Griffith Era' because of his many contributions and efforts to integrate research with practice (Gould & Pick, 1995). Whether the epithet 'the father of American sport psychology' is warranted or not can, of course, be discussed, but it is supported by among others Kroll and Lewis (1969).

What Griffith did was three things that differentiated him from his predecessors: (1) he devoted a major part of his time to research in sport, (2) he directed a research laboratory mainly focused on topics related to sport psychology, and (3) he worked closely with coaches and athletes, building the link between research and practice. Others before him clearly touched on topics related to sport and exercise psychology, but not with such a long-term commitment as Griffith. In that respect, he was indeed different from his forerunners and a first of his kind—at least in the United States.

Another perspective is offered by an article in the *Journal of Applied Sport Psychology*, with the title 'The Russian origins of sport psychology: A translation of an early work of A. C. Puni' (Ryba, Stambulova, & Wrisberg, 2005) offers a non-Anglo-Saxon perspective. The authors describe how Puni performed research in Russia, at the P.F. Lesgaft Institute of Physical Culture in Leningrad (now St. Petersburg), at the same time when Griffith was active in America. Of course, Puni wrote in Russian and Griffith in English so their audiences differed—as did their impact on the future of sport and exercise psychology. Equally unknown to Anglo-Saxon sport psychology is Piotr Antonovich Roudik who performed his research within the walls of the Psychology Department at the State Central Institute of Physical Culture in Moscow. Whereas Puni's research was applied—he was interested in studying table tennis and the psychophysiological effects of training—Roudik's research was more politically influenced and aligned with the ruling party in the mighty Soviet Union. It may therefore come as no big surprise that it was Roudik that in 1925 founded the first sport psychology laboratory in the Soviet Union; Puni replied some 20 years later by creating a Department of Sport Psychology at the Lesgaft Institute (Ryba et al., 2005).

The article by Puni, translated and later published and commented by Ryba et al. (2005), is an excellent example of research conducted without the possibility to interact with international researchers outside—in this case—the Soviet Union. The references mentioned by Puni, and the research he described, all originated within the same strictly controlled Eastern European context. Consequently, most of this was not known outside the Soviet Union, thereby with limited impact on contemporary researchers elsewhere. It is noteworthy that two such different systems— the Soviet and American—could produce researchers with so many similarities. However, Ryba and colleagues conclude by offering an interesting perspective and a huge difference between Puni and Griffith:

> Finally, we should point out that Puni's effect on Soviet sport psychology appears to have been more robust and persistent in his country than was that of his counterpart, Griffith, in the U.S. While Griffith was in many ways the model scientist-practitioner, he failed to train or stimulate others to follow in his footsteps and thus the field of sport psychology remained fairly dormant in the U.S. from around 1940, when Griffith ceased working with professional sport teams (the University of Illinois had shut down his laboratory in 1932), until the late 1960s. Puni, on the other hand, continued to shape the development of sport psychology in the Soviet Union for over 50 years and his influence persists to the present day in Russia and other East European countries (p. 167).

Whether Griffith failed, as alluded to by Ryba et al., to stimulate others to follow in his footsteps is not certain; what is certain is that there were no graduate degrees offered by Griffith's academic affiliation. Students wanting to pursue an academic career at that time had therefore to look elsewhere—to the dismay of Griffith, one may assume.

As for the University of Illinois closing Griffith's Research in Athletics Laboratory, their reason must at least to some extent been financial, namely the Great Depression, which had a mighty impact on western society as a whole. But as suggested by Gould and Pick (1995), another reason may have been that Robert Zuppke, football coach at the University of Illinois, lost faith in Griffith's research as contributing to the players' performance. This is, of course, an interesting suggestion, given that the link between research and application sometimes is fraught with conflict as soon as theory meets practice (this is also something we will return to in Chap. 8). Maybe this becomes even more obvious and visible within sport where athletes and coaches strive to win competitions, whereas researchers struggle to win knowledge. A clash between ultimate goals that still explains why researchers battle to gain access to elite athletes and teams, because their question 'what is in it for us now?' can be difficult to answer. Not because research cannot be applied, but more a simple matter of timing. Whereas a coach may want immediately usable results that can be implemented 'today', a researcher may be somewhat reluctant to release the results until data has been properly analysed and presented in a scientific journal.

Griffith, however, was no stranger to applying his knowledge to sport for the benefit of athletes and coaches; not always appreciated though as evidenced by coach Zuppke's decision to separate his team from Griffith. In a widely cited article, entitled 'Psychology and its relation to athletic competition', Griffith (1925) offered his view on applied sport psychology:

> The more mind is made use of in the athletic competition, the greater will be the skill of our athletes, the finer will be the contest, the higher will be the ideals of sportsmanship displayed, the longer will our games persist in our national life, and the more truly will they lead to those rich personal and social products which we ought to expect of them. Because of these facts, the psychologist may hope to break into the realm of athletic competition, just as he has already broken into the realms of industry, commerce, medicine, education, and art (p. 193).

As described above, Griffith's Laboratory for Research in Athletics closed down in 1932, after seven productive years with Griffith as its director. Baseball, basketball and football were often the sports investigated and resulted in 20-something articles published alongside two books: *Psychology of Coaching* (1926) and *Psychology of Athletics* (1928). After the closing of the Athletics laboratory, Griffith authored two more textbooks, but not specifically related to sport (*Introduction to Applied Psychology*, 1934; *Introduction to Educational Psychology*, 1935).

But Griffith's contributions to applied sport psychology did not finish there; in 1938, he was hired by Philip Knight Wrigley, the owner of the successful baseball club Chicago Cubs to help improve team-performance (Green, 2003). The story told by Green is recommended to anyone interested in applied sport psychology; Griffith and his assistant John E. Sterrett built a scientific training programme supported by filming and measuring the players' baseball skills. Between 1938 and 1940, Griffith delivered reports, totalling over 600 pages, to Wrigley and the team. Little, however, was used or implemented in their daily training as the coaches and players seemed either threatened or uninterested—to the disappointment and increasing frustration of Griffith who in his reports did not hesitate to conclude that one particular coach 'was not at all a smart man' or that the players were lazy. It seems that the stint with the Cubs concluded Griffith's work within sport psychology and he assumed other academic roles at the University of Illinois. Again, one may assume that coach Wrigley expected immediately implementable results and when he failed to detect that—although obviously not too keen to try either—he dismissed Griffith.

Griffith's influence, however, was not over. In fact, he was instrumental in creating a Sport Psychology Laboratory in the 1950s. Not by actually reopening the laboratory that was closed in 1932, but as provost of the University of Illinois supporting the proposal submitted by Alfred W. Hubbard. The laboratory was officially opened in 1951 and Hubbard continued to make important contributions for many years to come. Griffith as a researcher in the 1920s and 1930s had a significant impact, and his influence can further be seen in the publications originating from the new Sport Psychology Laboratory during the 1950s and 1960s. Many journal articles, master and doctoral theses investigated the same topics as Griffith had many years before. For example, blindfolded practice, peripheral vision and basketball free throw shooting (publications that frequently cited Griffith's earlier research). In 1969, Hubbard presented a 10-year plan for the continued development of sport psychology at the University of Illinois (Kornspan, 2013); a plan that created an environment that attracted notable researchers such as Rainer Martens, Daniel Landers, and a few years later, Glyn Roberts, Daniel Gould and Robin S. Vealey.

Smocks and Jocks in the Box

In 1979, Martens published an article entitled 'About smocks and jocks' in which he refutes his laboratory 'smock' to his more fitting sport 'jocks'. Martens argues that sport psychology researchers need to leave their confined laboratories to fully enter the fields of sport, thereby being closer to the action when performing sport relevant research; this will also ensure a satisfactory degree of external validity. This call was surely heeded by some contemporary researchers, but did Martens forget that Griffith already in the 1920s and 1930s worked in the field, while at the same time leading a sport psychology laboratory? Martens' former doctoral student Robin S. Vealey remembers this and states: 'Indeed, what made Griffith the model pioneer for the field [sport psychology] were his abilities not only as a researcher and teacher, but also as a practitioner in applying knowledge in an attempt to enhance the performance of athletes and coaches' (Vealey, 2006, p. 136). That much of that knowledge was obtained in the field and outside of the laboratory seems to have escaped Martens, but not Vealey.

Nevertheless, Vealey 25 years later followed up on Martens' article and voiced the question: 'Have smocks and jocks escaped the box?' (Vealey, 2006, p. 128). The term 'box' was used to represent the dominant 'paradigm' (we will return and discuss the definition of a paradigm in Chap. 5) for doing research and applied work. In the opening paragraph, Vealey describes how she one day, while 'busy testing psychological theory, safe inside my paradigmatic box', was asked by a graduate student 'What are we trying to discover?' which led her to realise that she—in her own words—might have 'lost sight of the meta-questions that take precedence over all others. Why do I do research? What makes my work relevant and meaningful? What *am* I trying to discover?' (p. 128).

Inspired by the graduate student, Vealey encourages all her fellow researchers to regularly ask themselves 'what are we trying to discover?'— a call to rethink why and what we do as a collective. Because it is not only what we as researchers are trying to discover but also very much how we go about this process. Vealey herself discusses these questions, but from the perspective of sport science in the United States, exemplified by her statement that 'it was not until the 1970s that sport and exercise psychology was formally established and recognized as a subdiscipline of kinesiology' although it 'obviously has close ties to the discipline of psychology' (p. 130).

Maybe this applied perspective, and close link to kinesiology/human movement, focusing on practical solutions immediately usable in sport and exercise practice, to some extent explains the accusation that sport and exercise psychology at times has been unsystematic and even atheoretical (Landers, 1995). Perhaps sport-related topics, when researched from a kinesiology-focused perspective, are performed without realising that the same topics—albeit not sport-focused—may already have been well researched within the discipline of psychology. This would also explain the on-going conflict between theoretically based research and experientially based applications in real-world sport settings (e.g. Landers, 1983) —or in the words of Martens (1987), the science–practice dualism (see also Chap. 8).

Another box proving difficult to escape is the positivistic and nomothetic one with quantitative measurements at its core. Although, qualitative methods are finally becoming more common, they are still trailing quantitative methods (Sparkes, 2013). There is no way we can escape the history that has shaped modern day sport and exercise psychology, and the words voiced by Vealey (2006) more than a decade ago are still worth repeating:

> .....we can be critical of the 'box' used at various points in history, it is hypocritical to criticize previous research traditions as ineffective. All our research traditions were effective in showing us the way, similar to working through a maze where at times backtracking and rethinking is required (pp. 147–8).

Vealey thus suggest that by backtracking and rethinking our past, we may indeed succeed in 'building doors' to the future so that the boxes open up to allow us to aim for 'practical theory' and not 'theoretical practice' (p. 148; also see Chap. 9 on the *Myth of the Framework*). This also 'requires individuals to leave their comfort zones and develop research agendas that are less familiar and require extra preparation and training' (p. 146). Vealey further describes how the box has 'moved from positivism to what seems to now be a post-positivistic, modernist era with some movement toward constructivism' (p. 148). Remember that this decade-old text only saw the early stages of constructivism that now—thanks to sport and exercise psychology researchers such as Brett Smith and Andrew C. Sparkes—has come a long way in a relatively short period of time (e.g. Sparkes, 2002, 2013, 2015; Sparkes & Smith, 2009, 2013; see also Chap. 5).

Concluding Remarks

We conclude this chapter by reiterating what Martens suggested already in 1979: that sport psychology should work more closely with sport sociology to properly acknowledge the relationship between the individual athlete, coach or team and their environment, physical as well as social. This is actually one reason that the three authors of the book you are currently reading stem from these two related, yet distinct disciplines. We believe this to be an additional strength on our part as we endeavour to rethink sport and exercise psychology. The next chapter will focus on building the knowledge base and the importance of creative and critical thinking while doing this.

Which brings to mind an article published in 1990 by a research ecologist, Craig Loehle, on the topic of creativity. Loehle refers to Popper (1963) and his call to generate alternative hypotheses, but Popper never suggested how researchers should go about creating them, which Loehle instead have some thoughts about. However, the prevailing 'publish or perish' climate is not, according to Loehle, conducive to creativity (and for venturing outside the paradigmatic box). The focus on quantity instead of quality may also explain the bulk of 'normal science' (Kuhn, 1970) and lack of paradigm shifts: most researchers simply do not have time to think, creatively. Loehle (1990, p. 125) follows up by posing an intriguing question: 'What would have happened if Darwin and Einstein as young men had needed to apply for government support?' His answer, 'Their probability of getting past the grant reviewers would be similar to a snowball surviving in Hell.' The current audit culture (further discussed in Chap. 5) does not encourage unconventional thinking, as this will most likely lower productivity (quantity is more important than quality). That it will also hamper creative new ways to research problems and extend the knowledge base seems to be a much smaller concern—the need to critically assess and rethink our ways seems urgent.

3

How Do We Know That We Really Know?

Everyone in today's society is constantly exposed to advertisements and infomercials extolling the virtues of something or other. Sometimes 'research' is said to prove that a remedy is working, or the effectiveness of some new and innovative method or gadget. Sport and exercise psychology as a field is not exempt; there are numerous books on the market extolling how the mind can overcome anything and make everyone perform at a level you only could dream of—until you buy and read a particular book. The interested reader can use the search terms 'mental training' and 'peak performance' to see which books are currently available on any given online book retailer.

Likewise, to 'Google' a question has become the norm with the Internet making any type of information available without restrictions around access or content. Nowadays, almost everyone has access to more information than is humanly possible to digest, and this also permeates the world of science. The careful reading of peer-reviewed scientific journal articles can sometimes be viewed as an unnecessary chore for sport and exercise psychology students. Because the Internet provides easily accessible, colourful, highly produced and often interactive and visually

© The Author(s) 2016
P. Hassmén et al., *Rethinking Sport and Exercise Psychology Research*,
DOI 10.1057/978-1-137-48338-6_3

appealing content, content that is easier to access and grasp than ever before and that does not require prior knowledge to understand—at least on the surface.

This would all be fine, *if* all available information on the Internet and in books (other outlets) were accurate and reliable, which we will argue is not the case. Good and reliable information sits beside the unreliable, the misleading and even dangerous ideas for individuals and society alike. The gullible or simply uninformed person is worse off than ever before because it takes astute and highly developed critical faculties to evaluate claims, and to distinguish between the good and the bad. At the same time, an open mind for new knowledge is necessary; only because something has not been researched thoroughly does not mean that it is inaccurate. Sagan (1995) expands on this:

> Science involves a seemingly self-contradictory mix of attitudes. On the one hand, it requires an almost complete openness to all ideas, no matter how bizarre or weird they sound, a propensity to wonder…But at the same time, science requires the most vigorous and uncompromising scepticism, because the vast majority of ideas are simply wrong, and the only way you can distinguish the right from the wrong, the wheat from the chaff, is by critical experiment and analysis. Too much openness and you accept every notion, idea, and hypothesis – which is tantamount to knowing nothing. Too much scepticism – especially rejection of new ideas before they are adequately tested – and you're not only unpleasantly grumpy, but also closed to the advance of science. A judicious mix is what we need (Sagan 1995).

People, however, are not always sufficiently critical: a 2005 Gallup survey revealed that 73 % of all Americans held at least one paranormal belief. Astrology as a science, communication with the dead, extrasensory perception, faith healing and beliefs in ghosts and haunted places are readily discussed on the Internet; many swear by their accuracy and occurrence. Systematic evidence is, however, sadly lacking—or is provided in the form of anecdotes and testimonials by purportedly reliable witnesses, but rarely holding up to scientific scrutiny. We are also prone to look for easy solutions, such as the secret performance-keys of successful athletes or coaches. When an athlete or team succeeds, despite being considered the underdog: what is their secret weapon? It is easy to believe that the answer may also help us perform better, so we buy the books, listen to the stories and hope for the best. The healthy scepticism that Sagan (1995) speaks about, and the ability to critically consider alternative explanations, seems to be rare commodities.

Critical Thinking in Sport and Exercise Psychology

An exercise psychologist recruited 10 patients diagnosed with major depression. After four months of jogging three times per week, their average score on an established depression inventory was significantly lower than at the pre-test. The researcher concluded that exercise is a reliable treatment for those suffering from depression.

Do you see any flaws in this conclusion, or in the design of the study? For example: are spontaneous changes over time considered (a control group would have enabled the researcher to compare those who exercised with those that did not)? How depressed were the participants to begin with (a diagnosis only stipulates that certain symptoms are present)? Were there other differences among the exercisers (gender, age, weight, height, etc.)? How many—if any—did already perform some form of regular physical exercise (frequency, duration, intensity, mode)? If you voiced some of these questions, you did indeed use your critical thinking skills; that is 'a purposeful reflection that requires logic' (Behar-Horenstein & Niu, 2011: p. 26). You have thereby demonstrated that, on this occasion, you have not fallen prey to naïve realism: that is, the belief that the world is exactly as we see it (Ross & Ward, 1996). To naïvely presume that an observed change in average depression scores is a direct result of the intervention is a logical error of thinking ('post hoc, ergo propter hoc': which translates to 'after this, therefore because of this'). We can assume that the exercise psychologist was not aware of this risk, which would have been significantly reduced by including a non-exercising comparison group and better control over the intervention and background variables. There are indeed many potential explanations for the reduction in depression scores over time. First and foremost, the simple passage of time is an important variable in the spontaneous remission of depression symptoms, and this is evident not only in research evaluating the effect on depression, but of just about anything studied over time. People get older, more experienced, and in the case of something like depression—it's not very nice, so there is an inherent strong motivation to 'get better'. Spontaneous physical activity also differs over the year, with most sedentary people being more active during the warmer months when there is more daylight, compared to the darker and colder months of the year. Without a control group, it is therefore impossible for the exercise psychologist to ascertain whether time or the exercise led to the observed reduction in depression scores or, for example, whether exercise helped *more* people get better than time alone. Similarly, the attention received by the patients, in any shape or form, may induce change whether it is an effect due to the novelty of the activity (non-exercising patients starting to exercise), a placebo effect (patients expecting change, as is the exercise psychologist) or merely the Hawthorne effect (behaviour change as a result of being observed). We also know that a statistical artefact, namely regression to the mean, may be the cause as extreme scores at pre-test are more likely to become less extreme (rather than even more) at post-test.

The only way to rule out most random and systematic errors is through well-designed studies—and that is not to say there is only one 'true' way of designing a study (often the 'randomised control trial' springs to mind), but that the careful design of studies is key to establishing causal links, relationships and so on. Study design is something we will consider later in this chapter: the following discussion focuses on the topic of critical thinking. To counteract the proliferation of unsubstantiated beliefs, one would imagine that critical-analytic thinking is a skill taught from pre-school to university. Regretfully, it is not (Marin & Halpern, 2011). Although it should be—at least at the university level—as most tertiary curriculums state that students are supposed to develop their ability to think critically during the course of their studies (Behar-Horenstein & Niu, 2011). The American Psychological Association (APA), in their Guidelines for the Undergraduate Psychology Major (Version 2.0, 2013), describe five comprehensive learning goals including 'Scientific inquiry and critical thinking'. What is interesting, however, is the lack of definition of what this constitutes. APA instead chooses to focus on skills related to scientific reasoning and problem solving, for example, Goal 2.1B: 'Develop plausible behavioural explanations that rely on scientific reasoning and evidence rather than anecdotes or pseudoscience' (p. 20)—pseudoscience will be discussed at length later in this chapter.

The problem with the approach taken by APA—as discussed by Schmaltz and Lilienfeld (2014)—is that learning the virtues of scientific reasoning and the nature of science is not sufficient to help students develop their critical thinking skills, and therefore their scientific thinking skills are also underdeveloped. The same line of (critical) thought is expressed by Kirschner (2011): 'Teaching critical thinking thus becomes synonymous with finding ways to operationalize (and as much as possible, to quantify) phenomena of interest, as well as with fostering sensitivity to such pitfalls as confirmation bias, not confounding correlation with causation, and other sound and important, but quite circumscribed, tenets of critical appraisal' (p. 176). The latter is of course one facet of critical thinking, but critical thinking involves so much more (e.g. Kirschner, 2011), and it needs to be addressed directly, and repeatedly (Schmaltz & Lilienfeld, 2014). Science with pseudoscience will later be contrasted, thereby focusing on critical issues and warning signs to counteract that 'All of us are prone to errors in thinking' (Lilienfeld, Ammirati, & David, 2012: p. 7). As a field, sport and exercise psychology may be (even more) at risk for errors in thinking, for example, the athlete or coach that becomes convinced that a certain training regimen is the key to optimal performance. The evidence? One athlete succeeding by winning an Olympic Gold Medal. Or why not a sport psychologist claiming that an athlete succeeded entirely because of the psychological skills programme devised by the psychologist (subsequently described in a bestselling book with a photo of the athlete on the cover). Elite sport is, in many respects, unique in that performance is measured with a high degree of precision, but there is little scientific control in the form of control groups or random allocation of athletes to different treatments. So it is easy to claim that a certain result is a consequence of this or that, and when the scientist point out alternative explanations this is not always well received or even appreciated. We must also remember that elite sport often involves substantial amounts of money—professional soccer alone is a billion dollar industry—so when a sport psychologist can claim that an athlete or team has benefitted from their involvement, this can also mean big business for the sport psychologist. Consequently, critical thinking is a skill that is necessary to develop for everyone—including those procuring the services of sport and exercise psychology practitioners—not only academics in search for reliable knowledge.

These are some attributes suggested to distinguish critical thinkers from non-critical thinkers; the former will tend to: '(1) be capable of taking a position or changing a position as evidence dictates, (2) remain relevant to the point, (3) seek information as well as precision in information, (4) be open-minded, (5) take into account the entire situation, (6) keep the original problem in mind, (7) search for reason, (8) deal with the components of a complex problem in an orderly manner, (9) seek a clear statement of the problem, (10) look for options, (11) exhibit sensitivity to others' feelings and depth of knowledge, and (12) use credible sources. Critical thinkers generally use these skills without prompting' (Behar-Horenstein & Niu, 2011: p. 27). Being open-minded yet search for alternative explanations and consider the 'precision in information', not merely accepting any available information, is also in line with what Sagan voiced earlier. The final point (use credible sources) is worth stressing, given the previous discussion and the abundance of information available to us. To develop the skill to identify weak arguments, unwarranted conclusions and unsubstantiated claims is imperative for a critical thinker. Thus, critical thinking is about *how* to think, not about *what* to think (Daud & Husin, 2004).

Critical Thinking About Sport and Exercise Psychology

The preceding discussion adopts the viewpoint of considering critical thinking *within* sport and exercise psychology. Separately, it is reasonable to attempt to apply critically thinking *about* sport and exercise psychology. For example, returning to the idea of randomised control trials, a popular view (one propagated by Boring, 1929) is that there is a hierarchy when it comes to scientific methods, with experimental research at the pinnacle. He reasoned that: 'The application of the experimental method to the problem of mind is the great outstanding event in the study of the mind, an event to which no other is comparable' (Boring, 1929, quoted in Kirschner, 2011: p. 176). In fact, much of what is written about critical thinking in psychology is based on the experimental method, and with randomised controlled trials (RCT) forming a gold standard to which all other forms of research are compared and judged. Boring made his statement nearly 100 years ago. It still seems to be held as true—by some at least—and while it does an important job of emphasising experimental design, there are certainly threats and problems that can undermine the integrity of a formal experiment. For example, inappropriate or invalid measurements, inappropriate samples, lack of clear instructions about the 'intervention'—among other things. There is no doubt that the experimental method was indeed central for the development of psychophysics as an area of research and measurement (psychometrics). The experimental method is also evident in the work of the early sport psychologists, not the least the work of Coleman Griffith in his Athletics Laboratory that followed in the tracks made by Wundt and his predecessors and contemporaries in Germany.

Boring (1929) was not, however, thinking very critically about psychology, or the methods used to study psychological phenomena. For him, the experimental method was by far the best and probably the only one that he would regard as sufficiently objective to produce reliable and valid results in a jungle where so many subjective and unreliable methods exist—a standpoint that seems to lack some critical thinking on his part. As noted by Teo (2011), 'tradition is the source of knowledge but also limits knowledge' (p. 193). Considering the development of psychology and sport and exercise psychology (see Chap. 2), the early dominance of the experimental method may, for a long time, have hindered other methods and designs to be used to the extent they otherwise would have.

The discussion above focuses on different ways of viewing what constitutes reliable and valid knowledge; a completely different framework is offered by agnotology, or the cultural production of ignorance (Proctor & Schiebinger, 2008). Another way of describing this is offered by Frankfurt (2005) who labels a lack of concern with truth and reality as 'bullshit'. Teo (2011) again: 'Tobacco industry scientists (including psychologists) are bullshitters in the sense that arguments such as 'correlation not causation', 'no one really knows', 'nothing has ever been proven definitely', 'we have to understand the times', and so on, misrepresent what actually went on without being false' (p. 197).

We may extend this thinking to sport and exercise psychology where claims are made such as 'you can do whatever you set your mind to, so reach for the stars'. And when an athlete reaches the pinnacle of sport, with an Olympic Gold Medal, is that because the mental training was successful, or despite the mental training? Some sport psychologists propagate the former view since this may attract new clients, without any firm evidence ('post hoc, ergo propter hoc')—an error of thinking that we previously labelled naïve realism. Whereas claims can be made without any substance on the Internet, scientific journals are held to a higher standard; this is one reason that sport and exercise psychology journals rely on peer reviews.

Peer Reviewers, as Gatekeepers

When a manuscript is submitted to a scientific journal for publication, the editor will most likely ask two or three experts—or peers—in the field to review the manuscript. This sometime lengthy review process is in place to ensure that every manuscript is scrutinised for accuracy and content, so that the editor knows that the manuscripts subsequently accepted for publication conforms to the highest scientific standard. This in turn assures the reader that an article published in a peer-reviewed journal is a trustworthy source of information. Most of the time, this process succeeds in rejecting questionable manuscripts and allowing well-designed and well-presented studies to be published. Most of the time...but not always, as history has shown repeatedly when even the most highly ranked and prestigious journals have to retract published articles, for example, Nature (http://www.nature.com/nature/journal/v511/n7507/full/nature13598.html). A possible record was set in 2014 by SAGE publication Journal of Vibration and Control: it retracted 60 published papers after having revealed a 'peer review ring' with at least 130 fake email accounts (http://jvc.sagepub.com/content/20/10/1601.

abstract). What then can we learn from this? Probably that there are bound to be published papers—including those that have survived the strictures of peer review—in sport and exercise psychology journals that must be treated with caution. Even outside the blatant fraud described above, there are phenomena such as publication bias (e.g. only publishing manuscripts that show statistically significant results), p-hacking (selecting analyses that generate statistically significant results, a.k.a. selective reporting) and salami-slice publishing (writing two or more manuscripts instead of one comprehensive) which skew the truth behind the data. Overall, this knowledge should highlight the necessity of being a critical and informed reader, not blindly accepting something as the truth solely on account of it being published in a scientific journal.

The above has always been a risk with the traditional process, which is the 'post-submission pre-publication' review by a small number of peer reviewers. An alternative is the post-publication review, made much more feasible when on-line publications are rapidly taking over from the printed academic journals (also see Chap. 9). The thought being that questionable research will be detected when many experts in the field are able to scrutinise a published paper; although as pointed out by Schuklenk (2015), this requires that experts chose to read a certain paper and also out of free will are willing to offer constructive and unbiased feedback. Schuklenk also queries who should be considered 'qualified' to act as a peer reviewer. His conclusion seems to be that the traditional peer-review process is still the best, even when considering its weaknesses. With the advent of open access publishing, the media landscape has forever changed and that may have consequences not only for researchers and reviewers, but more importantly, for consumers of scholarly research.

Open Access Publishing

The Internet has changed most things in society, not the least how science is disseminated. Open access has revolutionised the publishing market and there are now more than 10,000 open access journals in the Directory of Open Access Journals. From this website: 'We define open access journals as journals that use a funding model that does not charge readers or their institutions for access. From the BOAI definition [http://www.budapestopenaccessinitiative.org/read] of "open access" we take the right of users to "read, download, copy, distribute, print, search, or link to the full texts of these articles...or use them for any other lawful purpose" as mandatory for a journal to be included in the Directory.'

However, the cost of publishing has to be covered by someone, and most open access journals therefore demand a fee from the author. This fee can be rather steep and approach several thousand US dollars; as a consequence, the publishing business has become a highly lucrative market and created a foundation that predatory open access journals now can thrive on (see Beall's List below). Because the more manuscripts these journals accept, the more money they will make. Even though open access publishing is a relatively new occurrence, there are already several thousand predatory open access journals hunting for unsuspecting researchers. And the number of predatory journals increases every day as some publishing houses now have hundreds of journals in their stable. Cunning as they are, it is difficult to differentiate between a legitimate and predatory open access journal/publisher. Because the predatory publishers use the same language, often have similar (or even identical) names that reputable journals have (with a preference for 'International' in their title), and also a named editor in chief and editorial boards that on the surface looks as impressing as those associated with a legitimate journal. When scratched, what presents under the surface may, however, differ substantially. For example, a predatory open access journal often have unknown doctors and professors on their editorial board, people that rarely have published themselves in reputable journals although their personal publishing lists may be both long and impressive, until scrutinised.

To differentiate a legitimate, long-standing journal from a fraudulent one can be reasonably easy. However, some of the new and predatory open access journals have skilfully emulated established journals and even an authority as Dr. Jeffrey Beall, a librarian at the University of Colorado, who regularly updates his list of questionable publishers (Beall's List: https://scholarlyoa.com/publishers/), uses the heading 'Potential, possible, or probable predatory scholarly open-access publishers'. He also lists hundreds of questionable standalone journals, that is, single journals that do not belong to a publishing house. Taken together, Beall presents a disturbing picture that every student and researcher needs to be aware of. For the consumer of research, this translates to even greater demands on awareness and scepticism, not automatically accepting claims simply because these have been published in scholarly journals—because the journals may be everything but scholarly. Critical thinking skills are essential, as well as general science literacy to avoid becoming prey to the predator.

Scientific Literacy

The old saying 'there are lies, damned lies, and statistics' implies that 'you can prove anything with statistics'. And that is indeed true, at least if the receiver of the message is not statistically 'literate'. Similarly, a scientifically illiterate person may be unaware that the earth orbits the sun; 74 % of all Americans believe this to be the case while 26 % believe it is the other way around (National Science Foundation, 2014; https://www.nsf.gov/). Scientific literacy is thereby not only for the research oriented, it relates to everyone in every society. Or as expressed by the National Science Education Standards, 1996; see https://www.nsf.gov/):

> Scientific literacy means that a person can ask, find, or determine answers to questions derived from curiosity about everyday experiences. It means that a person has the ability to describe, explain, and predict natural phenomena. Scientific literacy entails being able to read with understanding articles about science in the popular press and to engage in social conversation about the validity of the conclusions. Scientific literacy implies that a person can identify scientific issues underlying national and local decisions and express positions that are scientifically and technologically informed. A literate citizen should be able to evaluate the quality of scientific information on the basis of its source and the methods used to generate it. Scientific literacy also implies the capacity to pose and evaluate arguments based on evidence and to apply conclusions from such arguments appropriately (p. 22).

To become scientifically literate is thereby one way of reducing the risk of being fooled by unsubstantiated claims, which rests on the ability to think critically about science and research. Consequently, we may all need to become more sceptical, but refrain from becoming cynical, in line with Sagan's (1995) suggestion at the beginning of this chapter: there is a clear need for a 'judicious mix' between openness and scepticism. Too much openness makes you gullible—you will believe anything, especially when psychobabble accompanies the claims, that is, the use of 'words that sound scientific, but are used incorrectly, or in a misleading manner' (Schmaltz & Lilienfeld, 2014: p. 1). At the same time, becoming a cynic and not accepting any novel claim unless it has been tested and verified on numerous occasions is being too close-minded, as it will stop any effort to expand the knowledgebase. The above can also be discussed in terms of believing or knowing something, which reminds the first author of this book about something his father said to his then very young son: 'you must always know what you speak about, beliefs are fine as long as they remain in church'—we cannot know for sure whether this affected the author's career choice, but we might believe so.

A somewhat more scientific distinction between believing and knowing is made by Daniel Kahneman in his book *Thinking, Fast and Slow* (2011). For many of us, it is difficult to think of Kahneman without Amos Tversky; they wrote many highly cited research articles and books together that dealt with judgement and decision-making. A body of research so successful that Kahneman received the Nobel Prize in 2002 (in Economics, as there is no Prize in Psychology). Had Tversky not died in 1996, the Prize would most likely been shared. In his book, Kahneman distinguishes between two systems related to our thinking. The first is automatic and fast, the second controlled and slow. Another way of describing these systems is to label the first as intuitive thinking and the second as scientific thinking. Both are active all the time, with the first typically in automatic mode and the second typically in energy-saving mode.

> System 1 continuously generates suggestions to System 2: impressions, intuitions, intentions, and feelings. If endorsed by System 2, impressions and intuitions turn into beliefs, and impulses turn into voluntary actions. When all goes smoothly, which is most of the time, System 2 adopts the suggestions of System 1 with little or no modification. You generally believe your impressions and act on your desires, and that is fine—usually (Kahneman, 2011: p. 24).

The downside of this rapid automatic processing is that it is highly dependent on heuristics (mental shortcuts; Tversky & Kahneman, 1974). As a consequence, System 1 is also more prone to bias—or systematic errors of thinking.

Heuristics and Bias

Using heuristics (mental shortcuts) is important for processing a lot of information rapidly; without this ability, cognitive overload would soon develop. So in some circumstances, heuristics can be viewed as very useful, because it protects one of our most precious assets (critical/analytical thinking) but it also makes us vulnerable. For example, by making us focus on information or evidence that are consistent with our beliefs, and similarly to dismiss anything that goes against those beliefs, a form of confirmation bias. And to complicate things, once a decision is made and a belief is considered valid, then it takes a lot to change it even when conflicting evidence emerges, a form of belief perseverance, which in turn depends on an anchoring heuristic (initial information is weighted more heavily compared to information acquired later)—first impressions are indeed important and people are generally not very good at adjusting them later.

Researchers are not exempt, as described in Chap. 2, although it was not labelled as bias then, more like inflexibility. As you may recall, Popper, Lakatos and Feyerabend all considered the dogmatic scientist a necessity with an important role to fill; Stevens (1961) on the other hand was less convinced judging from his dismissal of Fechner ('It was asking too much, perhaps, to expect a professor to change his mind after two decades of devotion to an ingenious theory': p. 80). The German theoretical physicist Max Planck, who in 1918 received the Nobel Prize in Physics, once said that science advances one funeral at a time (Boudry, Blancke, & Pigliucci, 2015). It is thereby only logical that Steven's critique of Fechner was voiced about 100 years after the publication of Elemente der Psychophysik (Fechner, 1860). Popper suggested that deliberately trying to find the opposite to what we expect could reduce the risk for confirmation bias and belief perseverance. Popper's mundane example famously included swans: if we believe that all swans are white, confirming this in numerous studies will never be sufficient. What we should do instead, according to Popper, is to look for black swans. As soon as one single black swan is detected, the belief that all swans are white is falsified. The subjectivity can then be balanced with some objectivity, although as David Hull (1990) notes, this may not come in the form of one individual scientist:

> The objectivity that matters so much in science is not primarily a characteristic of individual scientists but of scientific communities. Scientists rarely refute their own pet hypotheses, especially after they have appeared in print, but that is all right. Their fellow scientists will be happy to expose these hypotheses to severe testing (pp. 3–4).

Indeed, this explains why Fechner vigorously defended his pet-law, and why Stevens so eagerly refuted it. This balance between confirmation and falsification, between proponents and opponents, can be translated into all forms of research, not the least sport and exercise psychology research.

One bias that may play an increasingly important role is groupthink, because research nowadays is often performed in groups, sometimes disciplinary groups and sometimes interdisciplinary. One example of a safeguard, still predominantly used in qualitative research, is the 'critical friend' (or devils advocate), who is to question the other researchers interpretation of, for example, an interview. By questioning the analysis and trying to find faults, the hope is that this will reduce the risk for confirmation bias and groupthink. The same can be applied when working in teams: One individual can explicitly take on the task of trying to identify weaknesses or lapses of logic in order to weed these out before they influence the results. There is also the 'not me fallacy' (or bias blind spot): everybody else except me is at risk for making errors in thinking. Unfortunately—and when under uncertainty—we all are. So the important message is then that nobody is protected against various forms of errors in thinking, regardless of whether these are called bias, overreliance on heuristics, naïve realism or simply illusions or prevailing myths.

Myths in Sport and Exercise Psychology

Weinberg and Gould (2015) in their highly acclaimed book *Foundations of Sport and Exercise Psychology* describe some prevailing myths about psychological skills training (PST). Some of these myths are directly related to issues we have previously discussed; for example, PST is not useful for improving performance, or PST provides a 'quick-fix' solution (p. 254). If a sport psychologist agrees to meet with an athlete immediately prior to an important competition, and the athlete after a brief talk exceeds everyone's performance expectations, then it is easy (but incorrect!) to infer a cause and effect relationship. Which may exist, but it is also possible that the result would have been exactly the same without the brief intervention. We simply don't know, given that no comparison with an athlete not receiving the intervention is possible. Had the result been reversed, the meeting occurred but with no discernable effect, the conclusion could have been that the intervention was useless (or even detrimental, had the athlete underperformed). The same line of reasoning can be extended to longer mental training regimens, because in elite sport there are rarely any control groups. So it is easy to draw unsubstantiated conclusions, which is one distinguishing feature of pseudoscience.

Science Versus Pseudoscience

When grappling with the difficult questions of how one can truly 'know' something, versus developing irrational or baseless beliefs, it is important to contrast science with pseudoscience. Pseudoscience is not, however, the same as non-science. Whereas non-science lacks every distinguishing feature of science, pseudoscience is trying to mimic science and the scientific method, but ultimately failing in so doing.

Occasionally, people try to reason that science is 'simply' the application of common sense thinking. It turns out, however, that what is 'common' to some people is not to others. Lilienfeld and his colleagues (2012) even considered science to be uncommon sense: 'science is unnatural, because it often requires us to override our gut hunches and intuitions about the natural world, including the psychological world' (p. 13). The bounty of books devoted to research methods also support the notion that thinking in the scientific sense must be learned (textbooks), practised (assignments/exercises/research) and maintained (regularly used) to become ingrained and to protect against errors in thinking and the various forms of biases discussed previously.

Another way of conceptualising the above is to return to Kahneman's (2011) framework: fast thinking is associative and intuitive, whereas slow thinking is analytical and structured. System 1, in Kahneman's words, operates quickly and is basically automatic, thereby requiring no conscious effort or need for control; it helps us manage everyday life and it is active all the time. In contrast, System 2 is the slow, deliberate, conscious, mental activity that requires effort and deliberation; it is necessary for making sure we avoid the common fallacies that otherwise will impede on what is learned and—as a consequence—believed to be known. System 2 must be wilfully activated and applied, but its contribution is necessary for a scientist and when research is attempted. In fact, science and scientific thinking are the only way to distinguish between what we do know and what we do not know, with any degree of certainty. Phrased differently: the first system makes us believe, and the second assists us in going from believing to knowing, at least with a greater degree of certainty although researchers tend to avoid such words as 'proof', 'conclusive evidence' and other words because scientific claims are tentative and open to revision (in fact, strong wordings such as these are another indicator of bad science and pseudoscience).

As pointed out by Kahneman, these two systems interact, constantly. When the automatic System 1 signals a problem, System 2 is scrambling to help with solving the issue by more elaborate and effortful processing. But, and this is an important reservation, if we accept the suggestions made by System 1—because this system constantly suggests solutions based on intuition, impressions and feelings—then System 2 will remain inactive and quiet. Or rather, System 2 will simply accept what System 1 suggests without raising the alarm. And it is then that inferences may be drawn that if scrutinised would have been detected as erroneous. Most of the time, this division of labour is working out just fine; we save a lot of effort and energy by allowing System 1 to help us quickly decide on a course of action instead of activating the slower and more cumbersome System 2.

Kahneman provides an illustrative example that shows what can happen when System 1 is given free rein, although he frames it in a slightly different way. Kahneman describes how he was teaching flight instructors, telling them that rewarding good pilot performance always works better than punishing bad pilot performance (p. 175). One of the more experienced flight instructors did not, however, agree with Kahneman's suggestions. In the flight instructor's experience, every time he praised a clean execution of an aerobic manoeuvre, the following one was less well performed. If he on the other hand screamed at a pilot making a bad manoeuvre, the next one in his experience usually was performed better. So praise did not work as well as punishment, according to this very experienced flight instructor, who based his claim on numerous empirical observations. There are probably many athletes that have similar experiences: coaches that are reluctant to praise a good performance but ready to loudly 'discourage' the first sign of underperformance.

Can you see any flaws in the reasoning described above? From a System 1 viewpoint, the flight instructor (or coach) came to a valid conclusion. If we enlist the help of System 2, we may instead realise that the pilots' (athletes') performance regressed towards the mean: meaning that a very good performance is more likely to be followed by a worse performance (than a very good to be followed by an even better one)—and this regardless of whether the feedback is negative or positive. Similarly, a poor performance is more likely to be followed with a better one, than by an even poorer one. At least if the person we are interested in is motivated to do as well as he/she can on the task, which we can assume both pilots and athletes are. Here we see how regression towards the mean has implications in real life, clearly showing that the solution offered by System 1 (punishment is better than praise) may lead us astray and fool us into drawing erroneous conclusions. Conclusions that then result in less than optimal feedback, potentially with dire consequences or at least inferior learning. So one take home message from the book by Kahneman is to treat anything that sounds too good to be true as just that, at least until System 2 is given a chance to falsify the claim. If it holds up to careful scrutiny, then maybe, maybe it is not too good to be true?

Signs of Pseudoscience

Science and pseudoscience are different entities, but not always complete opposites as one may first think. Or at least, there are nuances to the differences worth discussing, thereby hopefully making the reader better equipped to distinguish between good and bad science, and between science and pseudoscience. In order to do this, we need to become informed sceptics. Deliberately questioning our fast and automatic thinking (System 1), even though the alternative (System 2) requires more effort and time. Sometimes, it certainly is better to think slowly instead of quickly draw conclusions that later may prove wrong.

Below follows a list, in part, from Lilienfeld et al. (2012), highlighting some distinguishing features between science and pseudoscience. This is not to be taken as a comprehensive or definite checklist, merely as some suggestions as to how science and scientific thinking can act 'as safeguards against human error' (Lilienfeld et al., 2012: p. 7).

Claims Are Reasonable and with Boundaries

Would you buy and wear a magnetic bracelet if the seller claimed it to alleviate migraine, pain in general, repair broken bones, improve circulation, improve your concentration and sport performance, restore energy, prevent stress disorders and cure cancer? Well, some people must believe in the power of magnetism because such bracelets continue to be sold. Thereby seemingly disregarding that most claims within this area have few if any boundaries and are grossly exaggerated and/or untestable. For example, wearers of magnetic bracelets may believe that a magnet around their wrist will alter their bioenergetic fields and positively affect their life force (chi, or energy flow). Because that is what the infomercials are trying to convince us of. What chi or life force actually is, or how it potentially can be detected and measured is a question left unanswered. The National Centre for Complementary and Integrative Health in the United States are, however, not convinced: 'Scientific evidence does not support the use of magnets for pain relief' (https://nccih.nih.gov/health/magnet/magnetsforpain.htm). Research attesting to the impact on migraine, broken bones or cancer does not pass the tests offered by critical thinking.

Note, however, that it is possible to find an abundance of anecdotal evidence on most websites that are trying to convince unsuspecting customers of some gadget's extraordinary powers (we refrain from naming any particular website, but the interested reader will have no problem in finding examples on the Internet). There are even 'scientific' claims on the Internet, and some studies—albeit of questionable quality—have indeed presented results that attest to the effects of magnets and magnetism on the human body. The only thing these studies prove beyond a reasonable doubt is that some research claimed to be scientific is nothing more than pseudoscience dressed up to fool those that are satisfied with believing instead of knowing. Wanting to believe is human, but it is also something that some people take advantage of to sell often expensive gadgets that have no scientifically established effect, except as found in pseudoscientific studies that lack trustworthiness. Hence, as argued throughout the chapter, critical thinking is a skill well worth developing in all facets of life, not just the scientific part of it. A claim that is vague, seems exaggerated, or is untestable requires you to activate System 2.

Claims Can Be Reproduced

One of the cornerstones of science, and something discussed in almost every textbook dealing with research methods, is reproducibility. If replicating a study produces the same or very similar results, this strengthens the belief that an effect is really present. This, however, is not saying that studies should be replicated *in absurdum*—remember Popper and his white versus black swans. Replication is, however, warranted in order to verify claims from a novel study, to determine whether the first results were merely a fluke or if some real effects have been detected.

If results cannot be replicated, doubts are cast on the initial findings, which often happen to be the case with pseudoscientific results. These are mostly impossible to replicate, unless the (likely faulty) design or method used is also replicated. This in turn explains why replications by the same research group are less valued and trusted than if an independent research group present the same conclusions as the first did. In other words, inter-group reproducibility is more trusted than intragroup reproducibility. Pseudoscience researchers, however, avoid peer-reviewed journals as their outlet, both because the likelihood of publication is low, and because it would open up their findings to scrutiny from other researchers. Consequently, they write books instead or describe their findings on the Internet, where as we discussed earlier anything can be posted. More often than not they will also attack 'conventional science' for being narrow minded and not open enough to see when something really different and revolutionary surfaces (adhering to the principle that attack is the best defence).

To be fair, replicating scientific findings is not as easy as one may think. A recent study of the reproducibility of psychological science was published as Open Science Collaboration when 100 experimental and correlational studies appearing in three high-impact psychology journals were replicated (Science, 2015). Results showed that the mean effect size of the original studies (Mr = 0.403) was less than half in the replications (Mr = 0.197). Whereas 97 % of the original findings reached significance, only 36 % of the replications did. Not surprisingly, the conclusion was that 'this project provides accumulating evidence for many findings in psychological research and suggests that there is still more work to do to verify whether we know what we think we know' (p. 943). This also highlights another problem, namely, when science journalists report a novel finding to the public and mass media helps spread this information to all parts of the globe within hours. If the finding was a coincidence, and will later prove to be impossible to replicate, that will be too late to prevent an erroneous message being transmitted to unsuspecting recipients. So it is not only the public that needs to develop their critical thinking skills, this applies to journalists as well.

What then can explain the findings presented by Science? Suggestions include: selective reporting and analysis, and insufficient specifications of the methods and designs used to fully allow accurate replications. We can also consider publication bias, that is, results are more easily accepted for publication in scientific journals when they are statistically significant compared to when they are not. Consequently, of the 100 original studies published, less than half of the replications would probably have been accepted for publication. Solely on the basis of the replications not being statistically significant to the same extent as the original studies, and not making any judgement of the editors' preference for novel versus replicated findings. The latter is also discussed in the article: 'Journal reviewers and editors may dismiss a new test of a published idea as unoriginal. The claim that "we already know this" belies the uncertainty of scientific evidence. Innovation points out paths that are possible; replication points out paths that are likely; progress relies on both' (p. 943). Based on the findings presented in the Science article, it sounds like editors and reviewers ought to look more positively on replications so that we as scientists know more and believe less. As an additional benefit, replications made by independent research groups will help to weed out pseudoscientific claims.

Claims Are Falsifiable

Similar to the notion that claims can be replicated is that they also can be falsified (or tried to be). Popper and his white versus black swans again: it only takes one observation of a black swan to falsify the claim that all swans are white. Unfortunately, there are many examples where it is less obvious and thereby more difficult to falsify a claim. Popper used easily observed swans as his example, but what if the claim is for something invisible or unmeasurable? Like Qi?

We know that an increased level of physical activity results in an elevated heart rate, making the blood flow more rapidly in our bodies and can thereby have beneficial effects on the breakdown of stress hormones. This can easily be verified in simple experiments, and the rate of breakdown of adrenalin, noradrenalin and cortisol in the blood or saliva can be assessed in relation to the intensity of the physical activity.

But how about Qi, an allegedly invisible energy force? Believers in traditional Chinese medicine (TCM) are convinced that meditation and slow movements will positively affect Qi, although Qi has neither been measured nor verified scientifically (Schmaltz & Lilienfeld, 2014; Zollman & Vickers, 1999). Consequently, whereas the effect of meditation and/or physical activity on the body and mind can be studied scientifically, Qi remains an entity believed by some to exist but without any convincing proofs that it does. This in turn makes any claim of its existence pseudoscientific, as it is impossible to verify or falsify that such an invisible energy force rests within our bodies. Believers of TCM are, however, convinced and instead put the blame on the scientific method and available techniques as inadequate for detecting Qi. Because if it does not exist, 'why have so many been convinced that it does for so long', goes the argument. Another popular way is to discredit the scientists, because they are narrow minded and not open enough to see how the world 'really is' (cf. Sagan, 1995).

Another example of pseudoscience is astrology, which has been around for more than 2000 years despite the lack of any evidence that astronomical phenomena will affect humans on earth. In 2010, two-thirds of the American population said that astrology is 'not at all scientific'; in 2012, this proportion had shrunk to slightly more than half of those included in the sample. This percentage has not been this low since 1983 (Science and Engineering Indicators, 2016; https://www.nsf.gov/statistics/2016/nsb20161/uploads/1/nsb20161.pdf), meaning that more devotees than in a long time believe that they are influenced by the movements and relative positions of the Sun, Moon, and planets. Many newspapers and magazines continue to support astrologers by regularly publishing their horoscopes, and people continue to read them to find out how the future will be. Thanks to confirmation bias (and generally voiced and all-inclusive predictions), it is easy to believe that horoscopes present the future with some degree of accuracy (Munro & Munro, 2000).

Claims Are Cumulative

One of the reasons that researchers write Introductions in their scientific manuscripts that contain a multitude of references to previous research is to show how the present research relates to the past. Or in other words, how the present research builds on already existing knowledge. Without a thorough literature review with a logical rationale, few editors of scientific journals will consider a manuscript for publication.

Pseudoscience notably lacks this clear link to extant knowledge, which also explains why some claims can be unrealistically imaginative, such as the claim that magnetic bracelets will cure just about any ailment afflicting our human existence. Or that planets and stars will have a profound effect on us and by understanding how they line up, we can reveal the future. Conversely, this also explains why it is rare to find pseudoscience published in quality journals with a thorough peer-review process in place. But as alluded to before, accidents happen even in the world of science and pseudoscience dressed up with fancy words and psychobabble (see below) can at times slip through the net.

Claims Are Self-Correctable

Closely linked to the view that claims should be possible to falsify, and that new knowledge should align and build on previous knowledge, is the idea of self-correction. If a claim cannot be replicated, or if it does not link in with extant knowledge, the claim will most likely need to be adjusted, corrected or even discarded altogether. Logically then, claims are tentative. A hypothesis is never 'proven to be true'; it is merely accepted as representing how we currently see things. An alternative hypothesis can be voiced and subsequently tested and possibly supported. This will force the original hypothesis to be replaced—until potentially another change will become necessary. Most likely, however, the changes or adjustments will become smaller and smaller as the research process provides better and more convincing support.

In contrast, pseudoscientific claims are pervasive; they rarely change despite accumulating evidence that contradict them. Magnetic bracelets are a prime example. Although no well-controlled study can be found that reveals their healing power, of broken bones, for example, this claim is still out there. A quick search on the Internet will turn up some interesting results of the power of magnetism and how this power can be utilised by simply wearing a magnetic bracelet.

Claims Are Not Overly Complicated

We have all heard something along the lines: if something sounds too good to be true, it probably is (Sagan 1995). Using overly complicated terminology and hypertechnical language (technobabble) can, however, deliberately be used to legitimise practices that if scrutinised would fail to provide any proof of their effectiveness. Such practices are common in sport and have attracted the label 'scienciness' by Bailey and Collins (2013). When such claims are accompanied by smoke screens—or psychobabble if the discipline of psychology is involved—then it is time to sound the alarm, as this is often a defining feature of pseudoscience. The challenge then becomes to detect when a claim is complicated yet legitimate, and when it is deliberately made to be overly complicated to confuse and lure the unsuspecting into believing whatever fantastic claim presented. One way to recognise pseudoscience is to focus on the words used as these are not ordinarily found in everyday scientific language, buzzwords (jargon, psychobabble) such as: psychoenergy field activator, brainwave neurosynchroniser and others that are not generally found in peer-reviewed publications, only in texts that are trying to convince the unsuspecting reader that something new and revolutionary is for sale that will 'change your world'.

Concluding Remarks

This chapter started with a question: how do we know what we really know? The answer centred on the importance of critical thinking, which require what Kahneman labelled slow thinking (System 2). This is in contrast to energy saving and fast thinking (System 1), which relies on mental shortcuts (heuristics) that increase the risk of accepting incorrect answers. Myths are excellent examples—such as learning is faster when accompanied by punishment rather than praise—as they are easy to believe (accepted by System 1) but when scrutinised (using System 2) revealed as false. The same applies to pseudoscientific claims: they may seem trustworthy on the surface but fail when examined more closely using scientific methods. Balancing scepticism with openness towards new ideas are key attributes not only for researchers and students in the field of sport and exercise psychology but for everyone exposed to infomercials that necessitates a critical mind and an ability to separate the wheat from the chaff.

4

The Status of Theory

Four Views on Theory

In the three preceding chapters, we have taken a relatively wide-angle view of research in the field of sport and exercise psychology. The aim of this chapter is to mobilise some of the ideas introduced and explored previously in a much narrower and more critical analysis of the state of theory in current research practice. To this end, the chapter is very much focussed on describing the *present*. It begins with a brief reminder of the alternative views of theory explored in Chap. 1, before applying them in a critical analysis of the two most popular approaches to research in quantitative and qualitative traditions, respectively: (a) regression studies drawing on self-determination theory and (b) studies drawing on the methodology of 'grounded theory'. By selecting the two most popular research trends of the moment, we argue that our analysis is likely to be illustrative of similar practices in other domains. The chapter concludes with a brief critical assessment of the state of theory in the field—both received and created—and offers some positive and constructive ideas for moving research practice forward.

© The Author(s) 2016
P. Hassmén et al., *Rethinking Sport and Exercise Psychology Research*,
DOI 10.1057/978-1-137-48338-6_4

Chapter 1 introduced four different views of science, with concomitant views on theory. For Kuhn, theory is part of the furniture of a paradigm; it takes the form of metaphysical assumptions that guide the identification and solving of puzzles in periods of 'normal science'. On this view, a theory is uncritically accepted and defended by a community of scientists as it forms part of the very material that bonds them together, making scientific activity possible. Conversely, for Popper, a theory is a fallible solution to a problem which must be subjected to criticism in order to maintain progress. Well-defined scientific theories enable us to develop expectations (or make predictions) and are therefore testable, and those that survive criticism are maintained tentatively until harsher tests can be developed. Lakatos agreed largely with Popper but argued that only groups of theories—or 'research programmes'—can be considered scientific. He also suggested that criticism of theory is not so simple, since a research programme is made up of a 'hard core' of theory, often with a 'protective belt' of hypotheses that makes simple criticism and overthrow highly unlikely. Feyerabend's radical view, by contrast, holds that there are *only* theories, so scientists move forward by creating (or reviving) bold theories and putting them into competition with one another. There are no rules to method on this view, and progress is achieved, according to Feyerabend, by breaking received rules, violating accepted standards and inventing better alternatives.

So what of theory in the present moment in sport and exercise psychology research? Are researchers puzzle-solving in Kuhnian paradigms, doggedly defending theory come what may? Or are they subjecting theories to crucial experiments, as Popper might have compelled? Perhaps research activity resembles a progressive Lakatosian 'research programme'? Or perhaps researchers, in the spirit of anarchism, are proliferating theories and forcing them into fruitful competition? In order to find out, detailed case studies of research practice are necessary. In order to avoid bias in the selection of case studies, we surveyed the editorial boards of the four most popular journals in the field: *Journal of Sport and Exercise Psychology*, *Journal of Applied Sport Psychology*, *The Sport Psychologist* and *Psychology of Sport and Exercise*.

The survey findings offer a strong rationale for the first case study: motivation research drawing on SDT using cross-sectional questionnaires and correlation methods. This type of research (paradigm or research programme) was clearly the most popular in the field over the last 5 years according to our sample of editorial boards (see Table 4.1).

Table 4.1 Overview of responses to editorial board survey

Question	Most popular response
What is the most common theory used in the last 5 years?	Self-determination theory (60 %)
What is the most popular phenomenon studied in the last 5 years?	Motivation (60 %)
What is the most common methodological approach used in the last 5 years?	Regression (inc. correlation; 73 %)

There were 15 responses to the survey: 2 editors, 4 associate editors and 9 board members. The mean time spent on the editorial board was 5.9 years with a range of 1–13 years.

Theory as a 'Framework': The Example of SDT

In order to sample papers for the case study, we drew on systematic literature review principles and processes (CRD, 2009; Swann, Crust, Keegan,
Piggott, & Hemmings, 2015). We searched the SPORTDiscus database
between the years 2010 and 2015 using the following search phrase:

"self dete3rmination theory" OR "self-determination theory"
(ABSTRACT)

AND

correlation OR regression (ABSTRACT)

We then applied some limiters—accept only papers published in English
language and in a journal with an impact factor—to return a subtotal of
27 papers. After reading the abstracts, we removed a further three papers
from the sample (one review, one validation study, one non-sport paper)
leaving us with a final sample of 24 papers. We then read and re-read the
papers extracting passages that helped us to answer two main questions:

What is the purpose of the theory as conceptualised in the paper?

How are the findings reported vis-à-vis the theory?

The relevant passages from papers were copied into a table for analysis
purposes and then analysed and coded into categories derived from the
four philosophical positions identified earlier in the chapter. The purpose
of the review, therefore, was *to determine the extent to which researchers in
this highly popular sub-field are following an identifiable philosophical tradition.* However, prior to exploring the findings from the review, assuming
some readers are unfamiliar with SDT, a brief review of the main tenets
of the theory seems necessary.

SDT, as conceived by its founding authors (Ryan & Deci, 2000, 2002), is a rather complex two-levelled set of ideas. At its most abstract, it is claimed to be a 'metatheory': a coherent collection of mini-theories united by a common set of assumptions about human behaviour. Specifically, these assumptions are that human agents are active, goal-seeking, resourceful organisms which occupy a social world that can both support and thwart the nutriments required to satisfy their basic needs, and thus their development. This is known as the 'organismic dialectical perspective' (Ryan & Deci, 2002: p. 5): essentially an ontological theory of psycho-social interaction and behaviour. One of the claims made by the proponents of SDT, then, is that its postulates are universally applicable, irrespective of age, sex or culture (Ryan & Deci, 2000).

At a substantive level, however, the mini-theories that describe the relationships between basic psychological needs and the environment, the general orientations of individuals, and intrinsic and extrinsic motives are argued to be predictive of many kinds of specific behaviour and also of general well-being. The slightly cumbersome arrangement of interacting mini-theories[1]—cognitive evaluation theory (CET), organismic integration theory (OIT), causality orientations theory (COT), basic psychological needs theory (BPNT)—were generated piecemeal through an inductive or 'Baconian' process (Ryan & Deci, 2000, 2002) over a period of 25 years but are held together by the common metatheoretical string. We outline briefly the main propositions of each mini-theory in turn below, based largely on the authoritative account offered by Ryan and Deci (2002):

Cognitive Evaluation Theory (CET)

- Motivation for sport and exercise is controlled by perceptions of autonomy (locus of causality) and competence
- Tangible rewards undermine motivation by shifting the perceived locus of causality from internal to external (i.e. individuals feel they are being controlled)

---

[1] We do not explicitly differentiate Goal Contents Theory (GCT) and Relationships Motivation Theory (RMT) in this brief outline as they are relatively new (and minor) additions to the SDT canon and did not feature significantly in the papers we reviewed.

Table 4.2 Overview of some SDT mini-theories

Type	Amotivation	Extrinsic motivation				Intrinsic motivation
Regulatory style	Non-regulated	External regulation	Introjected regulation	Identified regulation	Integrated regulation	Intrinsic regulation
Perceived locus of causality	External			Internal		
Quality of Behaviour	Non self-determined --- Self-determined					
Outcome	Less persistent --- More persistent					

Adapted from Ryan and Deci (2000)

- Positive feedback (about competence) only enhances intrinsic motivation when accompanied by a sense of autonomy
- Increases in perceived autonomy and perceived competence lead to greater levels of motivation and increased persistence

Organismic Integration Theory (OIT)

- Extrinsic regulators (and values) can be internalised and integrated with self to produce more self-determined behaviour over time
- Types of extrinsic regulation can be placed on a taxonomy, ranging from 'amotivation' (no intention to act) to 'integrated regulation' (extrinsic factors are congruent with personally endorsed goals and values) (see Table 4.2)
- Supporting competence, autonomy and relatedness is crucial for internalisation (i.e. introjected, identified and then integrated styles of regulation)

Causality Orientations Theory (COT)

- People possess different degrees of three broad motivational causality orientations: autonomous, controlled and impersonal
- Autonomy orientation leads to a tendency for intrinsic and integrated regulation of behaviour which relates positively to indicators of well-being (e.g. exercise adherence)

Basic Psychological Needs Theory (BPNT)

- The basic psychological needs for autonomy, competence and relatedness are 'motivating forces' that have a direct relation to well-being
- Basic psychological needs are innate and universal, though may be interpreted differently across cultures (i.e. the same behaviour may satisfy a need for one group, while thwarting it for another)
- There is a positive relationship between goal satisfaction and well-being only insofar as the goal contents foster basic psychological needs (i.e. intrinsic aspirations such as affiliation, personal growth and community engagement)

Table 4.3 Overview of findings from the review of SDT papers

Question	Category	Papers[a]
What is the purpose of the theory as conceptualised in the paper?	'Framework' (for understanding) or 'Perspective' (or 'theoretical base')	1, 3, 4, 5, 6, 9, 10, 12, 14, 16, 20, 21, 22, 24 **(14/24)**
	Model/theory for prediction and/or testing	2, 7, 8, 11, 13, 15, 17, 18, 19, 23 **(10/24)**
How are the findings reported via-a vis the theory?	Findings supported/confirmed/verified SDT	3, 5, 8, 9, 10, 11, 13, 14, 15, 17, 18, 19, 20 **(13/24)**
	'Partial support' for SDT (unexpected findings explained by recourse to auxiliary hypotheses e.g. context, individual diffs.)	2, 4, 6, 7, 21, 24 **(6/24)**
	'Partial support' for SDT (unexpected findings explained by methodological errors e.g. sample, questionnaire, analysis)	1, 12, 16, 22, 23 **(5/24)**

[a]A full reference list of the papers included in the review can be found in appendix A.

In summary, the SDT mini-theories represent a rich source of hypotheses for understanding and predicting human behaviour in a range of sport and exercise domains. It is no wonder, then, that SDT has become the 'go-to' theory in the field in recent times, given its claimed explanatory power and range. Moreover, with a metaphysical theory at its centre, a cluster of substantive theories to guide the setting and solving of puzzles, and a set of accepted measurement tools, SDT certainly looks and smells like a Kuhnian paradigm, at least on first inspection. But is this how current research in sport and exercise has conceived of, or represented, SDT?

Returning to our review, in response to the first main question—what is the purpose of theory?—two basic positions were apparent (see Table 4.3). The first and most popular position (14 of the 24 papers) conceptualised SDT as a 'framework' or perspective from which to conduct research. The second position (10 of 24) tended to describe SDT as a 'model' for making and testing predictions. As noted above, both positions are consistent with Ryan and Deci's (2000, 2002) claims for SDT as a metatheory and a collection of substantive mini-theories, yet none of the papers made this distinction clear. The 'framework' position is most obviously representative of Kuhn's idea of a paradigm. It was often understood as simply a way of looking at the world: equipping researchers with a set of handy concepts and tools with which to explore motivation (often for exercise). The 'model testing' position, by contrast, was slightly misleading insofar as these authors all claimed to be testing a model, or hypotheses derived from a model, yet none of them specified the conditions under which the model would be rejected. The commitment to 'testing' SDT-based models in these papers, then (at least in the Popperian sense), could certainly be questioned, and was arguably little more than a semantic slip.

With respect to the second question—how are findings reported vis-à-vis SDT?—three basic positions emerged. The first and most common approach (13 of 24) was to simply state that the findings supported SDT. Authors typically claimed that findings 'supported or confirmed hypothesised links' (Bortoli et al., 2014; Inoue, Wegner, Jordan, & Funk, 2015) or tended to follow 'predictions or expectations' derived from SDT (Fortier et al., 2011; Rottensteiner, Tolvanen, Laakso, & Konttinen, 2015). Another common claim was that these studies 'provide additional evidence' (Chin, Khoo, & Low, 2012) or 'further support' for SDT (Gaston, Wilson, Mack, Elliot, & Prapavessis, 2013; Guzmán & Kingston 2012). The extent to which these studies add anything new to our understanding of motivation can therefore be questioned. At best, they fall into a Kuhnian category of progress by extending the paradigm in very small, piecemeal steps (e.g. applying the theory to new sample groups, in new subdisciplines, in combination with other theories). Such behaviour was perhaps to be expected, however, following Deci and Ryan's (2002) call for research to 'extend and refine the tenets of SDT… applying the concept to new domains' in order to make SDT more 'exhaustive and precise' (pp. 432–433).

The second and third positions were similar (see Table 4.3) in that authors often claimed 'partial support' for SDT but also noted unexpected findings. In the second position (6 of 24), these anomalies were explained away with reference to cultural, contextual or individual difference factors (i.e. ad hoc hypotheses are developed or utilised to 'save' SDT from criticism). Stellino and Sinclair (2013), for example, claim that their 'study provides evidence, grounded in the contentions of SDT, that prediction of physical activity motivation and behavior is not explicable by the exact same mechanisms for all children' (p. 175). In a similar yet contrasting vein, Edmunds, Duda and Ntoumanis (2010) invoke a cultural explanation for their anomalous findings:

> [the findings] may intimate that relatedness need satisfaction is derived in a different manner for individuals of Asian/British Asian origin. That is, relatedness, or a connectivity with significant others, may be satisfied when individuals from this ethnic group are being told what to do by someone they value. (p. 459)

In suggesting that definitions of relatedness and autonomy may change across cultures and therefore account for anomalous findings, researchers could effectively explain *any* result in terms of SDT. And without deliberate follow-up investigations—for example, qualitative explorations of the hypothesised reasons—such ad hoc hypotheses are likely to continue to protect SDT from criticism (or even refinement).

The third position (5 of 24) also attempted to 'save' SDT from unexpected findings but this time by claiming methodological error on the part of the researchers. The unexpected results in these studies are variously explained away with reference to 'statistical artefacts' (Adie, Duda, & Ntoumanis, 2012); a lack of subtlety or precision in measurement tools (Guzmán, Kingston, & Grijalbo, 2015; Van den Berghe et al., 2013) or the timing of data collection and sample characteristics (Martinent, Decret, Guillet-Descas, & Isoard-Gautheur, 2014). By effectively ignoring these anomalous results—some small, some large—the five studies in this final category were able to maintain a strong positive stance towards SDT, with recommendations for further research and practical application made in the context of the theory. As Kuhn (1962/1996: p. 80) averred, it is a poor normal scientist who blames their paradigm!

A further common refrain seen in these final two categories of papers is that future research—typically involving experimental or longitudinal designs—needs to be conducted to account for the unexpected findings. Brunet and Sabiston (2011), for example, claim that 'future research is warranted to understand the mechanisms that explain the inconsistency between SDT's postulations and empirical evidence before conclusions can be drawn' (p. 103). Zarrett, Sorensen and Cook (2015) call for future research to explore the observed sex differences in the way that autonomy and competence needs are met in their study of physical activity (in spite of SDT's claimed universality). In other words, the responsibility for checking out the unexpected findings is passed onto other researchers, a practice that is legitimate in the academic publishing tradition, but potentially dangerous if nobody ever follows-up.

So what, in summary, are the conclusions from our review? First, it is clear that most authors treat SDT as a paradigm, explicitly or implicitly, in the Kuhnian sense: it provides a conceptual language and toolbox for studying a wide range of motivation phenomenon. It simply does not occur to these authors to 'test' the theory. After all, following Kuhn's analysis, why would it? These researchers have presumably been trained in sport and exercise psychology where SDT provides some of our most basic assumptions and conceptual tools on motivation (e.g. the very basic distinction between intrinsic and extrinsic forms). Moreover, they are likely to be following in the footsteps of their doctoral supervisors who have created 'exemplars' for papers with well-trodden routes to publication. SDT also reflects a relatively low-risk position from which to publish, given its wide acceptance, which presumably extends to journal editors (see Chap. 9 for an extended explanation). Given these forces, then, it would be a brave (or foolish) researcher who set out to criticise SDT, if the thought ever occurred to them in the first place (recall Kuhn's point in Chap. 1 about the 'immense restriction of vision' that accompanies a paradigm, resulting in 'an inability to see phenomena that do not fit').

If we can agree that SDT may be understood as a paradigm—at least according to the cases we reviewed—the activity we see is also characteristic of normal science. The specific nature of the 'mopping-up operation' in SDT seems mainly to involve the extension of the paradigm with new sample groups (e.g. pregnant women), new problems areas (e.g. fan behaviour) or by synthesising it with complementary theoretical perspectives (e.g. achievement goal theory). And, as we have seen in all of our 24 cases, SDT is used to both define *and* solve the puzzles in question, without consideration of possible alternative perspectives. So much is to be expected, of course, according to Kuhn's descriptive view of science. Indeed, the increasing speed and depth with which puzzles can be framed and solved within the SDT 'framework' is, from a Kuhnian point of view, the very definition of progress. The conceptual precision and detail that SDT mini-theories can offer a researcher undoubtedly expedite the conduct of research. Indeed, this was the very point made by Deci and Ryan (2002) in the preface to the *Handbook of Self-Determination Research* (see Chap. 1).

A Popperian would be appalled by such a definition of progress, and would no doubt point out the way in which our example cases dealt with anomalies symptomatic of 'pseudoscience'. Again, as we saw in Chap. 1, Kuhn was evasive about anomalies, both in terms of how they were spotted in the first place (i.e. researchers are trained not to notice them) and also with respect to how accumulations of anomalies eventually come to be seen as representing a 'crisis' in the paradigm, pre-empting a revolution. The specific 'tipping point' is unclear. The extent to which the 11 papers citing 'unexpected findings' constitute a crisis is therefore difficult to determine. As we have seen, when treated as individual anomalies, it is easy to dismiss rogue data as either the result of a methodological mistake, or by mobilising ad hoc hypotheses to explain them away. However, a meta-analysis or systematic review focussing on anomalies *across* a range of SDT studies might provoke an interesting debate about the extent to which they *really* are the result of methodological errors, or how far ad hoc hypotheses can be stretched to account for them.

Astute readers will recall that these are the types of questions to which Lakatos addressed himself, as a Popperian with a realistic and pragmatic view of the sociology of science. A Lakatosian 'research programme', to repeat, is a series of theories which is simultaneously defended and attacked (but never overthrown due to simple falsification) by members of a research community. Constructive criticism is mobilised from the perspective of rival programmes, and 'progressive' programmes are classified insofar as they invite and survive criticism while also explaining more facts than rivals (Lakatos, 1970). Degenerating research programmes, by contrast, do not make novel predictions and simply explain what is already known, while saving theories from criticism with the invention of ad hoc hypotheses (Khalil, 1987). Our review of a small and limited sample of studies from the last five years seems to point in the direction of degeneration, for three main reasons:

1. There is a lack of serious consideration of rival programmes (i.e. positions from which to launch constructive criticism);
2. There is an absence of bold and novel predictions;
3. There is a tendency to overlook anomalies and undertake 'patching-up' procedures with the invention of ad hoc hypotheses.

Based on a Lakatosian (or even Feyerabendian) assessment, it is therefore possible to argue that the defensive element of SDT has become too powerful in recent times with 'tenacity' outstripping the 'proliferation' of new ideas. And while staunch defence is necessary to increase the stability of a 'budding programme' in the early stages, according to Lakatos (1970), it represents a hindrance to the growth of knowledge as long as it persists in the face of anomalies. Moreover, given that Deci's seminal work was published 40 years ago, it is hardly possible to classify SDT as a 'budding programme' any longer. The question remains, then, as to what might be done to cause a 'progressive shift' in the SDT research programme (or paradigm). We consider this question in more detail following the second part of this chapter where we review the state of theory (or theory generation) in the qualitative tradition of sport and exercise research.

Generating 'Grounded' Theories

Grounded theory (GT) is a methodological approach to generating substantive theories which are grounded in empirical data. In this respect, it represents a legitimate but opposite approach to the more dominant deductive (or theory-driven) approach reviewed in the previous section. GT is often claimed to be the most popular and widely used qualitative methodology in the social sciences (Bryant & Charmaz, 2007). It has also become increasingly popular in sport and exercise psychology in recent years as methodological approaches, especially qualitative methodologies, have grown more diverse (Weinberg & Gould, 2015; Smith & Sparkes, 2016). Specifically, following a basic search for papers claiming to apply GT in the field, we found 38 papers published over a 22-year period.[2] As

---

[2] We searched using EBSCO database with the phrase 'grounded theory' (in abstract) and 'psychology' (anywhere in the paper) and then added a limiter of only peer-reviewed papers. We then

Years	Number of papers
2011–2015	18
2005–2010	15
2000–2004	3
1995–1999	1
1990–1994	1

Table 4.4 Number of GT papers published in leading journals between 1990 and 2015

shown in Table 4.4, there has been something of an explosion in GT-based papers in the last 10 years. Yet with this increasing popularity, it is perhaps inevitable that criticism has followed. In this subsection, we initially focus on describing the methodology of GT before exploring the critical debate that featured in *Psychology of Sport and Exercise* between 2009 and 2010. We conclude the section with a critique of this debate and some philosophically informed constructive suggestions for a way forward.

GT's founding authors (Glaser & Strauss, 1967) espouse an iterative and inductive approach to theory 'discovery' in the Baconian tradition; not unlike the methodological approach attributed to the generation of SDT's mini-theories by Ryan and Deci (2000). The roots of GT stretch back beyond the training of its founding authors, with a symbolic interactionist interpretive element coming from Anslem Strauss who trained with Herbert Blumer at Chicago (i.e. the 'Chicago School' sociological tradition), and a more positivist, middle-range theory element coming from Barney Glaser, who trained under Paul K. Merton at Columbia (Charmaz, 2000; Hammersley, 1990). The contrasting backgrounds have since led to a philosophical split between the founders and their students, leaving us in a position where at least three different versions of GT are now recognised: Glaserian, Straussian (based on his work with co-author, Juliet Corbin) and Constructivist (based on Kathy Charmaz's revision) (Holt & Tamminen, 2010a). Notwithstanding these philosophical differences, which we return to later, there are a number of common features of GT on which most authors agree (though specific interpretations can differ), and therefore constitute a basic description of the methodology.

GT studies begin with, and are continuously influenced by 'theoretical sensitivity'. Derived from Blumer's notion of 'sensitising concepts'

---

selected only papers appearing in journals with impact factors (i.e. 8 journals: JSEP, PSE, TSP, JASP, PE&SP, QRSEH, IJSP, IJSEP) to reach a subtotal of 42 papers. Finally, we removed 4 discussion papers to finish with 38.

(Blumer, 1969), theoretical sensitivity is GT's answer to the question of induction. It suggests that researchers inevitably bring prior knowledge to investigations which naturally influences the kinds of questions they ask and how they interpret data. Although GT is often classed as an 'inductive' approach, the founding authors understood that the richness of a researcher's theoretical sensitivity—their awareness of formal concepts, professional experience and training and so on—ultimately enhanced their insightfulness, so long as they did not become 'wedded' to (or stifled by) a particular theoretical approach (Glaser, 1978; Glaser & Strauss, 1967; Strauss & Corbin, 1998). Theoretical sensitivity, therefore, is a slightly slippery concept that tries to explain how researchers might respond to the question of *how* (not if) to use existing knowledge during an investigation. In short, it implies a critical difference between 'an open mind and an empty head' (Strauss & Corbin, 1998: p. 47).

Once a broad area of interest has been identified (it is considered poor form to begin with a specific question), a GT study begins proper with 'theoretical sampling', or sampling based on a desire to check out an emerging theory or hypothesis. Again, different authors place a slightly different spin on this idea—some emphasise the verification of a theory, while others advocate looking for counterinstances—but most agree that the goal of theoretical sampling is to develop, flesh-out and refine concepts and categories (Charmaz, 2006). Put another way, the emerging theory *controls* an iterative process of data collection and analysis, helping the researcher identify 'what groups or sub-groups to turn to next in data collection' (Glaser & Strauss, 1967: p. 45).

At the very heart of GT, then, lies the idea of a 'constant comparative' method, arguably its most fundamental feature (McCann & Clark, 2003). Unlike many other qualitative approaches where data collection and analysis are separate sequential processes, GT demands that they proceed in tandem. As initial data collection begins, data are compared (with each other and with theoretical sensitivity) which leads to the development of concepts; then, as a study progresses, new data are compared to existing 'grounded' concepts. The aim of comparison is the generation of mutually exclusive concepts that have clearly defined properties and dimensions. Over time, and with further theoretical sampling, concepts are compared in more abstract analysis processes in order to generate core categories which eventually form the basis of a substantive theory (Strauss & Corbin, 1998).

It is this feature of GT that lends it a natural sense of rigour, as the developing theory is constantly checked against the data, establishing a degree of 'credibility, plausibility and trustworthiness' (Kvale, 1996: p. 242).

To the thorny question of when to conclude a study, GT also has an answer: 'theoretical saturation'. This concept is intended to describe a point at which 'gaps in a theory are almost if not completely filled' (Glaser & Strauss, 1967: p. 61). It is the point at which new data no longer add anything to the emerging theoretical picture, and nothing further can be learned about the substantive phenomena under investigation. If GT processes have been followed diligently, this point also signals the emergence of a final 'substantive theory': 'A set of well developed categories that are systematically interrelated through statements of relationships to form a framework that explains some specific social phenomena' (Strauss & Corbin, 1998: p. 22). The theory should also explain all of the variation in the data above which it sits; it should be explicitly anchored or 'grounded' in the data (Charmaz, 2006). The final fundamental feature of GT relates more explicitly to such quality assessment criteria. Specifically, the concepts of 'fit', 'work', 'relevance' and 'modifiability' are offered as post-hoc criteria for evaluating the substantive theory within a GT approach (Glaser, 1978: pp. 4–5). That is to say, a theory should fit the data; it should work for and be relevant to the research participants; and it should be modifiable through the writing and redrafting of papers so as to increase vividness and clarity (Charmaz, 2006).

Having described the main features of the methodology—theoretical sensitivity, theoretical sampling, constant comparative method, theoretical saturation, substantive theory, quality criteria—we turn to the question of why it has become so popular in recent times in sport and exercise psychology. Weed's (2009) critical review, which appeared in a special issue of *Psychology of Sport and Exercise* on 'research quality', offers an interesting suggestion:

> The grounded theory label is being adopted by sport and exercise psychology researchers because it is fashionable… and confers *legitimacy* on qualitative approaches, about which there is a widespread lack of understanding (p. 510) (emphasis added)

The search for a 'legitimate' methodology after the so-called 'postmodern turn' is a recurring theme in social research more generally. Indeed, it was

Popper, Kuhn and Feyerabend (principally), as we have seen, who demolished ideas such as individual objectivity, theory-neutral observation, certainty and truth (Cf. Stove, 1982), leading to what Schwandt (1996) called 'cartesian anxiety': a motivating force in the quest for new definitive criteria to justify theories. Writing about GT in particular, Thomas and James (2006) echo this point, arguing that its popularity is a product of the misplaced desire for 'epistemic security'. Similarly, and more directly in the field of sport and exercise, Sparkes and Smith (2009) have cited the so-called 'crisis of legitimation' as a driving force for the desire to remove uncertainty. And in sport psychology, in particular, it was Martens (1987), we recall, who pointed out that 'orthodox science'—his caricature of naive positivist science—had perhaps had its day but left little by way of viable positive alternatives. If this is true, and sport and exercise psychologists are indeed desperately searching for methodological legitimacy (or security) in a sea of doubt, then GT, with its tools, techniques, procedures and processes arguably represents an attractive solution.

This, however, was only the opening salvo of Weed's (2009) critique. His principal criticism was that only 2 of the 12 papers he sampled from the previous 10 years met his criteria to *earn* the label of GT (he had a list of 8 'core elements' similar to ours, above). He accused the authors of the 10 'pseudo-GT' papers of 'dabbling' and having 'no real commitment to the appropriate application of GT' (ibid: p. 503) and claimed that GT is a 'complete package' or 'total methodology' and not a 'pick and mix box' of techniques that can be selected piecemeal to application in any old qualitative study (ibid: p. 504). In his bold conclusion, Weed (2009) claims that 'the label of grounded theory should only be applied to studies that meet the sufficient conditions [the eight elements] outlined in this paper' (p. 509). Such statements were always likely to cause a stir, and Holt and Tamminen (2010a)—among the authors accused in Weed's paper—duly responded with a spiky riposte.

First, Holt and Tamminen (2010a) took issue with Weed's sampling process and broadened their search to include 17 papers. Second, while they 'tended to agree' with Weed's eight core elements as a 'fair list of characteristics' (ibid: p. 407), the basic yes/no categorisation was too simplistic and they problematise Weed's classification in a number of cases. They do this in order to undermine (legitimately) Weed's 'fundamentalist stance' as the 'methods police', arguing instead that 'there simply cannot be a single gatekeeper or viewpoint that does justice to such a diverse methodology' (ibid: p. 410). In a conciliatory conclusion, Holt and Tamminen (2010a) offer some constructive (not prescriptive) 'tips' for researchers which include the advice to 'stick with one approach' (i.e. Glaserian, Straussian or Constructivist) and to show 'how the approach was appropriate to the research question' (ibid: p. 412). The two following papers in the debate (Weed, 2010; Holt & Tamminen, 2010b) do little more than make small conciliatory moves back towards a middle ground—both agree on the eight elements and on the issue of sticking to a philosophical stance—while making claims for a productive and quality debate with double meaning (i.e. a debate *of* quality, *about* quality). However, the extent to which this debate was productive or sufficiently critical can certainly be questioned.

There are two main problems with the *PSE* debate that are relevant to our subject in this chapter: (1) the agreement over the 'essential elements' of GT (the micro-issue) and (2) the suggestion that researchers choose a specific internally consistent variant of GT (the macro-issue). We deal with each in turn.

First, the implicit assumption of both parties is that, with the faithful application of the eight elements of GT, a *quality* substantive theory will emerge. The so-called 'pick-and-mix' approaches that appear common in sport and exercise psychology (i.e. 83 % of the papers reviewed by Weed, and arguably 50 % of the papers Holt and Tamminen reviewed, depending on interpretation) do not represent robust theories. Yet, as both authors point out, a number of alternative lists of characteristics (or elements, or whatever) have been offered (Cf. Strauss & Corbin, 1994; Lingard, Albert, & Levinson, 2008; Piggott, 2010a), so agreement over what they present as a definitive list can be questioned. Moreover, as Piggott (2010a) points out, at least four of Weed's (2009) eight elements—induction, theoretical sensitivity, sampling and saturation—contain serious philosophical problems and can be revised, or jettisoned entirely, by applying a Popperian stance. Piggott (2010b) also repeated and widened the two original reviews, finding 25 papers between the years 2000 and 2010, and applied a more minimal 'critical rationalist' criteria (similar to Lingard et al., 2008) to assessing which deserved the GT label. In this analysis, 19 of the 25 papers applied GT processes *only* at the data analysis stage; they did not carry out the iterative constant comparative process, bringing into question their GT credentials. In summary, debates about 'who has the *real* GT?' (Charmaz, 2000: p. 513) are useful and continue to be productive and should not be shut down by the likes of Weed and Holt and Tamminen who conservatively defend lists of 'essential' elements.

The second issue—the notion of choosing a variant of GT—is also highly problematic insofar as all of the variants contain significant philosophical misunderstandings. To this day, Glaser remains staunchly positivist in his approach (Cf. Glaser, 2015), clinging onto outdated mantras like 'trust in emergence' and arguing that researchers 'enter the field in abstract wonderment of what is going on' (Glaser, 1992: p. 22). This makes his variant hard to take seriously given the formidable philosophical critique of positivism, as outlined in Chap. 1 (also see Bryant, 2003). Both the Straussian and Constructivist variants are slightly more sophisticated, with more honest and realistic views on research practice. However, where Charmaz (2000, 2006) claims to be a constructivist, she often writes from an implicit (critical) realist stance. Weed (2009) quotes a series of passages showing this to be the case. Strauss and Corbin (1998) claim an interpretive position, but they also fail to deal with the problem of induction and often fall back on positivist-sounding practices derived from the original 1967 text (Thomas & James, 2006).

For both Weed (2009) and Holt and Tamminen (2010b) to simply recommend 'selecting an appropriate philosophical stance' is to evade the tricky problem of having to argue that one variant may be better than another. It is, in short, a recommendation for a Kuhnian brand of relativism: if you feel like a positivist, choose the Glaserian approach (or paradigm), remain consistent and nobody can criticise you. The Popperian view is that a *better* variant of GT can be developed, contrary to Thomas and James (2006), but that this involves the modification of a number of the 'essential elements' drawing on critical rationalist principles (Piggott, 2010a). To take just two related examples, we shall briefly consider the related concepts of theoretical sampling and theoretical saturation.

Under a critical rationalist revision of GT, sampling would take a very different character: where researchers currently search for *verifications* of their emerging theory, a Popperian would look for harsher tests—cases where they expect the theory to fail. The conventional GT researcher, having found some data to verify the theory can easily declare that saturation has been reached as nothing new is learned. After all, if you look for data that agree with your theory, you will more than likely find it. The Popperian, on the other hand, would point out that a theory can never be saturated since new data depend on the kinds of questions you ask, or the tests you apply. Theory is always tentative, never certain, but is improved through corroboration which, we recall, is a product of the number and harshness of tests it has faced (Popper, 1959).

The *PSE* debate, in summary, was too narrow because both parties accepted the two problematic premises concerning the eight essences and choice of variant, inadvertently closing down debate about more fundamental philosophical issues with the methodology in general. Moreover, in doing so, both parties were 'hung by their own petards' since their own analyses of micro-quality issues in GT were positivist in nature (i.e. inductively generating a list of essential elements; assuming this list to be a true and definitive criteria). The suggested critical rationalist revision, by contrast, is internally consistent (at a macro-level) and solves or circumvents the philosophical problems that have plagued GT thus far (at the micro-level). It also argues that continued debate about *what is a quality grounded theory* is only possible under two conditions: (1) lists of 'essential elements' or criteria need to be offered *and* open to challenge in order to improve them; (2) we must be prepared to accept that some variants of GT are simply wrong, or worse than others (e.g. on the basis of philosophical naivety or confusion). So, while we agree that the application of GT in sport and exercise psychology papers may often be flawed or incomplete, neither Weed's (2009) hard line policing nor Holt and Tamminen's (2010b) prescriptive advice is likely to lead to meaningful advances in the field without a deeper philosophical critique.

Conclusion: Theory, Dogma and Progress

In this chapter we have reviewed the state of theory in sport and exercise psychology through the specific lenses of the two most popular approaches to theory use and theory generation in the field. The two approaches are linked in that Ryan and Deci (2000, 2002) claim that SDT's mini-theories have been developed following processes similar to those espoused by grounded theorists (also in the development of the overarching 'formal theory' following the application of substantive theories in across a range of contexts). We also concluded that SDT as a theory of motivation and GT as a theory of how to generate theory are similar in that both have come to be applied dogmatically in the field. In this final section, we briefly recap the main points and offer some suggestions for ways forward, based on normative theories of science. We keep this section brief as Chaps. 9 and 10 offer more in-depth general recommendations for moving the discipline forward in the future.

Our review of recent papers applying SDT in sport and exercise psychology showed that the theory is often understood as a 'framework', akin to a Kuhnian paradigm: a rich and highly productive set of concepts (and assumptions) that are used to set and solve puzzles, providing exemplars for the conduct of research. Paradigms are irrational and dogmatic in that critical discussion between paradigms is held to be impossible (incommensurability), and adopting one paradigm over another a matter of faith (relativism). We also considered how research findings were reported vis-à-vis SDT. The papers we reviewed either supported SDT (adding more evidence to the pile) or explained away unexpected findings (anomalies) by recourse to either ad hoc hypotheses or methodological mistakes. Based on a Kuhnian analysis, it can be argued that this research represents a type of progress, as the SDT paradigm is being gradually extended and deepened. But Kuhn was never clear about the normative value of his ideas (Feyerabend, 1970; Fuller, 2006) so reading his work in a prescriptive capacity is dangerous. We therefore applied Lakatosian thinking to critique SDT as a 'degenerating' research programme given how anomalies are treated by researchers. In the final analysis, we posed the question of how a 'progressive shift' might be stimulated.

In response to this question, and based on a hybrid Popperian/Lakatosian sophisticated falsificationist approach (see Lakatos, 1970: pp. 109–110), we make the following constructive recommendations for researchers applying SDT in their studies:

1. Consider rival theories from the outset (e.g. Temporal Motivation Theory—Steel & König, 2006) setting them up as viable alternative frameworks;

2. Develop clearly testable hypotheses with statements explaining the conditions under which the theory would be rejected (make the theory 'stick its neck out');
3. Avoid the use of correlation-type designs (i.e. it is hard to test a theory, see 2, without being able to comment on causality);
4. Where unexpected results are found, consider whether rival theories provide better explanations, rather than inventing or appropriating ad hoc hypotheses;
5. Journal editors and reviewers should avoid publishing research where unexpected results are attributed to avoidable methodological errors.

Finally, given Lakatos' point about the slow and gradual nature of criticism—'purely negative criticism must not kill as fast as Popper imagined' (Lakatos, 1970: p. 179)—piecemeal assessment of anomalies may be ineffective. We therefore suggest that occasional meta-analyses and systematic reviews of SDT research, focussing purely on anomalies, may be a fruitful method of appraising the extent to which the paradigm is in 'crisis', or the extent to which shifts may be deemed progressive (predicting novel facts) or degenerating (patching-up with ad hoc hypotheses).

In the second section of the chapter, we showed that recent debates in GT have become similarly irrational and dogmatic, with prominent authors declaring a fixed list of essences which must be applied in order to 'earn' the lauded GT label, and advocating the adoption of internally consistent but incommensurable variants (i.e. a Glaserian may not engage in a constructive discussion with a Constructivist). These essentialist and relativist arguments make for strange bedfellows. Nevertheless, the *PSE* debate intended to protect (Weed) or promote (Holt and Tamminen) quality in GT studies. Both parties in the debate agree that GT presents a potential route out of the 'crisis of legitimation' (Sparkes & Smith, 2009), *as long as the eight essential elements are applied within an internally consistent approach.* Holt and Tamminen (2010b) go further and offer three bits of advice for young researchers: (1) read the original texts, (2) attend GT workshops and conferences and (3) seek experienced supervisors. At first glance, this sounds like sensible advice but could also be considered perfect training for socialisation into a paradigmatic way of thinking. We have tried to show that there are fundamental philosophical problems with the so-called eight essential elements which could only be identified (and tentatively solved) by researchers who have taken pains to gain critical philosophical distance from the GT literature.

As a way forward, we applied Popperian thinking to criticise the tendency to close down debates in GT in the name of 'quality assurance', and to modify some of the more problematic ideas in the GT canon (e.g. theoretical sampling and saturation). The critical rationalist revision of GT (Piggott, 2010a) attempts to put the methodology on surer philosophical footing, while also demonstrating that there are more than three games in town. Others have gone further (Thomas & James, 2006), invoking Feyerabend's anarchism to advocate for the dismantling of GT and its philosophically flawed, mechanistic, recipe-like approach to social enquiry. While this critique has merit, we would argue that this amounts to 'throwing the baby out with the bathwater'. GT can be 'reinvented' and should continue to be used by sport and exercise psychologists, *as long as they engage with it critically*. The critical rationalist revision is but one path researchers might take, but, we argue, a better one insofar as it contains fewer errors and ambiguities than other variants.

We set out in this chapter to explore the status and use of theory in sport and exercise psychology research. Our rather narrow but in-depth investigations have demonstrated that dogmatic attitudes towards theory use and theory generation currently prevail. We have specified some of the techniques used to protect theory from criticism, and to close down debates about the quality of substantive theories. It is probably clear by now that we favour a Popperian/Lakatosian normative idea of progress and this has motivated our suggestions for ways forward. Ultimately, however, it is up to the readers of this chapter to accept (or decline) the challenge posed by critical rationalism: to make theories testable; to create harsher tests and search for anomalies; and to engage in higher-level debates about the quality of theories and the criteria used to make such assessments. We do not disguise the difficulty of this challenge; after all, if it were easy, everyone would already be doing it.

5

Research Paradigms, Methodologies and Methods

This chapter is focused on the research process and factors influencing it. Initially, with a focus on paradigms, followed by a discussion of preferred methodologies and methods that follows from the paradigm subscribed to by the researcher. First, a definition:

> A paradigm may be viewed as a set of *basic beliefs* (or metaphysics) that deals with 'ultimates' or first principles. It represents a *worldview* that defines, for its holder, the nature of the "world," the individual's place in it, and the range of possible relationships to that world and its parts, as, for example, cosmologies and theologies do. The beliefs are basic in the sense that they must be accepted simply on faith (however well argued); there is no way to establish their ultimate truthfulness (Guba & Lincoln, 1994: p. 107).

A paradigm by this definition is thereby neither objective nor easily defined, rather 'a set of basic beliefs' but nevertheless with immense implications for how research is performed. Because make no mistake, all research throughout history has been affected by what the performing researcher either personally or collectively considers 'good' research. The approach favoured by Wundt in Germany influenced Griffith in his

© The Author(s) 2016
P. Hassmén et al., *Rethinking Sport and Exercise Psychology Research*,
DOI 10.1057/978-1-137-48338-6_5

Athletics Laboratory, so it was not surprising that early sport psychology research was performed in the laboratory and not in the field, using quantitative methods instead of qualitative. There is no such thing as an undisputable formula for good research—if we by this mean how the research process is conducted, from a question in need of an answer to actually providing that answer to external parties. The worldview, or the researchers' basic set of beliefs, will without a doubt influence the decisions made and thereby also the knowledge obtained. This is why it is important to consider how research in sport and exercise psychology originated, because the foundation laid in the early days continues to influence present day research. And possibly even more important, it will form future research as well, which is fine as long as the decisions made are informed and researchers well aware that there is no such thing as objective research that can be accepted as such by everyone.

In order to discuss and criticise these decisions, it is illustrative to consider a common vision of the research process, see Fig. 5.1. The process starts with the initial question, for example, 'why do some athletes

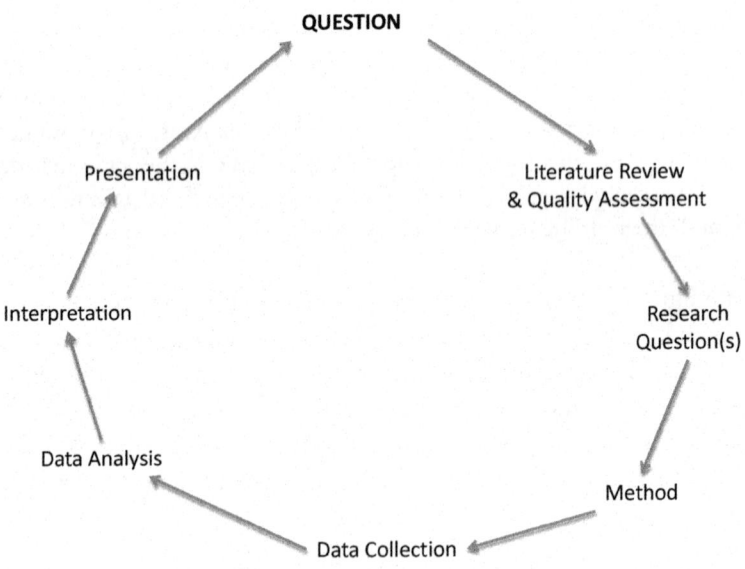

Fig. 5.1   An example of the research process

struggle to cope with competitive pressure?' The answer is subsequently and most often presented in the form of a scientific article, published in a peer-reviewed journal. In this way, the findings can be communicated to the relevant audience, contribute to the existing knowledgebase, but also be judged on its merit and whether the findings presented hold up to rigorous scrutiny. Secondary dissemination in the form of conference presentations and popular scientific texts are also common, although often not subjected to a careful review process. This is one reason why university students are so often encouraged by their supervisors to focus on accessing primary sources of information. That is, peer-reviewed journal articles published in high-quality scientific journals; articles that are authored by the researchers that actually performed the research. Although secondary sources such as textbooks are, for the most part, good sources of information, but ultimately their quality depends on the selections made by the authors, and further how these authors interpret and report research performed by others. In a way, textbook authors act as peer reviewers, selecting and rejecting what research to include and what does not in their mind merit inclusion. Also remember that not only *what* will be included is decided by the textbook-author, but also *how* the research will be presented. The textbook you are currently reading is also an example of what we as authors believe to be important to include, and what is not. Judgements open to discussion, of course.

Peer reviewers enlisted by scientific journals are, as discussed in Chap. 3, gatekeepers trying to weed out research that is not on par with acceptable scientific criteria. These criteria are not—unfortunately—as objective as one may initially hope for; this is because acceptance or rejection of a submitted manuscript is also influenced by the worldview of the reviewers as well as the editor in chief (not to mention other contributing factors, such as 'boy-clubs', a topic discussed in the next chapter). Included in this chain from manuscript to finished article is also the publisher that ultimately decides on the faith of submitted manuscripts. With the advent of online outlets, the numbers of publishers and their journals have increased exponentially. This has also led to an increasing specialisation; we now have journals that only accept research that uses one particular method stemming from one particular worldview. For example, *The Grounded Theory Review*, an international peer-reviewed online journal aimed at advancing Glaser's specific version of grounded theory (www. groundedtheoryreview.com). The advent of method-specific journals is noteworthy, because it puts the emphasis on the *method* rather than the research *question*. Of course, this does not mean that the research method is allowed to determine the research question, merely that the journal only accepts research stemming from one paradigm, using one methodology, and one particular method. So if anything, paradigms, methodology and methods are becoming increasingly important, not less as one might believe given the constantly changing nature of science.

However, the worldview —or paradigm, to use Kuhn's terminology— does not constitute anything more than basic beliefs as to what is considered acceptable research. Consequently, different paradigms exist and believers and non-believers have for a long-time struggled to win what has been labelled the 'paradigm wars' (Gage, 1989: p. 4). Proponents and opponents of existing paradigms (worldviews) sometime take the discussion to the extreme; which may not be surprising when the foundation is built on beliefs and subjective preferences instead of indisputable facts.

In the early days, when Gustav Fechner developed psychophysics as a scientific discipline, there was basically only one acceptable paradigm: positivism; at least if we distinguish between empirical sciences and philosophy. Wundt and the early sport psychology researchers Scripture, Fitz, Triplett and Griffith (see Chap. 2) were all positivists, or possibly postpositivists—a distinction to be made soon. But before that, a word of caution: 'paradigm' as a concept is in itself laden with meaning and interpretation. It has through history been used interchangeably with other concepts in science, such as perspective, discourse, theory, discipline, school, methodology and method (Hassard, 1988). Kuhn's own use of the word paradigm was allegedly rather inconsistent: Masterman (1970) detected at least 21 different uses. As can be imagined, if Kuhn as the first person to use this concept with a scientific focus then uses it inconsistently, it is no wonder that those that follow will add to the confusion rather than lessen it. It also explains—at least to some extent— why the paradigm wars have raged for many years. Some even believe that they still do (e.g. Denzin, 2009), but this chapter is not intended to create peace among dissidents or to help identify a 'winner'. Rather, the following text will discuss, highlight, and critique some of the prevailing controversies. Our proposed solution—one that has been offered by others before us—is to encourage, facilitate, permit and celebrate pluralism. Not merely 'tolerate'—which would still imply resentment and disagreement. Rather, we must value and proactively foster pluralism.

Philosophical Differences Between Paradigms

A paradigm is thus a worldview or a set of general assumptions upon which research is based and developed. Guba and Lincoln (1994) suggested three fundamental questions; the answers reveal the basic beliefs that make it possible to distinguish between paradigms.

The *ontological* question is focused on the nature of the world, or more specifically, what can we as researchers gain knowledge about in the world that surrounds us? A related but different question is the *epistemological*: what is the relationship between the researcher and what is being researched? The *methodological* question is focused on the how: how do we gain or go about getting knowledge of the world? The beliefs held by the researcher as to the very nature of the world to be studied (*ontology*) and whether it is possible to obtain objective knowledge or if knowledge by its very nature is subjective (*epistemology*) influences the researchers' choice of methodology, and subsequently which methods are deemed appropriate. *Axiology* has been added more recently to account for the values underpinning ethics, aesthetics and religion (Guba & Lincoln, 2000); from a researcher's viewpoint, an axiological question would be: what is the value of knowledge itself?

What Kuhn did in his book *The structure of scientific revolutions* was to suggest that science can be divided into normal science, when one paradigm rules, interspersed with a period of revolution, until another paradigm can take over and become (the new) normal science. Kuhn referred to this as a paradigm shift; his ideas—although appealing with its digital notion of 'either this or that'—can easily be criticised, at least in the social sciences; Kuhn himself even acknowledged this and stated that his thoughts about paradigms were less relevant for the social sciences. In contrast, the natural sciences have seen many paradigm shifts; for example, Albert Einstein's theory of relativity (1916) effectively challenged Isaac Newton's theory of mechanics that for 200 years had been the ruling paradigm. In the social sciences, paradigms instead can and do exist in parallel. Maybe it is therefore more productive to discuss 'research traditions', as suggested by Laudan (1977). This makes particular sense if we regard paradigms or research traditions as nothing more than a researcher's assumptions and beliefs that form how research is performed.

Paradigms (a.k.a., Worldviews, Research Traditions)

One way of beginning to understand and represent the different paradigms in social sciences is to capture the two most diametrically opposed viewpoints; which have been labelled positivism and constructivism, respectively. Guba and Lincoln (1994) suggested that two more paradigms were relevant: postpositivism and critical theory. The following text will consider these four paradigms or research traditions—although we acknowledge that more have subsequently been suggested and that subcategories of each clearly exist. The aim of the following is not to merely describe these four paradigms but to critically discuss how they affect research questions, designs, analyses, interpretations, and how research is communicated to the intended audience. This is an important consideration, because, in the words of Lincoln (2010):

> Paradigms and metaphysics *do* matter. They matter because they tell us something important about *researcher standpoint*. They tell us something about the researcher's proposed *relationship to the Other(s)*. They tell us something about what the researcher thinks *counts as knowledge*, and *who can deliver the most valuable slice of this knowledge*. They tell us how the researcher intends to *take account of multiple and contradictory values* she will encounter (p. 7, *emphasis* in original).

So paradigms are influencing the way research is performed, and to have an understanding of their respective strengths and weaknesses may indeed be important. Not the least to offer an understanding when it comes to the methodologies and methods used to perform the research. The issue was also emphasised by Keegan (2015), who offered a model of core philosophical 'traditions' underpinning applied psychological practice.

Positivism is the classic way of viewing research. Proponents of this paradigm assume that it is possible to study a single external reality objectively and to draw conclusions and make generalisations that are independent of context and time. The researcher is believed to have direct access to the real world and is a detached and external observer that neither influences nor is influenced by what is studied. Being able to manipulate the independent variable(s) is highly valued, preferably in an experimental setting where hypotheses can be tested, thereby making it possible to draw conclusions about cause and effect. Measurements are at the core, the methodology usually quantitative, and statistical analyses the way to determine whether significant relationships or differences exist. Positivism has been associated with naïve realism. That is, a belief that there is but one single reality that can be studied independently without bias by an objective researcher may be considered naïve at best. Research within this paradigm is said to be both reductionist and deterministic, meaning that researchers try to reduce existing complexities by studying one or a few variables at a time, and further that independent and dependent variables are causally linked. Today, few if any researchers are positivist-purists in this classical meaning. Although the early sport psychology researchers appeared to be, many of them were deeply interested in timing issues, for example, athletes' reaction time, which they carefully measured in laboratory settings. There were little room for interpretations, and the results were seen as objective and undisputable.

Postpositivism is sometimes described as an evolution from positivism—which is the way we will discuss it here (occasionally the same term is used to refer to what we are terming constructivism—Cruickshank, 2012; Guba & Lincoln, 1994). Postpositivism can be viewed as a more subdued and flexible form in comparison to positivism. Postpositivistic researchers still study reality, but are aware that their study can never be fully unbiased or objective; observations are considered both time- and context-dependent (instead of independent). As a consequence, the researchers mind-set must be critical, hence the notion of critical realism (instead of naïve realism). Postpositivistic researchers often focus on measurements and to operationalise concepts; consequently, reliability and validity are considered critically important and are often discussed at length in journal articles stemming from within this paradigm. The methodology is often quantitative and with a preference to control extraneous variables in order to determine if the independent variable(s) is causally related to the dependent variable(s). Most of the researchers in sport and exercise psychology that are using standardised measurement instruments would probably, if asked, describe themselves as postpositivistic researchers.

Critical theory is an umbrella-term for ideas that are influenced by ideology. That is, knowledge is never considered objective, value free or completely free from bias. Findings are instead shaped by values—or value mediated (Guba & Lincoln, 1994)—stemming from cultural, economic, ethnic, feminist/gender/queer, political and social issues. The most important ingredient is the critical framework that all critical theorists adhere to and their striving to be a force of change that can have a positive impact on people's well-being through an understanding of power dynamics, as they affect the individual or society as a whole. Although new knowledge is valued and sought, it is the facilitation of social change that is critical theorists' primary concern regardless of their ideological viewpoint (Kim, 2003). It is further believed that orthodox research—most often construed as research stemming from within a positivistic or postpositivistic paradigm—never questions but instead reinforces the superiority of a certain class, race and gender (Kincheloe & McLaren, 2002). Critical theorists deliberately question the status quo and strive to uncover injustices and inequities that otherwise are unnoticed due to the uncritical acceptance within other paradigms of the dominant culture. If we scrutinise sport and exercise psychology journals—both in regard to what they publish and who are on their editorial boards—men are overrepresented, as is researchers from English speaking, western and industrialised nations. This issue is increasingly important across all of science and is addressed in more detail in Chap. 6.

Constructivism (or as it is also labelled: *interpretivism*) is fundamentally different to positivism, and also different from postpositivism in the way we will discuss paradigms. As indicated by the name, constructivists believe that reality is not an objective entity; the individual instead constructs it (Hansen, 2004). If this is the case, then as many realities as there are individuals will exist. But athletes' or coaches' 'lived experiences' are not created in a vacuum; the surrounding environment and society also have a significant impact (Cronin & Armour, 2015; Hollings, Mallett, & Hume, 2014). This means that lived experiences are both created intraindividually (within the person) and interindividually (between persons). In both cases, the researchers try to create an in-depth understanding, which necessitates a hermeneutical (interpretative) approach to unravel meaning otherwise being hidden. The article by Cronin and Armour is particularly noteworthy as it stems from semi-structured in-depth collaborative interviews with one community coach. This in turn encouraged a close interaction between the researcher and the coach that together through dialogue jointly created and uncovered the lived experiences of the coach as these have been formed by both internal and external factors such as parents, carers and teachers.

This subjectivity can be interpreted in different ways: a positivist/post-positivist may think that qualitative researchers who are interested in lived experiences are merely involved in writing fiction, not performing science as there is no objective truth to reveal, only subjective and thereby 'unreliable' experiences as reported by athletes or coaches. The narrative format often used lends itself to this interpretation; consequently Cronin and Armour directly address this risk when describing the 'life-world' of the coach. Because individuals have had different experiences in their lives, their lived experiences will also differ. A constructionist will therefore consider the idiographic approach as necessary to reveal what is the perceived truth for each individual, and to allow what is hidden to surface, meaning that constructionists also are interested in implicit and tacit knowledge; to merely look for nomothetic laws is thereby considered superficial, even naïve (Guba & Lincoln, 1994). Reality is considered relative, and influenced by the social context as well as by the individual's lived experiences, which thereby means that what can be conveyed to a researcher will constantly change over time; if the coach was to be interviewed some time later, say a year or two, then Cronin and Armour probably would present a slightly different narrative to the reader—as can be expected when the experience from living is extended or related to a different time period in life.

Nomothetic Versus Idiographic Approach

In the previous paragraph, two terms were mentioned without being explained: nomothetic and idiographic. The names in themselves reveal very little, unless you infer that their origin is from two Greek words; nomo stemming from *nomos* and idio from *idios*, the former meaning custom or law and the latter along the lines of 'proper to one'. Despite being Greek in origin, it was the German philosopher Wilhelm Windelband that first used the terms, subsequently adopted by the American psychologist Gordon Allport. The latter is most known for his influence on personality psychology, where he became known as both trying to understand what makes people uniquely different (an idiographic approach) and what are common traits among people (a nomothetic approach). That Allport used these terms in his book *Personality: A psychological interpretation* (1937) is therefore not surprising.

A nomothetically inclined sport and exercise psychology researcher is probably most interested in revealing universal laws or making generalisations of phenomena from a sample to the population it represents, such as elite athletes or high school coaches. Consequently, nomothetic research is often performed within a positivistic or postpositivistic paradigm, predominantly with a quantitative methodology. Much of the criticism voiced against traditional sport and exercise psychology research is focusing on the use of standardised measurement scales or instruments trying to establish whether statistically significant relationships exist between independent and dependent variables (e.g. Sparkes, 2015).

In contrast, an ideographic researcher seeks knowledge about what is unique and individual, thereby not striving to draw inferences from a single individual to a group. The methodology is often qualitative and it fits best within a constructionist or interpretative paradigm where each person's lived experiences can be revealed (e.g. Cronin & Armour, 2015). This approach is common when, for example, trying to understand why one particular elite athlete has been so successful in her/his chosen sport; it would make little sense to try to extrapolate the findings to a group of elite athletes (although case studies sometime also focus on commonalities between individuals).

As with most concepts, the use of the terms nomothetic and idiographic has neither been consistent over time, nor have these labels been applied uniformly. Krauss (2008), for example, describes three different uses of the term idiographic, showing that the original meaning of these terms has been watered down; he even suggests that the debate whether research is predominantly nomothetic or idiographic should be closed. This is not a new suggestion; already in 1981 Lamiell published an article with the title *Toward an idiothetic psychology of personality*. Calling for an 'alternative to the individual differences paradigm' (p. 276) and the need to incorporate facets of the nomothetic approach—hence an 'idiothetic' approach. It is noteworthy that Lamiell, in 1981, used the term paradigm when discussing individual differences and the need to distinguish between differential psychology and personality psychology, inspired by among others Allport (1937). Proving once again that paradigm as a term has been used with vastly different meanings.

So far in this chapter, we have discussed how different belief systems—paradigms—influence research. Belief systems that a researcher can keep to, which in turn influences the researcher's search for answers, whether they be valid for groups of people (a nomothetic approach) or framed more towards an individual's unique qualities (an idiographic approach) or a mix of the two (the idiothetic approach). The next decision involves the actual methods.

Quantitative Versus Qualitative Methods

First, one additional comment relating to the apparent difficulty to decide on the definition of a paradigm: in two recently published articles (Jackson, 2015; Landrum & Garza, 2015), the authors compare qualitative and quantitative 'paradigms'. This is something that Madill (2015) strongly refutes in her article 'Qualitative research is not a paradigm: Commentary on Jackson (2015) and Landrum and Garza (2015)'. Viewing the arguments, a case can be made for both positions: if siding with Kuhn, then the answer will be different than if a paradigm is merely considered to be a rudimentary belief system. And if you believe in qualitative or quantitative research as the best way to obtain reliable and trustworthy answers, then one can easily argue that what some researchers call methods others would call paradigms.

There is little need for prolonging the 'paradigm wars' (Gage, 1989: p. 4); in Chap. 1, we therefore argued for transcending them; a point we will make more forcefully in Chaps. 9 and 10. This does not mean that a perceived war between paradigms has ceased to exist, even though that has been suggested (e.g. Bryman, 2006). An alternative explanation is that articles published after 2006 are merely comparing apples with pears, or more specifically confusing paradigms with methods. This interpretation finds some support in a comment made by Griffiths and Norman (2013: p. 583), stating that what remains is a 'simple conflict between the practitioners of qualitative and quantitative research'. This actually fits well with the arguments put forward by Jackson (2015), Landrum and Garza (2015) and Madill (2015) because their discussion is more about the terms (paradigms vs. qualitative/quantitative research) and less about what the terms stand for. The sum of arguments actually boils down to whether one way of finding answers in superior or inferior to another way. In short, people may wish to ask: which is best… qualitative or quantitative?

As interesting as this question may seem at first, it is demonstrably inappropriate, like asking whether a hammer is better than the concept of ennui… *best at what?* Because different methods answer different questions; for example, if we are interested in how anxious an athlete feels before a competition, we can use a standardised scale (inventory) and the rating will tell us something about the intensity. The answer will be viewed as more accurate if the scale has been thoroughly tested and found to be both reliable and valid (more about these concepts in Chap. 7). But the scale only measures what it has been constructed to measure, and that depends on how well the researchers have operationalised the concept 'anxiety'. A standardised scale never offers an insight into what 'anxiety' is, which instead a qualitative method may do. Interview question: 'when you feel anxious before a competition, can you please describe how you feel and how that affects how you perform?' Such a question will not only tell us how the athlete perceives anxiety but also any effects this may have on behaviour or performance.

The above is a relatively simplistic way of approaching the question of whether qualitative or quantitative methods are 'best'—and yet it still illustrates the core issue. One can of course draw the conclusion that quantitative research methods are better than qualitative, because the former have been used to a much greater extent than the latter. In fact, quantitative methods have been dominating general psychology as well as sport and exercise psychology for many, many years. And they are still more common than qualitative methods in published research despite the influx of journals devoted to the new kid on the block. One reason—going back to the paradigm controversies—is the early dominance of positivist and postpositivist research paradigms. Lincoln and Guba (1985) argued that this was due to the influence of the likes of John Stuart Mill—who channelled Bacon's inductive and empiricist ideas—on nineteenth-century science and the great progress of the early twentieth century. The work of Weber, Fechner, Stevens and many others that was described in Chap. 2 thereby fits with Mill's positivist notion that the search for general laws that can help us predict and explain relationships is what distinguishes good from bad science (notably Weber's law, Fechner's law and Stevens' law). Social scientists should, according to Mill, emulate the 'hard' sciences; thereby real progress can be achieved even in a field that from the beginning was dominated by philosophers.

Maybe this actually constitutes the origin of the paradigm wars? That is, one line of research (the quantitative) dominated research for a very long time; when social sciences then slowly got traction, they tried to be perceived as 'a real science' (and real scientists) by following the lead from the natural sciences. The alleged incompatibility (ontology, epistemology) between the two methods was then held as proof that the researcher needs to choose one over the other. This in turn escalated into becoming a standoff between the ruling positivist paradigm and the challengers in the form of constructivists. By forcefully defending a positivist stance, and simultaneously undermining the opposing force with allegations of being too subjective or too unscientific, the hegemony could remain in place for many years despite being regularly challenged. This is also logical from a self-preservation viewpoint because researchers heavily invested in the positivist tradition may perceive anything based on a different foundation as a threat (for promotion, tenure, fame, recognition, etc.—see Chap. 9). Consequently, if threats are immediately met with force, this can indeed be considered a war between proponents of qualitative versus quantitative methods and positivist versus constructionist paradigms.

Either you are with us or against us, there is no middle ground—a stance taken throughout history to define who 'we' are in relation to 'the others'.

The above is one facet that may explain why textbooks dealing with research methods sometime describe one group of methods as incompatible with another group, instead of merely being devised to answer different questions. Another critical question when considering qualitative versus quantitative research methods is whether these terms are as unambiguous as we have treated them so far? Can a method really be deemed as purely qualitative or quantitative? Consider the following: A researcher interviews athletes. Does the interview constitute a qualitative or quantitative method? You may answer a qualitative method, thereby assuming that the interview is less structured, allowing follow up questions, and that the results are presented in a narrative form that also can be subjected to, for example, a content analysis. Now, if the researcher counts occurrences of words or themes, and then compares different groups of athletes, for example, individual versus team athletes—using a suitable statistical method—then there seems to be a mix of methods.

The Mixed-Methods Approach

Despite the problem of labelling a method as either strictly qualitative or quantitative (Allwood, 2012), mixed-methods research is becoming more common in many social science disciplines, not the least sport and exercise psychology. The acceptance of a mixed-methods approach accelerated when first the *Journal of Mixed Methods Research* was launched in 2007, and then the Mixed Methods International Research Association (http://mmira.org) was created in 2014, convincing even more researchers that it is all right to mix methods. The primary goal of either the Journal or Association is of course not to bring peace to the camps supporting either qualitative or quantitative methods simply by mixing them, but to make sure that research questions are not answered from a limiting perspective or a restricted belief system; instead the most comprehensive approach possible should be applied. Or as described by Johnson, Onwuegbuzie and Turner (2007: p. 123):

Mixed methods research is the type of research in which a researcher or team of researchers combines elements of qualitative and quantitative research approaches (e.g., use of qualitative and quantitative viewpoints, data collection, analysis, inference techniques) for the broad purposes of breath and depth of understanding and corroboration.

Mixed-methods research is thereby according to its supporters suitable for obtaining a more comprehensive picture, to increase validity and build a stronger case by allowing one method to enhance or facilitate the other. Alternatively, the aim is to use one method to reduce shortcomings of the other method (O'Cathain, Murphy, & Nicholl, 2007). Researchers subscribing to a multi-methods approach are often pragmatists; they believe that research methods can and should be combined, provided that this facilitates answering the questions at hand. In contrast, purists advocate mono-method studies; the researcher choses one method and sticks with it. Usually, a purist is skilled in either quantitative or qualitative research methods and remains faithful to one approach—these are also often the combatants in the paradigm wars, swearing allegiance to either the positivist/postpositivist view or the constructivist/interpretivist view.

A situationalist is still a mono-method researcher but chooses the method that will best answer the current question; they believe that some research questions are more suitable for quantitative methods, whereas others are better answered by qualitative methods (Onwuegbuzie & Leech, 2005). With the growing number of both qualitative and quantitative methods, few researchers master everything with the same level of expertise; collaborative efforts in which both multi-disciplinary and multi-methods research teams work together are therefore becoming more common. This in itself creates new challenges when researchers with different experiences, training and skill sets are trying to collaborate while struggling to find a common ground and language to communicate effectively both internally and externally. With the advent of new outlets for research, not the least in the form of online publishers, multi-disciplinary/multi-methods research will most likely continue to grow, and with that the foundation for fruitful collaborations (we return to expand in Chaps. 9 and 10).

Some may argue that the uptake has been slower among sport and exercise psychology researchers in comparison to many other fields (Culver, Gilbert, & Sparkes, 2012; Sparkes, 2015). This can possibly—at least in part—be explained by the pros and cons described by Culver et al. (2012) and the view held by some researchers that '…the mixing of quantitative and qualitative methods grounded in different epistemological foundations makes little sense at all given paradigmatic incommensurability. There is a wariness of ill-informed attempts to do so lest the methods tail end up wagging the dog' (p. 275). Considering that the first journal in sport and exercise psychology was founded in 1970, it may not be surprising, given the above, that the first journal in the field to be entirely devoted to qualitative research was founded as recently as 2009: *Qualitative Research in Sport, Exercise and Health* (*Health* was added in 2011).

The quantitative dominance in three leading sport and exercise psychology journals is also striking, although the gap between quantitative versus qualitative between 1990 and 1999 (83 % vs. 17 %: Culver, Gilbert, & Trudel, 2003) has closed somewhat between 2000 and 2009 (71 % vs. 29 %: Culver et al. 2012). Out of the articles classified as qualitative in 2012, about one third (31.1 %) were mixing methods, which was actually down from the 2003 review (38.1 %). Although not discussed in the latter review, this may be a result of more specialised journals emerging and online outlets being considered as more appropriate by mixed-methods and qualitative researchers in sport and exercise psychology.

Sparkes (2015) offers a number of 'critical reflections' that may explain why mixing methods is still controversial in some camps and not as pragmatically clean as one possibly could expect given that this practice has been around for some time. For example, one might consider the confrontational stances taken by purists at one end of the continuum and pragmatists at the other. While not siding with either side, Sparkes nevertheless stresses the importance of making informed and deliberate choices. And further that it is necessary to judge the quality of the research using appropriate criteria: 'Judging a quantitative study using qualitative criteria and vice versa is wholly inappropriate. Any form of inquiry needs to be judged using criteria that are consistent with its ontology, epistemology, methodology, and use of methods for specific purposes' (Sparkes, 2015: p. 54).

The use of quantitative criteria to judge qualitative research can be explained by 'methodological orthodoxy' (Hesse-Biber, 2010), or the continuing inequality in power between qualitative and quantitative methods. Even when they are mixed in the same study, they are seldom given equal footing; instead mixed-methods research often 'subordinates QUAL methods to a secondary position to QUAN methods' (Teddlie & Tashakkori, 2011: p. 295). This is also the case in sport and exercise psychology research, according to McGannon and Schweinbenz (2011), claiming that qualitative research methods are only deemed valuable as long as they support the dominating quantitative component.

Difficulties of forming a productive research team, by bringing qualitative and quantitative researchers together, are vividly described by Lunde, Heggen and Strand (2012); power struggles, strained relationships, disempowerment and feelings of being of less value were contributing to alienation and distancing by the qualitative researchers. Sparkes (2013) conclude that this situation would:

> ...draw attention to the difficulties of bringing together teams made up of researchers who hold different positions with regard to ontology, epistemology, methodology and how various techniques should be used for specific purposes. Simply bringing researchers from different backgrounds together does not guarantee a successful mixed methods project. (p. 55)

This makes sense if we consider the power perspective and value attributed to the different methods—instead of focusing on the findings. What if the findings are contradictory? This is discussed by Lunde et al. (2012) based on an empirical case study, which included both quantitative and qualitative methods related to athletes with knee injuries. Whereas the quantitative findings indicated a successful rehabilitation process, the qualitative findings questioned this. These disparate results proved impossible to publish in one article, instead the quantitative and qualitative findings were published separately. One of the researchers interviewed summarised the complications with these words:

> Doing mixed methods research requires a common understanding, and it has not been like that. We thought that it should work out by itself. We

have thought we knew what research is. And it is first in retrospect that we became aware of all the differences that we have not been explicit about. It is not just about what kind of questions you ask – it is about a completely different understanding (Lunde et al., 2012: p. 209).

The challenges described by Lunde and colleagues seem insurmountable, which at least in part may be due to a power struggle between paradigms. It may also be a consequence of an emerging audit culture.

Methodological Backlash

The paradigm wars were—as described above—largely fought in the 1980s (Gage, 1989), although Denzin (2009: p. 14) spoke of the 'the new paradigm war' suggesting that a resolution and peace was never really reached. And one reason for this is—according to Sparkes (2013)—the continuing power struggle between biomedical models of research and qualitative research performed in the social sciences and humanities.

Up until now, mixed-methods research has been discussed only as something that combines qualitative and quantitative methods within one discipline, for example, psychology or sport and exercise psychology. That is, one discipline incorporating multi-methods research and the potential for conflicts originating when researchers from within one discipline but with different skill sets try to answer interrelated questions. What we have discussed to a lesser extent is when multi-disciplinary and multi-methods researchers try to collaborate. Although this is really what Lunde et al. (2012) describe when they relay the clash between quantitative and qualitative researchers, one subheading is actually 'The knee project: Interdisciplinary research on knee injuries in athletes' (p. 199). The quantitative researchers were physiologists and physiotherapists, and their intention was to measure physiological and biomechanical improvements during a rehabilitation programme. In contrast, the phenomenological researchers were interested in subjective experiences, both from living with and rehabilitating from knee injuries. Consequently, this brings into play power inequality from two perspectives: firstly quantitative versus qualitative methods, and secondly natural versus social sciences. We have already discussed the privileged position that positivistic and postpositivistic paradigms have over constructivism (interpretivism), both because of their historic roots where measurement and quantification was highly valued, and the fact that even modern textbooks on research methods lean more heavily towards the former than the latter. Sparkes (2013) expands on this from a sport and exercise psychology perspective by also considering what he refers to as 'the neoconservative backlash and the rise of methodological fundamentalism' (p. 442). Specifically, the unbalanced support of biomedical models of research, and a climate in which one type of research (quantitative) is acknowledged more by the audit culture than another type (qualitative).

The Audit Culture

The above focus on measurement, quantitivism, favouring certain methods and publishing as much as is humanly possible is—according to Sparkes (2013)—a result largely driven by an emerging audit culture. To expand, there is an apparent necessity for measuring the performance of academics by which university life is transformed from academic freedom and the search for knowledge to striving to achieve individual and institutional targets. Most universities in Western countries have clearly articulated 'performance expectations' that are used to review and assess the performance of their academic staff every year. Overlooking the fact that this management approach has been undermined by the findings of scientific research, and abandoned by many world-leading multinational companies, the practice continues unabated in tertiary education. If such evaluative practice is applied regardless of discipline, the system will advantage some and disadvantage others. It will also adversely impact disciplines such as Sport and Exercise Science because they are by definition multi-disciplinary. Within the same walls, sport and exercise perspectives from disciplines such as anatomy, physiology, physiotherapy, biomechanics and sports medicine try to co-exist with sport psychology, sociology, pedagogy and sport history.

In an audit culture where a journal's impact factor (IF) becomes ever more important, along with the sheer number of publications; it is no wonder if researchers start to feel that they are valued differently.

University of Queensland's 'Q-index' is one example where each researcher is ranked based on research income, number of publications weighted by their respective IF, completions of higher degree by research students, along with supervision load (www.uq.edu.au). So more is always better. Thereby making it possible to rank order researchers from the worst to the best performers. This practice is hardly conducive to academic freedom or intrinsic motivation; it may instead further demoralise academics (e.g. Tourish, 2011). Another increasingly important force in Australia is the rankings provided by Excellence in Research for Australia (ERA), driven by the Australian Research Council (http://www.arc.gov.au/era). The objective of ERA is to promote and reward excellence in research—a worthy endeavour. However, Field of Research Code 1106 is 'Human Movement and Sports Science', an area that is multi-disciplinary and incorporating different paradigms as well as research methods.

An interesting question then becomes: what criteria are used to judge the quality of research? As can be suspected, publications in high-impact journals and substantial external funding are considered signs of excellence. Funding should preferably stem from Category 1 granting bodies, which in Australia translates to Australian Competitive Grants Research Income. Proof of these ingredients—publications in high-ranking scientific journals and Category 1 funding—are subsequently rewarded when ERA assess research within a discipline as belonging to one of five categories: Well above world standard (5), Above world standard (4), World standard (3), Below world standard (2) and Well below world standard (1).

To be ranked as a four or five, a discipline such as Human Movement/ Sport and Exercise Science must present their best work, which each institution self-select from their researchers and then submit to ERA for ranking. The question then becomes: how does ERA take into account that many submissions are from multi-disciplinary institutions? The short answer is that they do not. It is up to respective institution to decide whether to include or exclude certain publications and data. High-impact publications are thereby more valuable than low-impact publications, and Category 1 grants more valuable than Categories 2 and 3 (publications in journals without impact factors are in this environment considered of minimal value).

In the Sports Science field, articles published in sport medicine journals are more often than not valued more highly than articles published in sport psychology journals; and the likelihood that a sport medicine researcher successfully can compete for Category 1 funding is significantly greater than a sport psychology researcher. The real world consequence of this is simply then that areas belonging to the natural sciences are more valuable for a multi-disciplinary institution compared to contributions from social and humanistic sciences. This trend towards an audit culture and some of the negative consequences resulting from it has been noted before. Darbyshire (2008), for example, wrote the following lines:

> Somewhere in a university, at this moment a memorandum is surely being written, 'advising' staff only to publish in journals with an IF of 'X' or above, pointing out that a failure to achieve this level of 'publication excellence' will be deemed to 'demonstrate' a level of performance that is unacceptable and in need of remediation. That such epistemological fundamentalism could even be considered, let alone tolerated will scarcely raise a ripple of concern as the memo will be couched in the soporifically comforting context of being an 'initiative' designed to show the institution's 'commitment' to 'improved quality' and to 'ensuring' that all staff are suitably 'on message' about this (p. 38).

Surely, we are not alone in having seen such a memo and heard the discussions that inevitably follow suggesting that resources should be allocated to where they 'do most good'. But not 'most good' for building knowledge or targeting areas in greatest need of research; 'most good' is always phrased in terms of increasing the standing of the institution, by having more disciplines achieve high ERA rankings. This strategy, in turn, is believed to increase their market value, that is, it will help attract more students and increase the likelihood of securing external research funding; because universities are now more than ever before business enterprises, not pillars of knowledge.

From the above follows that some disciplines will be deemed more valuable than others, simply because of their potential for research output and funding input. Indeed, this can already be seen in many universities where STEM subjects ('hard' sciences, technology, engineering and mathematics) are pushing out the 'soft sciences' such as arts, humanities and social sciences (Sparkes, 2013). When ERA in 2010 was introduced in Australia, Haslam and Koval (2010) raised a flag of warning, stating that these rankings will:

> ...create powerful incentives for researchers to target high-ranking journals and for departments to hire and direct resources towards researchers who do so successfully. For these incentives to be effective in promoting quality research it is vital that the rankings capture journal quality validly and fairly. This task is difficult in a diverse field such as psychology. Research and publication practices in the "softer" areas of the discipline lean towards the social sciences, whereas "harder" areas lean towards the biosciences. This soft–hard dimension is reflected in citation-based indices of journal quality, such as the impact factor (IF), with journals in harder fields tending to have higher IFs. (p. 112)

This may—at least in part—explain the differences observed between the 39 Psychology Schools and Departments ranked in 2010 and again in 2012 (Crowe & Samartgis, 2015) as some lean more heavily towards biomedical psychology research, whereas others focus more on phenomenological research. Consequently, one easy way for any institution (not only those offering psychology or even sport and exercise psychology) to improve their rankings in future research quality exercises is to prioritise the biomedical areas. In a world of restricted resources, this ultimately means that areas within any discipline deemed 'softer' would lose ground and eventually become extinct. If knowledge is the body, and the audit culture the tail, the tail is ostensibly wagging the dog. Or perhaps more—perhaps picking it up and putting it in an entirely different place.

There are several options forward. One of these would be to realise that quality has many facets and that operationalising quality by calculating impact factors and external grant income may have more negative than positive consequences, at least compared to what was originally intended. A system change and return to the drawing board thereby seem pertinent (e.g. Sparkes, 2013). Another way forward is for the 'softer' sciences to mimic the 'harder' ones; this would then acknowledge that Mill was on the right track when he wrote *A System of Logic* (1843/1906).

To test this empirically, an enlightening set of experiments was conducted and reported (Fernandez-Duque, Evans, Christian, & Hodges, 2015). The researchers included superfluous neuroscience information to boost explanations of psychological phenomena. As can be expected, participants in the four experiments found the presented information more compelling when superfluous information was added. The authors offer several explanations, such as the 'prestige of the "hard" sciences' and that 'people believe that biological explanations are more complex and more scientific than psychological explanations' (p. 926). This may not be an example of the paradigm wars, but it explains why even researchers active in the same discipline, but with different focus (hard-soft), may at times feel underappreciated or that the bias that has existed for a very long time will most likely survive and thrive also into the foreseeable future. To avoid a resurgence of the paradigm wars, Denzin (2010) calls for a more nuanced approach, or in his own words:

> There needs to be a greater openness to alternative paradigm critiques ... There needs to be a decline in conflict between alternative paradigms proponents ... Paths for fruitful dialogue between and across paradigms need to be explored. This means that there needs to be a greater openness to and celebration of the proliferation, intermingling, and confluence of paradigms and interpretive frameworks (p. 40).

So instead of a continuing war between paradigms, is the simple solution a dialogue between paradigms? If so, the dialogue needs to be initiated within single-subject disciplines, such as Sport and Exercise Psychology. Because then the dialogue can focus on intradisciplinary challenges to determine how the knowledgebase best can be expanded. But not even a fruitful paradigm dialogue within single-subject disciplines, or even multi-subject disciplines such as Human Movement and Sport and Exercise Science, will be sufficient. As soon as different fractions within one discipline, or several disciplines within a multi-discipline institution, are at risk of fighting for limited resources—which is the case for all tertiary education providers nowadays—then there is a need of both an intradisciplinary and interdisciplinary dialogue. If performance-based evaluations are allowed to continue expanding their influence, such as ERA in Australia, the Research Excellence Framework (REF) in United Kingdom, the Hong Kong Research Assessment Exercise and the Denmark Bibliometric Research Indicator exercise, then the war will be won eventually. But can we afford the consequences? Is the only solution a paradigm-shift? Driven by a desire to rethink the prevailing belief system and change it into something that is focused on what we can learn from our research, instead of only accepting knowledge gained in a particular way and from using certain methods.

Concluding Remarks

The current research climate in sport and exercise psychology—influenced as it is by the audit culture, neoliberalism, new public management, methodological fundamentalism and a preference for biomedical models of research (Sparkes, 2013)—will be difficult to change. As long as individuals trained in the dominating paradigm dominate research councils worldwide, the current climate will not change; it will merely grow in strength and broaden its impact. The old adage 'publish or perish' may soon be substituted—as a result of the information revolution—by a new mantra: 'get visible or vanish' (Doyle & Cuthill, 2015). Citations are still important, as evidenced by the Times Higher Education World University Rankings. The calculated index for each university is to 30 % influenced by citations attributed to its researchers during the previous 6 years. This has increased the importance of being cited, as widely and frequently as possible (Dowling, 2014). To market one's own research is therefore as important—or possibly more important (e.g. Dowling, 2014)—as it is to perform good quality research. Various citation indexes (such as the *h*-index) are becoming increasingly important, but not as previously only for the individual academic wanting to promote her/his career; now universities worldwide compete for students and funding, thereby further supporting the audit culture. A consequence is that universities now are starting to rank their academics, from most to least valuable (and culling those that do not measure up).

This increasing reliance on counting citations and valuing quantity over quality encourages 'over-publication' (Doyle & Cuthill, 2015: p. 672) and increases the risk of producing 'mediocre, forgettable arguments and findings' (Bauerlein, Gad-el-Hak, Grody, McKelvey, & Trimble, 2010: p. A80). It also encourages 'boys-clubs' (see next chapter) and clusters of sport and exercise psychology researchers working to promote both their own and each others research (Lindahl, Stenling, Lindwall, & Colliander, 2015). To break 'the tyranny of the natural sciences' (Bairner, 2012: p. 102) and the emerging philosophy of 'get visible or vanish' (Doyle & Cuthill, 2015), there is a need to rethink the overreaching purpose of tertiary educational institutions. Maybe it is also time to rethink the current business model where research excellence is reduced to a number game instead of being judged by its quality and contributions to society.

6

Norms, Culture and Identity

Thomas Kuhn's highly influential book—*The Structure of Scientific Revolutions*—contains 13 chapters, only 2 of which attempted to detail how scientific advances are approached: paradigm shifts. As we saw in Chap. 1, he termed this process 'extraordinary science'. In contrast, the majority of the book details the ways he believed science is *actually done*, which he termed 'normal science'. In detailing the ways that 'paradigms' develop, propagate and dominate research topics, Kuhn's analysis comes to reflect the introductory quote to this chapter: 'The more things change, the more they are the same.' This is how Kuhn was able to trace recurring patterns across the history of science: while the topics, trends and methods may change, the basic 'rules' never do.

The rules contained within each paradigm typically prescribe: (i) what is to be observed and scrutinised; (ii) the kind of questions that are supposed to be asked and probed for answers in relation to this subject; (iii) how these questions are to be structured; (iv) what predictions made by the primary theory within the discipline; (v) how the results of scientific investigations should be interpreted; (vi) how is an experiment to be conducted; and (vii) what equipment is available to conduct the experiment (Kuhn, 1970).

© The Author(s) 2016
P. Hassmén et al., *Rethinking Sport and Exercise Psychology Research*,
DOI 10.1057/978-1-137-48338-6_6

Try to think, for a few moments about how much freedom a researcher has, and how much scope there is for new discoveries, when these considerations (i–vii) are predetermined, and extremely difficult to change, or challenge. There is an added layer to this problem, because even if we wanted to challenge the rules of a prevailing paradigm, who should we speak to? Who is in charge? The answer is that, in most instances, there is no formal system for determining such things and, instead, a more insidious system is in place—time and again, as observed by Kuhn.

Now insidious is a strong word, why use it? Well the fact that no one person, committee or organisation is 'in charge' of each paradigm makes it look like nobody is to blame: as if the status quo is entirely natural and even 'right-and-proper'. As a colleague of ours often argues 'That's just the reality'. This has led to many heated debates, however, because we tend to respond: 'No that's not right. That's the reality *we* are creating, permitting, and perpetuating'. Fundamentally, it leads us right back to the philosophy-of-science and the differences between 'hard' sciences (where reality is pretty consistent and difficult to redefine) and more social sciences where reality is a social construction: a construction that we participate in. If someone defines gravity as 'the force that attracts a body towards the centre of the earth, or towards any other physical body having mass, *that's just the reality*', then it's hard to argue. But if someone claims 'the system we operate in supresses new ideas and approaches, favours males over females, whiteness over non-whiteness, and Western cultures over all other... that's just the reality'; we need to say 'No that's not right. That's the reality we are creating, permitting and perpetuating'. Even if no single person seems to be to blame. Even if an individual has never knowingly been discriminatory in any capacity, it's still morally and ethically wrong. It can be 'correct' in terms of accurately describing a state-of-affairs, but that is all. It is not 'right-and-proper'.

Now for the hard question: could sport and exercise psychology exhibit similar properties and patterns? In this chapter we will undertake the difficult task of looking inwards at the world of sport and exercise psychology and attempting to capture, and reflect on, our own prejudices, discriminative practices and regressive tendencies. We will jointly consider the influence of dogma and paradigms alongside issues of discrimination of equal opportunities because of similarities between: (a) the underlying mechanisms (implicit, cultural norms/expectations and stereotypes) and also (b) the effects (regressive tendencies, impediments to progress, prevention of diversity and many justifiably upset people). As a clue to how the discussion might conclude, consider the following: issues of paradigms and impediments to scientific progress have been demonstrated across all of science—historical and contemporary. The physicist Max Planck once wrote 'Science advances one funeral at a time'—that is, as each 'gatekeeper' finally drops their opposition to change. Is sport and exercise psychology likely to be different? Likewise, issues of gender inequality, racial and cultural discrimination have always permeated human societies—do we have any special measures in place to prevent these in sport and exercise psychology? If not, then should we expect to magically have avoided these issues in our own discipline? The chapter will separately consider (a) paradigmatic dominance, and then (b) issues of discrimination and equality, in each case taking lessons from other areas of science and checking to see if they might apply to sport and exercise psychology. We will intersperse some personal stories, reflections and exercises with a view to illustrating key points and at least attempting to alleviate some of the discomfort generated by such issues.

Paradigmatic Dominance in Sport and Exercise Psychology

There are important reasons for the evaluation of ideas, methods and findings through the peer-review process, usually before they are 'published' and broadcast for public viewing. Peer review should allow for some evaluation of the quality and merit of an idea, method or finding; it should seek input from various perspectives and reduce the risk of bias stemming from the preferences of individuals or small groups; it should prevent misleading or unreliable findings from being published; it should reduce the sheer number of papers being published and reduce the likelihood of 'noise' when readers seek to learn about a particular topic. One only needs to quickly scan social media websites to quickly understand what sorts of claims and ideas can make it into the public debate without the quality assurance offered by peer review: nonsensical, impossible, misleading and even dangerous ideas and products are often promoted this way. Hence, processes such as peer review—by editors, reviewers and even examiners and supervisors—play a key role in science. But is there any scope for this reliance on peer opinions to contain problems of its own? Peer review often also informs the judgement of grant applications—which provide the funding and decide which research projects get to happen versus which do not—and even tenure/promotion panels at many universities. The problem is that humans are invariably prone to our own biases and fallibilities, and when such a premium is placed on the judgements of human peer reviewers, it can occasionally have unintended negative effects. Just imagine, for a moment, that you have a particular idea or theory to explain some aspect of sport or exercise psychology. Imagine that your idea was the main thing you researched and constituted the substantive work of your PhD and published papers. Now imagine someone pointed out a problem with your idea, suggesting it might be wrong. How would you react? Now imagine you have a bunch of friends who are on your side, and prepared to defend you, and attack the doubter mercilessly. Would you let them? Would you encourage such behaviour? We are all human.

By: Richard Keegan

In 2006, in the second year of my PhD studies, I travelled to the annual conference of the Association for Applied Sport Psychology (AASP), in Miami, Florida. It was an exciting opportunity to go to the United States, seemingly the spiritual home of sport psychology, and to surround myself with all the big names from our field. I shared an elevator with Judy van Raalte, and I shared a taxi with Jean Williams. Ken Ravizza passed me in the foyer: 'Wow, did you see that!! It was Ken!' I was lucky enough to see the famous Burt Giges' dance moves. At the time, I had been grappling with various aspects of my research: theories, methodology, philosophy and more. I was tormented by the type of existential angst that perhaps only afflicts PhD students, when one finally begins to experience the limits of one's knowledge, understanding and capability. Specifically, when one's data starts to prove that your assumptions—and by association your whole world-view—are flaky. For example, I had recently had what I now refer to as the 'Oh shit' conversation (described in Chap. 8), where a supervisory meeting led to us realising our initial plans for data analysis were not going to work.

I recall it as a very stressful time—both personally and professionally, for example, I undertook supervised practice as a psychologist alongside my PhD studies—meaning I was quite vulnerable and 'unbalanced' given the problems I perceived with my PhD. I had a particularly unpleasant time at the conference, which I will describe briefly below. Looking back, however, I arguably needed this 'shock' to break me out of the funk I was in and prevent me from gravitating back to simply complying and fitting in—which at the time was all I wanted!

Several stories from this conference are seared into my memory, which is often taken as an indication that they were quite traumatic—or at least very personally meaningful. The most unforgettable of all these experiences occurred during my poster presentation, when I eagerly stood by my poster and sought to engage passers-by or answer any questions that were put to me. My poster sought to address the question of whether a new variant of achievement goal theory (the 2 x 2 approach described by Elliot, 1999) would lead to a different interpretation of motivational climate: the motivational influence exerted by key social agents resulting in a situational goal climate (the specific pragmatic and social situations in which the achievement task is defined; Ames, 1992). It seemed a reasonable question. After a few polite and forgettable (indeed, forgotten) conversations, I was approached by an eminent professor in the field of sport psychology, surrounded by an entourage of his PhD students and research associates. It didn't strike me as unusual that they were together, as they worked closely together. He proceeded to simply argue with me, quite aggressively, that I couldn't possibly believe in this new update to the theory: that it must be nonsense. The existing 'preferred' theory was just fine as it was. Other concepts and constructs, not commonly studied in achievement goals, were judged to explain any possible arguments in favour of the 2 x 2 approach, and there was no need to update it. I kept trying to respond that we had to at least entertain new theories, especially if they had shown promise in other areas (2 x 2 goals were largely developed in education, and the suggested to be useful for sport too). I found these few minutes extremely intimidating, not only because of the reputation and influence of my opponent but also because of the jeers of support that came from his entourage (one of whom had been a former colleague and friend of mine, which was also distressing). By having an entourage, and by explicitly arguing that most people in our field don't believe any new theory is necessary, there was a clear linkage to 'safety in numbers'; and intolerance for deviations from the 'norm'. Such was my fear of repercussions, I found myself apologising in the bar that evening, in case I had been too defensive (!). I was gruffly dismissed.

I was shattered by this experience. Tougher individuals would have simply moved on, but for me it was the proverbial straw that broke the camel's back. None of the conference's social activities were enjoyable to me, and I totally failed to soak in the beautiful surroundings that Miami offered. Further still, I began to notice a lot of other things I didn't like. Stung by the 'press gang' approach I had perceived at the poster, I began to notice how particular groups of researchers travelled around in groups: barely ever breaking away to go-it-alone, frequently presenting workshops and symposia together, socialising together, never going 'off-script' and largely advancing their particular idea or approach. It struck me that they can't all be right, especially when studying very similar topics (i.e. in the grand scheme of things, sport psychology is a relatively small topic). Even though these tensions and discrepancies seemed quite obvious, the groups seemed to be 'self-validating': if enough of us agree, we must be right. Scientifically, of course, there is nothing objectively true in a shared belief: truth is not democratic. I reflected that while social science, in particular, can be very difficult, we cannot simply resolve that difficulty by simply deciding to agree on certain short-cuts, frameworks, methods or conclusions. To do so is to effectively give up on science and begin a political process, or even a popularity contest. Ten years later, the existence of such groups is an obvious fact of academic life, as any experienced professor would attest. But at the time I was tied-in-knots by this realisation. The scales were falling from my eyes: it was painful, but I was beginning to see more clearly.

Two other conversations stood out to me, purely from this single conference: one repeated and one that occurred in isolation. First, having had a (what I felt was) bad experience at my poster, I wanted to show a little solidarity and offer my support to others in my position. On three separate occasions, speaking to PhD students after they had presented, I heard the following message: 'I wanted to study [Topic X] for my PhD, but my supervisor is _____, so now I have to study [Topic Y] instead'. I found this dumbfounding. Explanations included: 'If you get the chance to work with _____, you don't turn it down!' and 'You don't disagree with _____, you just don't!' Evidently, something other than science and truth was more important to these people: perhaps guaranteeing themselves a career, perhaps gaining favour and influence or perhaps—for the real forward thinkers—the better opportunities for citations and grant funding.

Second, following the meeting of a 'special interest group' I was interested in joining, I spoke with one tenured professor about what I perceived as an over-reliance on correlational methods. I joked that we were taught that correlation does not prove causation back in our first semester of university. His response—again—shocked me. 'You see, *for me*, correlation *is* causation... in fact for a lot of people it is'. He was really forceful about this.

It wasn't a joke. Technically, as any Year 1 research methods lecturer will tell you (with linear systems at least) correlation is a *necessary but not sufficient* condition for establishing causality. If two things are directly and causally connected, they should vary together in proportion, giving us a nice correlation. However, correlation is a quick-and-dirty statistical test, and it is possible to find correlations between variables that cannot possibly be causally associated (if you perform internet searches for 'spurious correlations' this will quickly become evident). Furthermore, correlations do not (cannot) tell us anything about the direction of causation: does A cause B, or vice versa? So once you find a correlation you need to use that as a prompt to begin a more robust experimental trial of whether changes to one variable cause the expected changes in the other. The only reason correlations appear to prove causation is because of our own assumptions—either the theory predicts a 'direction' (a prediction that needs to be tested!) or we mentally assume one must precede/cause the other. It is quite a powerful cognitive illusion exploited by newspapers and clickbait websites every day. But, of course, if your supervisors and direct peer group believe it does, perhaps that can make it seem okay. Perhaps if you can get people who believe the same as you to act as reviewers on journals, your papers will get published more easily. Too cynical?

These experiences certainly made me more cynical. But the story is reflective of resilience definitions: an adverse event followed by a positive adaptation. I was not broken by these experiences—well, not permanently at least, I was certainly affected. But I did not give up on sport psychology or postgraduate studies, and I did not simply decide to take the easy road and conform. Looking back, without this culture shock, I could easily have succumbed to simply 'fitting in'—it would have been a lot easier, and it would have felt 'right'. Nobody would have complained or criticised, and some of my papers would have had a much easier ride in peer review. However, my experience of the AASP conference in 2006 showed me exactly how I did *not* want to be, as a researcher. Now, that is notwithstanding the possibility that other people will definitely have had much better experiences! This is one person's narrative.

Most of the potentially unhelpful aspects of dominant paradigms and 'boys clubs' take place in private—they are subversive and difficult to bring to public attention. Peer reviews and journal editor decisions take place in private, and are often anonymous. There is rarely any recourse to appeal, or additional scrutiny—the editor's decision is final. The reviewers for key journals aren't particularly accountable to anyone—so long as they submit their reports on time. The editor is accountable in terms of ensuring readership, citations, impact factor and minimal errors or retractions. Nobody checks or assesses the quality of peer reviewers' reports as they are meant to be the quality assurance mechanism—so it is possible to act with some impunity in this position. If a reviewer has a particular bias, preference or axe-to-grind, they will not be assessed or criticised for letting their biases affect their review. 'Criticisms of peer review abound… knowing full well that there are many hardworking and discerning reviewers— critics of the peer-review system caricature reviewers as mean-spirited, lead-footed, capricious toadies and hacks who hide behind the cloak of anonymity.' (Suls & Martin, 2009; p.42). The problems generated by this peer-review process—despite it being widely recognised as the 'least bad' solution to offering quality assurance in scien/tific reporting—are increasingly coming to light. Even as far back as 1981, these problems were being recognised in psychology—for example, results of a survey of review accountability revealed that a majority of academic psychologists reported receiving reviews with obvious errors in fact (73 %), subjective reviewer judgements that were treated as objective truths (76 %) and other unconstructive and unscientific qualities (Bradley, 1981). In a more modern context, the website 'Shit My Reviewers Say' contains a number of such problematic reviews, and the phenomenon has led to a number of blogs and internet memes. Examples quoted on the site include:

(a) 'The reported mean of 7.7 is misleading because it appears that close to half of your participants are scoring below that mean'. [This misunderstands how 'means' work]

(b) '…by the time I had gone past Section 3.2, I lost interest because there was nothing that took me by surprise or wonder'. [Highly subjective judgement. Scientific papers are not supposed to fill us with surprise and wonder]

(c) 'There is a lot of terminology flung around such as "false negatives", "false positive" and "median", "first quartile", "third quartile."' [These are just normal scientific terms]

(d) 'I'm sorry, this topic is just not very interesting.' [This is a subjective judgement and irrelevant to whether a paper should be published or not]

(e) 'I am afraid this manuscript may contribute not so much towards the field's advancement as much as towards its eventual demise.' [Another subjective judgement and—assuming it was sent for review by a competent editor—unnecessarily harsh]

(f) 'The work that this group does is a disgrace to science.' [As above—and suggestive of some prior history with a rival research group]

(g) 'I am personally offended that the authors believed that this study had a reasonable chance of being accepted to a serious scientific journal.' [Again, highly subjective]

(h) What is disturbing is that the author was not adequately supervised or otherwise assisted by faculty at her institution. They failed her completely in providing oversight and input. Young and inexperienced researchers should never be placed in a position of subjecting themselves to the painful rigors of critical reviews without guidance prior to submitting. [This is suggestive of quite a poisonous cocktail of ageism, sexism and a blind acceptance that peer review is *necessarily* cruel and unpleasant—which is not the case]

To be clear, these problems are not specific to sport and exercise psychology, but we are certainly not above them. Examples in sport and exercise psychology are rarely made public, but some examples are personally known to us. Remember that the above examples were taken from reviewers' reports, which are rarely public documents. Thus, they were copied and posted from the emailed reports in most cases. Hence, for example, Keegan Spray, Harwood and Lavallee (2014)—which has been the most read and downloaded paper in its host journal since it was published—received almost identical comments to (e) and (g) above (in another journal, not the one where it was published). Essentially, one reviewer found their worldview to be challenged by the paper and get very angry about it. Similarly, Swann Crust, Keegan, Piggott and Hemmings (2015) were rejected by one journal simply for offering a 'different' viewpoint to the most popular approach in that area. Note that in each case, the papers were subsequently accepted elsewhere. It is possible for reviewers to be even more subversive and damaging than giving a bad review, and there are stories—spoken in whispers at academic conferences—of reviewers deliberately and 'tactically' taking an excessively long time to complete a review, demanding additional data be collected, deliberately misconstruing the findings or simply giving an intentionally 'destructive' review: intended to scupper a competitor's paper. As summarised by Suls and Martin (2009; p.43): 'Although an active researcher in the same domain will possess the greatest expertise, that person also is likely to be a direct competitor... This raises the possibility that limiting the dissemination of an author's findings could be in a reviewer's best interests'.

This problem has received analysis and critique in the wider literature—although arguably not (yet) in sport and exercise psychology. On the one hand, it may be the case that these bad experiences and lapses in standards could be quite random—perhaps all 'balancing out' in the end. On the other hand, there could be quite consistent biases, discrimination and detrimental effects if the system is permitted to play out unexamined, and without critical scrutiny. One clear and well-recognised effect of biases in peer review is that the effect can be extreme conservatism: prioritising pre-existing and recognised ideas, but suppressing new ideas and potential advancements (Suls & Martin, 2009; Trafimow & Rice, 2009). There is some evidence that controversial work is more likely to receive harsh reviews (Smith, 2006). Merton (1968) observed that Mendel's genetic discoveries were 'neglected for years' (p. 62). Horrobin (1990) documented 18 cases in the biomedical sciences where major innovations were initially blocked by the peer-review system (see also Garcia, 1981). Trafimow and Rice (2009) offered a particularly entertaining analysis of how social science reviewers would have responded to history's greatest scientific breakthroughs: spherical earth, the earth orbiting the sun, Einstein's special relativity and more. In each case, arguments for rejection focus on the new findings/ideas: (a) being inconsistent with currently accepted knowledge; (b) being too implausible; (c) not surprising or new enough; (d) offering their own (somehow more plausible) explanations for findings; and (e) deeming the suggested idea, theory or technique 'too complex'—we shall return to this particular issue shortly. In some cases, (f) methods and analyses were deemed too unconventional, and also there was a neat ability to classify an author's work as (g) either too 'applied' (i.e. not scientific and rigorous) or too sterile and controlled (i.e. lacking ecological validity): take your pick! In all of these cases, the prevailing paradigms—the currently preferred theories and methods—are preserved at the expense of potential advancements. This may begin to explain why peer review can become incredibly conservative. In all of the above cases, it is worth emphasising, that the judgements are highly subjective, and rarely objectively verifiable. Also—and here is where it gets tricky—it takes significant knowledge, experience, wordage/space and a sound knowledge of the philosophy-of-science to overcome some of these 'fatal criticisms'. As a potential exception, we recognise that that there is also a recognised strategy for some journals to 'take a bet' by choosing to accept papers containing 'weird' and unusual ideas, often simply in the form of narrative opinion papers. This approach—while much rarer—tips the balance the other way, and also leads to some problematic effects, so we are not simply arguing that peer review should be much more generous and positive. Recommendations for peer reviewing will be offered in Chap. 10.

Occam's Razor and the Principle of Parsimony in Achievement Goal Theory

As noted earlier, several of the key issues being illustrated here are only examined at the level of wider science literature, or perhaps sometimes psychology, but rarely in sport and exercise psychology. In the following section, we explore a slightly more fine-grained examination of one core argument in favour of the 'status quo' in sport and exercise psychology—one which has been used both in published accounts (where it can be exposed to scrutiny and critical appraisal) and also in anonymous peer reviews of submitted manuscripts.

The literature on achievement goals burgeoned between 1980 and 2010. The concept was adopted by researchers in diverse domains (e.g. education, sport, workplace), and the combined results of this research documented the correlates of different types of achievement goals (see summaries by Harwood, Keegan, Smith, & Raine, 2015; Hulleman, Schrager, Bodmann, & Harackiewicz, 2010; Kaplan & Maehr, 2007; Murayama, Elliot, & Friedman, 2012; Ntoumanis & Biddle, 1999; Van Yperen, Blaga, & Postmes, 2014). Reviews of this literature have noted excessive reliance on cross-sectional methods, with longitudinal and experimental methodologies being much less frequent (Harwood et al., 2015; Vansteenkiste, Lens, Elliot, Soenens, & Mouratidis, 2014). Most importantly for this section of the analysis, another trend that can be noted is the gradual increase in the number of achievement goals hypothesised: two (Dweck, 1986; Nicholls, 1984), three (Elliot & Harackiewicz, 1996), four (Elliot, 1999) and six (Elliot, Murayama, & Pekrun, 2011). Specifically, the dichotomous achievement goal perspective (e.g. Dweck & Leggett, 1988; Nicholls, 1984) was limited to the examination of two achievement goals: 'task' or 'mastery' goals (i.e. a focus on attaining task-based requirements or improvement) and 'ego' or 'performance' goals (i.e. a focus on outperforming others or avoiding doing worse than others). Our discussion will begin with that conceptualisation; we will in the next chapter return to this theory, but then with a focus on measurement.

Within the sport and exercise psychology literature, Nicholls' (1984, 1989) formulation of achievement goal theory has arguably served as the dominant approach in examining how performers perceive success or failure in achievement contexts (cf. Keegan, Spray, Harwood, & Lavallee, 2010). Achievement contexts are defined by the presence of some evaluative elements and so can include school, sports and sometimes exercise/ health (Roberts, 2001).

In the beginning, the 'breakthrough' in establishing achievement goals theory was based on a conception of goals that encompassed the entire achievement context. Hence, task, social and intrapersonal considerations were all contained within the parsimonious dichotomous framework. Nicholls (1984, 1989) asserted that an individual's internal sense of competence was pivotal in achievement contexts and that the subjective meaning of competence could be defined in at least two different ways (Nicholls, 1984):

> Achievement behavior is defined as behavior directed at developing or demonstrating high rather than low competence. It is shown that competence can be conceived in two ways. First, ability can be judged high or low with reference to the individual's own past performance or knowledge [termed either task or mastery goals]. In this context, gains in mastery indicate competence. Second, ability can be judged as capacity relative to that of others [termed either ego or performance goals]. In this context, a gain in mastery alone does not indicate high competence. To demonstrate

high capacity, one must achieve more with equal effort or use less effort than do others for an equal performance (p. 328).

Hence, individuals are task involved when improvements in, or the mastering of, a skill or task provide them with a sense of competence (and subsequent satisfaction). Alternatively, individuals are ego involved when their sense of competence depends upon demonstrating superior performance to others (e.g. genuinely superior or an equal performance to their competitor with less effort exhibited). These two definitions of competence were construed as applying across the involvement level of analysis, the contextual level (climate) and the pre-dispositional level (orientation)—as well as being two separate definitions in their own right. *How simple, how elegant!* Of course, by positing the same construct at all three levels, it raises the question of what an achievement goal actually is, and whether it really can exist at all three levels. Likewise, the relationship between orientations, climates and involvement states may also require further clarification.

In the late 1990s, Elliot and colleagues (e.g. Elliot & Harackiewicz, 1996) noticed that performance (or 'ego') goals were not always maladaptive and began a debate about how this might be possible. They proposed deriving two forms of performance goals: performance-approach and performance-avoidance goals. This version of achievement goal theory was termed the trichotomous perspective as it offered three different achievement goals: attainment of normative competence, winning or comparing favourably against others. Performance avoidance goals would focus on the avoidance of normative incompetence—for example, losing or comparing poorly versus others (Elliot & Harackiewicz, 1996; Matos, Lens, & Vansteenkiste, 2007; Skaalvik, 1997). Elliot's reconceptualisation of achievement goal theory therefore signalled the first steps away from the 'parsimony' of modelling two goals across all three levels of analysis.

Further evolutions in achievement goal theory involved applying the valence dimension—approach versus avoidance—across both performance and mastery goals, such that a 2 × 2 framework was developed (Elliot, 1999; Pintrich, 2000). Recently, debate has restarted as to whether an individual's attempt of surpassing an intrapersonal standard constitutes an adequate operationalisation of mastery goals (Martin, 2006; Van Yperen, 2006). From this work, a 3 × 2 model has been proposed, wherein individuals can focus on three different types of reference points for competence information: (i) the task, objective and absolute measurements such as time, score or similar; (ii) the self (i.e. how one is doing relative to previous performances); and (iii) normative comparisons (i.e. how one is doing relative to others). When adding the valence component with approach and avoidance considerations, individuals could focus on seeking to demonstrate success in each of these definitions of competence, or they can focus on avoiding the demonstration of incompetence: for example, failing to achieve a desired time/score, failing to perform to a level already achieved previously or comparing badly to others (losing or ranking low in a group). Research examining the 3 × 2 perspective is a relatively recent development and has focused primarily in educational settings, not sport or exercise.

One core argument *against* expanding the number of goal definitions has been that it undermines 'parsimony' and/or 'elegance' (Roberts & Treasure, 2012). Arguing against what he saw as unnecessarily complicating achievement goal theory, Roberts (2012) penned the following:

> In her profile of Nobel Prize winners, Zuckerman (1977) gave several attributes of the typical prize-winner, but one common attribute is particularly noteworthy: They see simplicity where other people see complexity. As an example, when Watson and Crick (1953) in their quest to discover the structure of the DNA molecule published their model of the double helix, Maurice Wilkins (a fellow scientist who was a rival in the quest) was surprised to see how simple the model was and is quoted to have said, "*How simple, how elegant*". The quest for expanded frameworks might be valuable because we may be able to provide a better description of the complexity of motivation processes, but a cost is often present, and part of that cost is a loss of parsimony! It is well for sport scientists to remember the famous saying of William of Occam (1285–1347): "Entities are not to be multiplied beyond necessity." Known as Occam's Razor, it is a call for parsimony, which is sometimes ignored.

To be clear, this is an argument that has captured many imaginations and inspired many critical reviews of papers and ideas. If it were a popularity contest, Occam's Razor would be winning right now. Nevertheless, detailed analyses of historical developments in different fields of science demonstrate that reality is not, in fact, parsimonious; and that applying parsimony as a key guiding principle does not offer any useful indication of quality in scientific theories (Courtney & Courtney, 2008; Gauch, 2003; Lee, 2002; Oreskes, Shrader-Frechette, & Belitz, 1994; Sober, 1996). Reviewing the parsimony argument in light of well-established debates in the philosophy-of-science, it is clear that the concepts of parsimony and elegance involve *highly subjective judgments* (Courtney & Courtney, 2008; Sober, 1990, 1996). Researchers examining the nature of science and scientific progress are clear that the principle of parsimony, in particular, should not be used as an axiomatic principle, but simply as one of many fallible heuristics (e.g. Courtney & Courtney, 2008; Gauch, 2003; Sober, 1996). Heuristics serve a purpose, of course, but are not capable of arbitrating in matters of truth and genuine 'advancement'. In fact, as noted earlier, one clear consequence of applying the parsimony heuristic in science is conservatism—that is, the notion of keeping things as they are (Courtney & Courtney, 2008). Sometimes, this can be good because it can prevent unnecessarily messy and unwieldy proposals from stealing effort and resources that should be devoted to promising theories. But, it can also actively inhibit progress (as Feyerabend argued). In the end, the parsimony heuristic does not decide which of several competing theories is better. Rather, progress is achieved when we are able to formulate theories into testable hypotheses and design experiments that actually compare competing theories (Courtney & Courtney, 2008; Popper, 2001). There is little, if any, empirical evidence that the world is actually simple or that simple accounts are more likely to be true than complex ones (Oreskes, Shrader-Frechette, & Belitz, 1994).

Overall, when examining the assumptions and hypothetical explanations required to support the 'parsimonious' dichotomous model of achievement goals, we see that the apparent parsimony of the model can be quite deceiving. Anyone wishing to become accepted as an 'achievement goal researcher'—welcomed into the paradigm by its gatekeepers and peers—is effectively required to memorise and rehearse a range of explanations, qualifiers and assertions in order to retain the simple 'dichotomous' model and still be able to tolerate accumulating contradictory findings. Often these qualifiers and explanations are stored across a range of texts, and some of which remain untested theoretical assertions or are supported only by correlational data—hardly axiomatic facts. The philosophers and historians of science—Duhem, Lakatos, Popper and others—have actually detailed this process, whereby a 'hard core' of theoretical assumptions is protected and maintained by a 'protective belt' of ad hoc hypotheses and corollaries, such that the core theory can never be criticised (we noted a similar situation in a section of the SDT literature in Chap. 4). On the one hand, the level of skill required to maintain the exclusive dominance of the original dichotomous model is impressive. On the other hand, through these manoeuvres, the paradigm is retained and defended; but at what cost?

We are generally quite resistant to having our worldview challenged, and we simply do not like feeling stupid (actually, this feeling is arguably central to conducting good science: Schwartz, 2008). Often times, this feeling can immediately lead to anger and hostility—for example, any of us who have received a challenging peer review from a journal (as above) would sympathise with such a reaction. Does it ever spill over into personal attacks, intolerance and insults? In the following section, we draw again from achievement goals research, as this has generated some interesting exchanges in the last 15–20 years. While many instances of anger and hostility may take place behind closed doors, and thus are not recorded for public viewing, they occasionally bubble up to the surface.

Ad Hominems, Straw Men and Exclamation Points

The above history of achievement goal theory gave rise to some interesting and noteworthy exchanges, some of which took place in published literature, some of which (unfortunately) are only recorded in memory, peer reviewer reports and email archives. Perhaps the most famous published example began with Harwood, Hardy and Swain (2000) and then progresses through Treasure and Roberts (2001) and then Harwood and Hardy (2001). This exchange may then have been reignited by a short passage in Harwood, Spray and Keegan (2008), which generated a further response from Roberts (2012). When reviewing these papers with the gift

of hindsight, it is possible to draw out a number of themes in the argumentation that neither advance science nor prove anybody right: ad hominem arguments, straw-man arguments, ridicule and exclamation points.
In order, we begin with 'ad hominem' arguments: An 'ad hominem' is recognised as a fallacious way of reasoning, in which a claim or argument is
rejected on the basis of some irrelevant fact about the author of or the person presenting the claim or argument. An example might be dismissing
another author, or group of authors, as 'young and arrogant' (e.g. Roberts,
2012; p.33). Ideas and theories exist independently of the person who
proposed them, and while we do reference heavily in science, this is more
a bibliographic exercise than a way of evaluating veracity. It works both
ways, such that (a) the most important theory or idea we ever hear might
be uttered by a serial-killing psychopath locked away behind bars, and
the source of the idea should be irrelevant to how good or bad the idea is.
Alternatively (b), if a scientific theory is proven to be incorrect, erroneous
or flawed, it actually does not reflect at all on the person who proposed the
theory. For example, the theories of Newton, Galileo, Curie, Einstein and
co. contain known flaws: flaws that have been detailed and written about
at length (Curie's mistake was unfortunately fatal). Does anyone think
any less of those scientists for not making their theory 'more perfect'?
Ostensibly not. Their new theories led science to a point where we could
ask new questions, and discover new problems. In fact, the people who
our collective memory does tend to forget are the ones who studiously
operationalised, tested and evaluated these new theories. Dismissing a fellow scientist's ideas on the grounds the person is judged to be young and
arrogant is as erroneous as dismissing famous theorists once their theories
are (inevitably) proven to contain errors and problems.

The technical definition of a straw man argument is an informal fallacy, based on giving the impression of refuting an opponent's argument,
while actually refuting an argument that was not advanced by that opponent or which is taken out of context. As an example, Roberts (2012)
appears to dismiss the paper by Harwood et al. (2008) by isolating and
criticising 600 words in a chapter of over 18,000 words. Similarly, a
section proposing that exclusively relying on one or two questionnaires
might become 'old hat' (Harwood et al., 2008) is mischaracterised as

dismissing *all* of Nicholls' (1984, 1989) work, and its derivatives, as 'old hat'. When reviewing the debates that surround achievement goal theory, and whether it should 'develop' or not, there are quite a few 'straw men' lying in tatters at the side of the road. As a writer, we get to look good by unceremoniously destroying an argument or idea that had been manufactured purely for the purpose of being destroyed—and which may have been taken totally out of context. It is difficult, if not impossible, to find an example of where such logic has contributed meaningfully to science or its advancement. As noted elsewhere in this text, such an argument is only likely to be fruitful in defending the status quo, and even then, only by circumventing the actual argument. The message of this chapter is that we must develop tests to allow for the discrimination between competing theories. Pure argumentation is likely to be unproductive, at best.

For our third argumentation 'habit', we can consider a collection of techniques that involve ridicule and exclamation points. Treasure and Roberts (2001) 'rebuttal' of Harwood et al. (2000) contained three exclamation points; Biddle, Duda, Papaioannou and Harwood's (2001) response to Pringle (2000) contained 7, and Roberts (2012) deployed 21 of them in 12 pages (pages 31–43). Perhaps no study of this exists, but in scientific writing, the average number of 'exclamation-points-per-article' is (almost definitely) zero: particularly using median values. There is little need to use exclamation points when considering observations, analysis, theorising and testing. Yet their proliferation in relation to achievement goals debates points to a number of 'argumentation techniques': including taking other people's logic to extremes and criticising the outcome (reductio ad absurdum); appeals to tradition and propriety (e.g. 'It's always been this way, so that must be right!'); and appeals to popularity and 'weight of numbers' (argumentum ad populum). For example, if a paper seeks to accrue a large authorship team with the intention of adding 'weight' or seeks to gain credibility by emphasising a large number of people/papers adopting a particular theoretical framework, these would be arguments based on popularity (and by association, authority). Remember again that the ideas of Copernicus, Gallileo, Curie, Darwin, Newton, Einstein and the like were all deeply unpopular when first proposed. In science, the truth does not submit to democratic votes or popularity contests (recall also Trafimow and Rice (2009), who offered up 'reviewer rejection letters' to some of the most famous and influential ideas in science: 'too different', 'too new', 'not like everything else we already do', 'simply unpalatable' and 'too complex' were all reasons that important ideas could have been wrongly rejected). Of course, exclamation points can also follow arguments based on straw-man argumentation, and ad hominem attacks.

What's the problem with debates involving exclamation points? Surely a bit of robust debate is central to good science? Possibly. But none of the above-listed techniques stand much chance of advancing science—unless one believes that the issue is already settled and advancement is the increasing of accuracy in measurement and more rigorous application of the idea. Arguably, none of the above-described approaches to a debate 'builds communities where controversy stimulates thought instead of enmity' (Nicholls, 1989; p. i). More likely, the existence of a group of gatekeepers who admonish and belittle anyone who questions a theory will actively discourage new joiners to the field, new ideas, and—ultimately—it will prevent advancement (by any definition). This may explain both the recent drop in papers published on achievement goals (detailed in Keegan, in press) and the conclusions of recent systematic reviews that we now have more than enough cross-sectional correlation-based papers (e.g. Biddle, Wang, Kavussanu, & Spray, 2003; Harwood et al., 2015). If the message is 'do achievement goals the right way (our way), or don't do it at all', are we not guilty of the same authoritarian leadership that our own research links to poor motivational outcomes (cf. Ames, 1992)—including superficial win-at-all-costs strategies, disengagement and dropout? (For a review of these associations, see Harwood et al., 2008).

To re-iterate, no amount of critical 'robust' argumentation will settle a debate between two (or more) fairly established theories competing for the same conceptual 'territory'. We need to develop fair tests that will allow us to discriminate between competing theories, perhaps even by collaborating. To achieve this, we must work to express each theory, or version of a theory, in a way that lends itself to such comparative testing. We must be brave enough to 'expose' our theories to testing and falsification. By contrast, we cannot expect new researchers joining the field to scour decades of sometimes contradictory and often confusing literature to find the 'right' hypotheses. It is not a new researcher's fault if they cannot find every detail and nuance of a debate that takes place: in diverse sources; from different people; in different fields (sport, education, exercise, PE); over a relatively long time; with different outcomes. This is not a reflection on someone's scholarship or 'literature reviewing skills'. In fact, the number of people capable of expressing each theory in truly parsimonious and testable frameworks—free of beliefs, presuppositions, opinions, auxiliary hypotheses and exclamation marks—is witheringly small and shrinking. Perhaps our research training, supervision, reviewing and publication preferences should reinforce such an approach?

If, by contrast, we want each new researcher to be given strict instructions on how to construe a theory, play with it 'correctly' and maintain/protect it, then we create an environment of expectation, anxiety and disengagement. We undermine independent thought and creativity. Ironically, one of the 'founding fathers' of achievement goals—John Nicholls (1989)—passionately argued this same point with regard to education. It was a founding principle of achievement goals research. Nicholls argued that instead we should treat each child, or in this case researcher, with tolerance, respect and unconditional support. It means permitting 'misconceptions' and 'confusions' because there is no objectively 'correct' way of construing and understanding the hypothetical construct of achievement goals—particularly when we consider the complex underlying phenomena that 'achievement goals' attempt to describe. Consider the following passages from Nicholls (1989):

> A 'scientific' orientation resists indoctrination and frees the individual from dependence on arbitrary external authority, but fosters an open-mindedness that is disciplined by observation and rational reflection and renewed by novel hypotheses... ...The progressive approach to education is based on the notion that development is most liberating and secure when students play an active role in the formulation of the questions they study. (p.166)
>
> When we reduce the concepts of education and inquiry to finding solutions for problems that textbooks or authorities pose, we become technocrats. When we [merely] stand ready to solve any problem we are presented

with, we have relinquished moral and political responsibility. When we encourage such a readiness in students, we cultivate the sort of person who would adopt the Nuremberg defense (p.167)

It is healthier for the scientist, and the interactions of the group, to assume that all our theories are wrong, and we are 'playing' by simply finding out how and why—so we can build better ones. Indeed, this approach represents the most cogent attempt to explain the history of advancements in science: replacing theories that are demonstrably wrong or unworkable with new ones that are less wrong and more readily operationalised. Hence, the outcome of permitting such pluralism and tolerating such diversity does not need to be 'anarchy': as might be the concern. Rather, if we can agree on ways of articulating coherent theories, deriving testable hypotheses and directly comparing each theory, progress is still possible. In this way, protecting the 'status' of a preferred theory (or author/researcher), or arguing over which is best, is comparable to becoming overly concerned about ego goals: one indicator of success, but a relatively unhelpful and unhealthy one. In fact, the approach being proposed here necessitates collaboration and co-operation, in exactly the way Nicholls might advocate. Researchers must work together to both express each theoretical framework, as our understanding evolves, and then to test them. Research does not have to be a 'winner takes all' competition. Such collaboration is evident if we look at the size of some authorship teams at the frontiers of particle physics (e.g. papers emanating from the CERN particle accelerator in Switzerland), genetics (Leung et al. [2015] included over 1000 authors) and medicine (e.g. large cancer trials and stem cell research). To turn a phrase, in cases such as these, the winner is science—not a specific theory or a specific researcher.

Diversity: Gender, Ethnicity, Disability and Culture

As noted in the introduction, there are also potential problems of discrimination and bias regarding gender, ethnicity, disability and culture. Such problems have been recognised to permeate society, and science, and there is no reason to expect that sport and exercise psychology would be significantly different. Nevertheless, the fact that these problems exist throughout Western societies and have a long history does not make them right: remember the earlier arguments that tradition and commonality are not indicators of correctness. In this instance, it is worth pausing to note that this issue is both one of objective truth and one of moral/ ethical correctness. Objectively, people who identify as any gender, any race and from any country are just as capable of contributing meaningfully to science, and in this case sport and exercise psychology. Diversity is defined as 'the degree of intra-organizational representation of people with different group affiliations of cultural significance' (Herdman & McMillan-Capehart, 2010, p. 40). Diversity in a group—of researchers, practitioners, athletes and so on—can serve as an important role in producing improved outcomes, by expanding of the plurality of workers' experiences and perspectives (Herdman & McMillan-Capehart, 2010). In fact, there is increasingly consistent evidence that when groups and team contain people from diverse backgrounds, *so long as this diversity is accepted and not resisted,* the group tends to perform better and generate stronger outcomes (Alesina & La Ferrara, 2005; Boone & Hendricks, 2008; Carter, D'Souza, Simkins & Simpson, 2010; Leslie, 2014; Pitts & Jarry, 2007; Umans, Collin & Tagesson, 2008). What that means is: if you find yourself conducting research or applied practice in a group of highly similar people, from similar backgrounds with similar training, you are likely to underperform and not even notice it. Does that sound like a paradigm, at all? Morally and ethically, people of any gender, race and location should be permitted to contribute to the debate, encouraged to, and rewarded equally for their efforts. Where structural barriers exist within systems and societies, those in power should proactively seek to remove and overcome them. That's the moral argument.

Despite the documented benefits of diversity in organisations, there are a number of barriers and challenges that limit progress (Fisher & Roper, 2015). Negative attitudes and discomfort towards people who are different, stereotypes, prejudice and bias have been found to greatly inhibit both diversity and its beneficial effects on performance/outcomes. Furthermore, organisations often form a hegemonic structure that serves to reinforce the cultural norms of the majority; for example, 'As organizations continue to adhere to various organizational practices, those behaviors become further embedded and perpetuated. Organizational members come to see those behaviors as the 'obvious' way to do things' (Cunningham, 2008, p. 137). Changing organisations to become more supportive of a diversity climate is likely to adversely affect the current dominant groups by altering the distribution of power and resources, and the dominant goals and values of the organisation (Cunningham, 2008). Thus, in a chapter about paradigms, self-reinforcing 'boys clubs' and their influence on sport and exercise psychology, we absolutely must consider the issue of diversity. Put simply, the strength of promoting diversity is to introduce different backgrounds, experiences, interpretive lenses and thus different ideas. Likewise, important ideas can be critiqued from additional perspectives that may not have even occurred to those 'within' the paradigm. According to the likes of Popper, this would be a good thing; it would lead to stronger and more thoroughly tested knowledge. From the perspective of a Kuhnian paradigm, the potential influence of diversity—new ideas, new perspectives, new and unanticipated criticisms—seems extremely threatening. Why would any Kuhnian paradigm ever embrace diversity within its researchers and practitioners?

Studies within westernised societies have been the norm for so long, much of the foundation knowledge within exercise and sport psychology reflects this. There is an increasingly acknowledged reliance of sport and exercise psychology on 'knowledge construction' prioritising the United States (and to a lesser extent, Northern Europe), Protestant, Caucasian, heterosexual, male, able-bodied experience (e.g. Bredemeier et al., 1991; Dewar & Horn, 1992; Duda & Allison, 1990; Duda & Hayashi, 1998; Fisher, Butryn, & Roper, 2003; Gill, 1994, 2001; Kamphoff, Gill, Araki, & Hammond, 2010; Krane, 1994; Martens, 1987; Martens, Mobley, & Zizzi, 2000; Naoi, Watson, Deaner, & Sato, 2011; Schinke & Hanrahan, 2009). Fisher and Roper (2015) quoted a former AASP president on this matter:

> There still remains a privileging of certain identities over others (e.g., male, White, heterosexual, able-bodied)… very few sport psychology researchers have critiqued sport psychology's own knowledge construction for its focus

on the United States, Protestant, Caucasian, heterosexual, male, able-bodied experience.

Rarely, it is argued that this has been a deliberate conspiracy to exclude other groups, but rather our field has unconsciously reproduced exclusionary stereotypes or practices—leading to a 'hegemony' that gives all the power and influence in our field to the male, able-bodied White Anglo-Saxon Protestants (WASPs—Fisher & Roper, 2015; Ryba, Schinke, & Tenenbaum, 2010; Schinke & Hanrahan, 2009; Schinke, McGannon, Parham, & Lane, 2012).

Steadily, however, the need for cross-cultural exercise and sport psychology has emerged and been acknowledged also by researchers (e.g. Blodgett, Schinke, McGannon & Fisher, 2015; Schinke, McGannon, Parham & Lane, 2012). For clarity, Ram, Starek and Johnson (2004) examined 982 manuscripts in the 3 leading sport psychology journals of the time: *Journal of Sport and Exercise Psychology* (JSEP), *Journal of Applied Sport Psychology* (JASP) and *The Sport Psychologist* (TSP). They found that 19.8 % of papers 'made reference' to race/ethnicity, but only 1.5 % adopted race/ethnicity as a substantive theoretical or empirical concept. They additionally examined sexual orientation and found that 1.2 % of papers 'made reference' to it, but only 4 papers (0.4 %) discussed sexual orientation as a substantive theoretical or empirical concept. Separately, Kamphoff, Gill, Araki and Hammond (2010) assessed the abstracts submitted to a prominent annual conference for sport psychology: the Association for Applied Sport Psychology. Of 5214 abstracts, 10.5 % made reference to cultural diversity in some way. Of this 10 %, over half was pertaining to gender, with 'almost no attention to race and ethnicity, nationality, sexual orientation, social class, disability or older adults' (p.231). Furthermore, their analysis suggested no significant changes in these ratios over time.

There is no reason to assume that findings generated using participants (mainly college students) from a straight, able-bodied WASP background will apply to people from completely different backgrounds, with their own rich and important heritages. Arguably, applying findings from Western, mostly white, and either US or Northern European groups to anybody else is extremely inappropriate. It might be appropriate to theoretically postulate some core psychological trait permeates all cultures, but you would absolutely have to test such an assumption before applying the findings from Westerners to people from elsewhere. To achieve this properly, we would need to properly engage with, even develop, researchers and practitioners in other cultures, countries and backgrounds. We would, furthermore, need to accept that this process will generate difficult questions regarding our theories and findings to date—and that is largely the fault of 'us' not those who have been excluded from the process for so long.

Exercise: On Privilege

If you're reading this, you're probably enjoying quite a few privileges that you may not even be aware of. You may even take what you have for granted: such is the nature of privilege.

It can be a hard thing to understand, even for adults. The following is a potential activity for the classroom, to be tried with students from high school through to university.

First, all the students received a piece of paper and crumpled it into a ball. Then, the recycling bin is placed in front of the classroom.

'You represent the country's population, and everyone has the chance to become wealthy and reach the upper class. All you must do is throw your paper balls into the bin while sitting in your seats.'

Of course, students in the back of the room had it worse than the ones in front, and complained about this unfairness. Everyone threw their ball and many (not all) students in the front made it, and only a few in the back made it, as expected.

'The closer you were to the recycling bin, the better your odds: this is privilege. Did you notice how the only ones who complained were in the back of the room?'

'But people in front of room were less likely to be aware of their privilege. They only saw 10 feet between them and their goal.'

From: http://www.boredpanda.com/lesson-about-privilege-awareness/

Gender

Most of our core textbooks offer information on the history of sport and exercise psychology offers, providing a general understanding of its past (Weinberg & Gould, 2015; Williams, 2001). Several analysis of this coverage have noticed an(other) important omission: these histories do not mention the roles women have played in the field's development. As Oglesby (2001) notes, 'awareness and appreciation of the women who were sport psychology pioneers is woefully lacking' (p. 375). Within the field of sport psychology, researchers have explored the career experiences of prominent professionals (Ploszay, 2003; Roper, Fisher, & Wrisberg, 2005; Statler, 2003; Simons & Andersen, 1995; Straub & Hinman, 1992). The majority of this research, however, has profiled the career experiences and perceptions of male professionals. Little attention has been directed towards the roles women have played in the development of the field. It was even suggested that female sport psychology consultants are not viewed as being as suitable for working in elite sport (Petrie, Cogan, Van Raale & Brewer, 1996; Yambor & Connelly, 1991)—even when coaches and athletes appeared to value such qualities as communication, counselling and trustworthiness and sometimes rated women higher on those skills. Straub and Hinman (1992) surveyed professionals in sport psychology and found that only one of ten of those identified as a 'leading sport psychologist' was female. Waite and Pettit (1993) found that men were paid 33 % more than females on average, even after accounting for career length and age. Roper, Fisher and Wrisberg (2005) focused on academic women in sport psychology, and made some interesting observations. In support of the above, one participant commented: 'So much of what we read, and our students read, is about our founding "father" and "grandfathers"; but we rarely learn about the mothers and grandmothers of our field'—note that we spoke of the 'father of American sport psychology' (Chap. 2). Likewise, it was noted that sport has historically been viewed as a macho world, dominated by males: 'Most of the work that is done in athletics is male-dominated and there is still a male jock mentality.' One of the more interesting points was that women may be more sensitive to ethi-

cal issues, and therefore benefit less from casually name-dropping the
famous athletes they worked for Table 6.1:

> So, I have never publicly said who I work with. Most of my male colleagues
> think of themselves as coaches, and they don't have a second thought about
> saying, "oh yea, I've been working with [name of high profile athlete]" or
> whoever it happens to be. So, it created a different sense of public acknowl-
> edgment I think of who people are working with, and I think that was
> partially because the women athletes were also less open to say publicly—
> "I'm working with a sport psychologist".

Typically, sport and exercise psychology has failed to recognise and promote the contribution—concrete and/or potential—that women make
to the field. Even now, despite typically training high proportions of
women to PhD level and beyond, the editorial boards of our leading
journals are largely male dominated, with 69 % males and 74 % male
at the editorial/associate editor level (see Table 6.1). Of course, there is
nothing inherently better about males that makes them more suitable for
refereeing and editing journal papers, so we do need to question this situation, while not necessarily blaming those at the helm: the issues are systemic. As discussed above, the issue is largely insidious, unconscious and
not a deliberate 'conspiracy'. Every so often, however, people do seem to
assimilate the values of the system they inhabit, and the ugliness inherent
in the system is explicitly expressed. Consider the following example, fortunately from an area outside of sport and exercise psychology (remember the questionable reviewer comments we raised earlier). In May 2015,
a reviewer for the journal *PlosOne* provided the following comment to

Table 6.1 Composition of editorial boards of main four sport and exercise
psychology journals (May 2016)

Journal	Editor	Associate eds.	Board
JSEP	Male	3M, 2F	29M, 8F
PSE	Male × 2	7M, 4F	28M, 12F
JASP	Male	5M, 2F	16M, 13F
TSP	Male	5M, 1F	21M, 12F
TOTAL	5 male	20 male, 9 female	94 male, 45 female

authors of a manuscript: 'It would probably also be beneficial to find one or two male biologists to work with (or at least receive internal peer review from, but better yet as active co-authors), in order to serve as a possible check against interpretations that may sometimes be drifting too far away from empirical evidence into ideologically based assumptions.' The rest of the review contained further sexist claims. Is it possible that certain influential figures within each scientific field presume males to be more objective, more hard-working, more productive and so on and make important decisions based on this assumption? Is it possible that women in a scientific field could perceive this bias, and unfairness, and be upset, disillusioned and angered by it? Roper et al.'s (2005) interviews certainly suggest that it can be perceived, understood and articulated for discussion. Two of the participants on Roper et al.'s study explicitly recognised this bias and rejected it, clearly expressing that they had more to offer academia than publications, citations and grants:

> I don't think of those things… and the reason I don't is that I fear that when one starts to think about those things like status and prestige and how many publications you have, that may lead to losing sight of why I got into this in the first place.

To a large extent in modern academia, deliberately rejecting publications, citations and grants as worthwhile pursuits would be 'career suicide'. Universities are measured on these things, and therefore academics are measured on these things. No 'points' in these columns can mean no job. But universities and academia do have a higher purpose, and it takes a different voice—in this instance, a female voice—to recognise and question that hegemony.

Overall, there are important considerations around gender equality, and important contributions being overlooked by not proactively ensuring that people of all genders are incorporated in the research, practice and discussion of sport and exercise psychology. The above section describes a problem, and its consequences, that urgently need to be overcome. Even if there is no immediately fault that can be ascribed to one person or group for this situation occurring, once you know about the problem doing nothing to fix it makes you complicit.

'Toughen up princess'

By: Richard Keegan

In recent years, there has been a proliferation of training courses and workshops promoting mental toughness, resilience and stress-management. As an academic teaching a course in resilience, I recently attended such a workshop.

Resilience, according to the definitions I was teaching, is a property of dynamic systems—meaning the individual is only part of that system. It is an ongoing process, not a stable trait/attribute.

I was disappointed then, to sit in a room full of eager people being told: 'Here are some skills and techniques you can use to cope with stress.' The entire workshop was focusing on what the individual can do differently when the system places them in difficult circumstances—for example, excessive workloads, workplace tensions and bullying, inappropriate work expectations and so on.

'If the system demands this of you and you cannot deliver it, you are failing.'

I politely put my hand up, and waited to ask my question.

'Theoretically, resilience is a dynamic process, emerging from a complex system. The whole workshop so far has given advice to individuals. I wondered what advice you give organisations to promote resilience?'

The answer:

'I don't believe in that.'

Translation: The system or organisation can demand whatever it damn well likes of you, and if you do not deliver it, you will be deemed to fail. Do not question the system. If there is a problem, it is you. You are the problem.

It turns out this is a relatively well-recognised criticism of workplace training programs seeking to promote toughness, and address 'stress'. They focus on the individual and do nothing whatsoever to address the systemic issues and imbalances that cause the stress. Actually, the core message I heard being presented was: 'Toughen up, princess'.

Obviously, I found it totally inappropriate.

Then I realised something.

This is what sport psychology has done for over 30 years.

'High performance sport demands a lot of you. If you cannot deliver it, you will have failed. High performance sport organisations can demand whatever it damn well likes of you and you must achieve it or else be deemed a failure. Do not question the system you are in. If there is a problem, it is you.... Luckily here are some skills and techniques you can deploy to help, and again, if they don't work it's on you. Toughen up princess.'

Not only that, but when sport systems heavily disadvantage non-White, non-male, non-Anglo-Saxon, disabled groups, we attempt to offer such

> individually focused 'toughening up' techniques based on White, Anglo-Saxon, male-dominated and able-bodied research. We are letting people down at both levels. The systems are often inappropriate, and our attempts to help are made of the same 'stuff' as that system.
>
> As an example, if a female, gay, indigenous, disabled athlete was pursuing her dream to race in the Paralympics but was experiencing difficulties due to only being offered an 'old school', male coach who has only worked with able-bodied athletes before.... would we really offer the same hackneyed advice from our core textbooks to 'breathe' and 'think positive'? Would we really simply tell her to 'toughen up'? *Sorry about your disadvantaged background, but still... if you fail to make it, the failure is on you....*

Disability

Finally, there is the issue of disability, which has received increasing research attention in recent years. Historically, however, both researchers and practitioners pursued either elite athletes (particularly practitioners), or highly generalisable findings (particularly researchers). It took a little too long, perhaps, for sport and exercise psychology to pay genuine attention to those seeking to participate differently—and there are perhaps reasons for this. Alongside the narrative that sport psychology, in particular, has tended to focus on elite sport—which may itself exclude a range of disabled athletes—people with disabilities are extremely diverse, pursuing extremely diverse goals. Hanrahan (2014) noted the ways that typical mental skills training had to be adapted for athletes with disabilities, and alluded to the requirement to adapt and respond. Fundamentally, every instance of disability can be quite different to the next, even if the same label or diagnosis is given. This has been the source of continuing controversy in Paralympic sports, where some athletes appear to gain significantly by having their 'classification' changed—that is, typically, they are moved into a category of more advanced impairment, gaining an advantage over any competition in that category who is genuinely more impaired. Even if one somehow ignores the significant political manoeuvring around this core issue, the variability in disabilities can place a significant demand on sport and exercise psychologists for (at least) three reasons: (a) little or none of our theories, findings and interventions have been generated in relation to this specific person's impairment, so we are having to adapt knowledge from the outset—not simply execute something that is well established; (b) almost none of the measures and needs analysis processes developed in sport and exercise psychology (notwithstanding the above critique of these) have been designed for a specific type of disability or impairment. Some such measures would simply break, or require 'revalidation' if they were to be adapted, so they become un-usable. The researcher or practitioner in this instance simply loses one of their favourite and most dependable tools; (c) communication, training and monitoring can also be different depending on the type of impairment, and this can be challenging to researchers and practitioners who have not been trained to adapt their style and systems accordingly.

Basically, anyone indoctrinated into following a specific approach (or methodology, or treatment model) and pursuing validity/reliability could be extremely uncomfortable in such a situation. There is an added layer of difficulty when it comes to ethics too. Certain types of disability may affect one's ability to give informed consent, and to stay across each ethical decision as applied service delivery or research projects develop. Ethics committees, professional regulators and supervisors/assessors all expect specific processes and considerations to be made, in advance, before undertaking work with people who may be considered vulnerable adults. Furthermore, certain type of disability affects an athlete's ability to perform certain classic mental skills—for example, blind athletes experience mental imagery very differently to others, and how would self-talk be experienced by somebody who was born deaf?

What might be the consequences of failing to properly represent people with disability in research, practice and in our ranks as academics and practitioners (e.g. a recent study in the UK reported that 80 out of 2460 academics in Sport Science and Leisure Studies reported some type of disability—3.2 %—Equality Challenge Unit 2015)?

If we avoid supporting those with disability, for example because measurement tools or particular intervention techniques are not readily compatible with the group or individual's disability, we are failing. We are either joining the long list of services, places and opportunities to which access has been denied, or we are creating an expectation and desire for a service that we cannot (or will not) deliver. Obviously that's unacceptable. If we fail to research key issues affecting people with disabilities as they participate in sport and exercise, then the above problem is exacerbated. Not only are we preventing ourselves, as a field, from being able to help people with disabilities, but we are failing to design approaches, measures, theories and knowledge of how to even try and help. We are effectively refusing to even try and help.

Furthermore, if we are failing to adequately study the psychological worlds of those attempting to participate in sport and exercise while experiencing disabilities, we are missing the opportunity to develop our approaches, methodologies, theories and knowledge in new and important ways. If an approach can be adapted to support someone with a disability, then that is potentially interesting and informative (even if n=1, it is still valuable knowledge). If a suite of approaches, or an entire theory for example, were to be unsuitable for helping an athlete with a disability then that would be extremely valuable knowledge. Knowing how the approach/theory fails and what may facilitate important improvements or revisions to the theory, equates to a new and better understanding.

Perhaps, worst of all, if and when our field fails to support, research or work with people experiencing disabilities, we are in breach of our own ethical codes. For example, the AASP code of ethics prescribes that members should: 'actively promote human diversity in research. Examples include studying diverse populations (e.g. ethnicity, sexual orientation, & disability)'. Of course it can be difficult—for the reasons discussed above—to adequately research, support and engage with disability athletes, but it is a moral and ethical imperative. Furthermore, following the same arguments that diversity strengthens teams and organisations by providing new ideas and different perspectives, properly engaging with disability athletes forces the field of sport and exercise psychology to expand its horizons—its methods, theories, practices and knowledge— and thus benefits the field itself. In response to any argument that it is too difficult, we must collectively respond that everything worth doing is difficult. The more important and worthwhile, the more difficult in many cases. But the investment is worthwhile, both morally and for the benefit of our field.

Conclusion

This chapter has provided an overview of how issues of norms, stereotypes and dogma play out in sport and exercise psychology—sometimes with documented evidence, sometimes with anecdotal evidence and sometimes observing the issues in the wider literature and inferring that they are very likely to affect our field too. We have spanned both the issues of research ideas, topics and paradigms, and linked that to the potential interplay with issues of diversity: ethnicity, gender, disability and more. We have signposted how particular processes can both select which ideas are considered 'valid' and 'worthy', and also exclude people from a range of backgrounds who could be contributing meaningfully to our discipline. It should be quite clear, following this review, that there are many opportunities to advance sport and exercise psychology by rethinking our approach. Rethinking the ways we evaluate ideas, theories and methods. Rethinking the way we interact with our colleagues already in the field, and substantially rethinking the way we interact with people and groups we currently exclude. In fact, if this chapter has not prompted at least some reflection, self-awareness and introspection, it has clearly failed. For the main part, the arguments detailed above apply across all human societies, all of science, or—where it has been studied—specifically in sport and exercise psychology. So in answer to the question, 'are we likely to be better than, or different to, these other settings, and immune to the problems discussed?': on balance, the answer must be 'highly unlikely'. Failing to recognise and respond to these issues is consequential: proving detrimental to the athletes, coaches and practitioners we seek to help as well as to people within the field, as well as to our knowledge, measures, theories and evidence. We must proactively address these issues. If ignorance is considered a potential defence by some people: well now you know. What is seen, here in this chapter, cannot be unseen. Quite the opposite for most people: once you become aware of these issues, you see them everywhere.

7

Measuring Constructs

One of the many consequences from the work of Weber, Fechner and Stevens (Chap. 2), together with repeated calls that social sciences should mimic natural sciences (e.g. Mill; Chap. 5), is that measurements are still a core feature of much sport and exercise psychology research. One prevailing belief—at least in some camps—seems to be that 'real sciences' do by default *measure* variables. Preferably, these measurements are performed in experimental settings where researchers can manipulate and control the independent variable(s) and determine if the intervention(s) has a statistically significant effect on the dependent variable(s). If pre- and post-scores are sufficiently different, the conclusion is that the experimental manipulation was successful, because the observed difference turned out to be statistically significant. The latter rests on the assumption that the methods chosen to (a) measure and (b) analyse the construct in focus are both reliable and valid. But before anything can be measured, it needs to be operationalised. We will therefore first discuss how constructs are operationalised, followed by reliability and validity issues.

© The Author(s) 2016
P. Hassmén et al., *Rethinking Sport and Exercise Psychology Research*,
DOI 10.1057/978-1-137-48338-6_7

In sport and exercise psychology research, a measuring device is often a rating scale or standardised inventory. Although commonly employed, they also suffer from some weaknesses—some of these they share with any type of measurement device, as expressed by a Nobel Prize winner (1932, in Physics):

> Since the measuring device has been constructed by the observer.....we have to remember that what we observe is not nature in itself but nature exposed to our method of questioning (Heisenberg, 1958, p. 25).

Operationalisation

Before any construct can be measured, it must be translated into quantifiable variables. Consider, for example, *physical activity*, which has been defined as 'any bodily movement produced by skeletal muscle that results in caloric expenditure' (Caspersen, 1989, p. 424). Is this definition sufficient to make it measurable? And then use this measurement to, for example, compare men with women, or athletes with sedentary people? Probably not, although we may be able to distinguish between individuals who do nothing (no bodily movement) and those who do something, thereby expending some calories, but it is difficult to make any fine-graded distinctions. For that we need more information. The word 'caloric expenditure' may offer a starting point—but how to measure it?

An exercise physiologist may suggest indirect calorimetry, which is measuring heat generated when a person exercises and uses oxygen and expels carbon dioxide as a waste product. Doubly labelled water is another option (Shephard & Aoyagi, 2012). Both methods are complicated and not suitable for quick measurements of energy expenditure in the field. This is the reason that accelerometers, pedometers, heart rate monitors and so on often are used to *estimate* energy expenditure as they help to distinguish between different levels of 'bodily movement produced by skeletal muscle'. The latter tools offer indirect measurements, that is, steps or heart rates are used to estimate how much energy the person is expending. And as with all estimations, both random and systematic errors will affect the precision of the estimations.

From the literature (e.g. Welk, 2002), we know that frequency is an important variable (how often the person is physically active) and also that intensity (higher intensity requires more energy) and duration (longer time requires more energy) provide important information. And more advanced accelerometers, pedometers and heart rate monitors will incorporate this information. Further, to know the type (mode) of physical activity will also help in determining energy expenditure (running requires more energy than cycling at the same velocity, at least on a level surface) and where the exercise is performed (environment, e.g. outdoors as compared to indoors in a lab).

Frequency, duration, mode and environment can also be ascertained by simply asking the person; alternatively by using a standardised questionnaire (e.g. International Physical Activity Questionnaire (IPAQ); www.ipaq.ki.se) or through a regularly kept exercise diary. Of course the difference between objective measures of physical activity and self-reported estimations remain a problem; self-reported figures often overestimate the actually performed activity (e.g. Lee, Macfarlane, Lam, & Stewart, 2011).

Intensity is more challenging, but with a reliable heart rate monitor or any of the newer apps available on smart phones, this information can also be gained. A sport and exercise psychology researcher will most likely also be interested in adding a perceptual measure of intensity, for example, in the form of ratings of perceived exertion: the RPE-scale by Borg (1970). The total amount of information makes it possible to compare the level of bodily movement between individuals with a reasonable degree of accuracy and repeatability. Although the suggestion to include a perceptual measure of perceived exertion is not uncontroversial, because: what is perceived exertion? And how is this construct operationalised?

Numerous researchers have voiced these questions ever since the Swedish Psychologist Gunnar Borg, notably in his doctoral dissertation from 1962, described this new construct. A related discussion emerged questioning Borg's (1978) suggestion that the 15-point RPE-scale, ranging between 6 and 20, for all practical purpose could be regarded as an interval scale (e.g. Gamberale, 1985). A property of interval scales is equal intervals between steps; otherwise it is merely an ordinal scale (Stevens, 1946). If the RPE-scale is regarded as an ordinal scale, then non-parametric statistics (statistics not assuming normally distributed data, etc.) is the only viable alternative. Few researchers seem to use non-parametric statistical methods; instead parametric statistical methods are often used, most likely following the reasoning by Graziano and Raulin (2010) that the RPE-scale is closer to being an interval than an ordinal scale. A single argument, however, cannot to be taken as proof that such a strategy is correct, at least not from a purely mathematical point of view. It merely shows that the majority of researchers using the scale have reached some level of *consensus*, or that a certain praxis has evolved over the years. Thus, it may simply be that the use and interpretation of RPE has become a paradigm, of sorts.

The RPE-construct itself is another issue; disagreement seems to prevail and even increase, and with that suggestions how to define and operationalise perceived exertion. Or should the term be perceived effort? The latter is a suggestion made by Razon, Hutchinson and Tenenbaum (2012) who uses perceived effort instead of perceived exertion: 'as it is believed to be a better term to describe an array of related perceptions, of which exertion is only one' (p. 265). It is outside the scope of this chapter to completely discuss all arguments put forward by Razon and colleagues; however, this appears to be an excellent example when one term is argued to be better than another simply because the researchers have a preference for one or the other. Anyone interested in semantics are encouraged to compare how various dictionaries define exertion versus effort (one example: 'exertion *noun* (effort) the use of a lot of mental or physical effort'; http://dictionary.cambridge.org). As a side note, both exertion and effort are translated into Swedish using the same term ('ansträngning'), which also happens to be the Swedish term Borg selected before a translation into English was ever made. Semantically, the difference is thereby small. Theoretically, however, a person might exert effort and subsequently perceives exertion from that—thereby arguing for a timeline where the effort precedes the exertion perceived; the opposite is of course also possible to argue. So depending on the researchers' frame of mind, operational definitions can become muddled and progress halted— unless the term in itself is actually more important than the construct? Or is this bordering to semantic idolatry (cf. methodolatry, a term we will discuss later in this chapter)? This is not our way of saying that semantics are unimportant; we merely question whether some researchers are keener on discussing the colour of the target than actually defining what the target is. Razon et al. (2012) reiterates what Noble and Noble stated in 1998:

Emphasis should be placed on understanding perception, not on studying the results of the Borg scale. Until that is done, the study of perceptual response during physical activity will reflect only what the Borg scale measures. (p. 356)

This is an interesting statement because this would seem to apply to most instruments. When researchers operationalise a construct—such as perceived exertion—they create a variable that can be used to quantify the construct. To measure perceived exertion, Borg created the ratings of perceived exertion scale (RPE-scale, or Borg scale for short). Borg did not claim to measure perceptual responses (or perceived effort), merely a construct he chose to label perceived exertion. To measure perceived effort, there seems to be a need for a new scale (preferably labelled RPES [ratings of perceived effort scale], to differentiate it from the RPE-scale).

The criticism voiced above is of course equally valid when considering burnout, mood states or achievement goals (or any other construct). Because these constructs have been operationalised and made measurable by such instruments as Maslach's Burnout Inventory (MBI; Maslach & Jackson, 1981), the Profile of Mood States (POMS; McNair, Lorr, & Droppleman, 1971/1992) and the Task and Ego Orientation in Sport Questionnaire (TEOSQ; Duda & Nicholls, 1992). To paraphrase Noble and Noble (1998), we should try to understand burnout, mood states and achievement goals before we try to measure these constructs; something that inevitable will include qualitative methods. We will return and discuss the MBI, POMS and TEOSQ later in this chapter, as examples of instruments that have both strengths and weaknesses, but first reliability and validity.

Reliability and Validity

Of the two options, it is relatively easier to determine whether a measure is reliable than to establish its validity. Although having said that, it is worth noting the word 'relatively'. Because neither reliability nor validity are terms that relate to only one thing, they are better regarded as umbrella terms, each with subdivisions and inherent complexities.

On the surface, the basic difference between reliability and validity is easy to grasp. Reliability deals with the question: how consistent (or reproducible) are measurements? Validity instead deals with the question: 'are we really measuring what we believe we are measuring?' Using an analogy from sport, an expert archer aims to reliably put the arrows in the centre of the intended target every time. A less reliable archer would spread the arrows, and even at times hit other targets than the intended one. We can assume that the first one would be more successful in competitions than the second one, and the same would apply to researchers and test-constructors within their field of expertise. Creating and/ or using instruments or psychological tests that produce very different scores over time—even when no changes have occurred—would not instil confidence that the results obtained are trustworthy. This explains why every textbook covering quantitative research methods devote much space to discuss reliability and validity; this also includes the *Standards* (Standards for Educational and Psychological Testing, 2014).

Reliability

In the *Standards*, the term used is 'reliability/precision' instead of merely reliability, this 'to denote the more general notion of consistency of the scores across instances of the testing procedure, and the term *reliability coefficient* to refer to the reliability coefficients of classical test theory' (p. 33). Reliability in sport and exercise psychology is often estimated by interclass or intraclass reliability, which relate to precision, stability and consistency of the test scores. Because that is basically what we are talking about: how precise, stable and consistent are the test scores? This can then be divided into stability of test scores over time (interclass), and consistency of test scores at the same time (intraclass). Administering a test twice (test-retest) and calculating the correlation between trials give an indication of stability: a high product-moment correlation coefficient is preferable to a lower one. Provided that an athlete's motivation has not changed between administrations, her/his scores should also remain the same. If they are not the same (or at least very similar), and this is a recurrent finding when other athletes' level of motivation is assessed repeatedly, the scale will not be deemed stable, or reliable—the measurement is said to lack consistency. Note that a test-retest coefficient can be very high when systematic errors exist. Variables that are prone to be inflated by social desirability may therefore produce high test-retest correlations, yet be far from a true reflection of what the researchers are trying to measure. Similarly, if the instrument used is not sufficiently sensitive to changes, the test-retest correlation between the scores may be significant but the informational value from them considerably less so.

Furthermore, many inventories used in sport and exercise psychology include subscales with several items each, supposedly measuring the same (sub)construct. The stability or consistency of scores within the subscales is consequently of interest. Cronbach's alpha (1951) is often used to establish whether all items tap into the same construct; α-coefficients $\geq$ 0.70 are deemed acceptable, a level dating back to Nunnally (1978). That most studies using an established instrument or test report Cronbach's alphas over .7 is not surprising. Because during the development process, each item with a lower correlation (<.70) to the other items (item-total) are most likely omitted or revised until the alpha-values are deemed satisfactory by the test constructor. This iterative process is aimed to increase the precision, but it only enhances the consistency of the instrument; it does not help us determine if we are actually measuring the intended construct or not—we may in fact consistently miss it. Neither can the alpha-value reveal if the construct is too narrowly defined, which later will be discussed in terms of construct underrepresentation.

Avoiding construct underrepresentation may, however, be detrimental to a high alpha-value as this value only indicates consistency of scores, not representativeness (Panayides, 2013). In fact, a low alpha-value may be a positive thing and indicate that a construct is broadly covered instead of narrowly, but researchers seldom discuss this alternative explanation. They are much more likely to dismiss the results and blame the instrument for being unreliable and inconsistent in the way it measures a construct. But if the construct is broad, a very narrow definition may produce consistently high alpha-values, yet at the price of merely tapping into a small part of the entire construct. This is but one example when the tool—the statistical calculation of a correlation—is at risk of becoming more important than the underlying message. Which indeed may be that we are on target; it is just that the construct is multi-faceted—but not multidimensional to warrant separate subscales.

Precision can also be discussed in terms of how close scores obtained on a test or inventory are to their respective true value—although this is actually impossible to determine. We nevertheless assume that there is indeed a true score—or more accurately a true level on whatever we are trying to measure. But as can be inferred from the quote at the beginning of this chapter, it is never 'nature itself' (or the true level of something) that we observe, merely a score influenced by the way the construct has been operationalised to make it measurable. It is of course assumed that a highly precise instrument will offer a score that is *close* to the true level (which is still unknown), and that the instrument will reliably produce the same score every time, provided that nothing has changed (test-retest) with a sufficiently high degree of internal consistency (e.g. measured by Cronbach's alpha).

Validity

In contrast to reliability and the precision of the scores obtained by measuring something, validity concerns whether we are really measuring what we believe we are measuring. Or phrased differently: do the test scores truthfully reflect the construct that they are intended to measure? And if so, do the test scores reflect the whole construct or only a minor part of it (construct underrepresentation)? If the aim is to measure motivation for physical activity, then a valid scale or instrument will do exactly that, and not measure something else (such as how confident a person is of becoming physically active). So a construct needs to be sufficiently covered, yet not 'spill over' into other domains.

As with many constructs in science, also the definitions pertaining to validity has changed over time. The earlier view was that construct validity was merely one type related to the test (inventory, instrument), along with related but largely independent types such as face, predictive, convergent, discriminant and content validity (Vaughn & Daniel, 2012). So when researchers discussed whether their instruments/tests were valid or not, they first discussed one type, then another and so on. Rarely did they discuss if, and if so how, the different types of validity were interrelated.

Nowadays, construct validity is regarded as the core attribute related to the test scores (not the test itself), surrounded by a number of interrelated facets or sources. In the words of the *Standards*: 'Validity is a unitary concept. It is the degree to which all the accumulated evidence supports the intended interpretation of test scores for the proposed use' (Standards for Educational and Psychological Testing, 2014, p. 14). So instead of discussing different attributes (or types) of validity, researchers are evaluating 'sources of validity evidence' (p. 13). These sources are grounded in the test content, response processes, internal structure, relations to other variables and the consequences of testing; these 'strands of evidence' are then integrated to thoroughly evaluate construct validity.

Much research in sport and exercise psychology still relies on standardised inventories, often presented online with the participants answering a considerable number of items with test scores subsequently subjected to statistical analysis. This type of cross-sectional collection of data rarely lends itself to causal interpretations, that is, it is difficult to ascertain if changes in the independent variable causes a change in the scores of the assumedly dependent variable—the scores of two variables are merely found to correlate. In validity terms, this would be considered to be a study with low internal validity. With an experimental design—including manipulation of the independent variable, a control group and random assignment of participants to the different treatments—it becomes possible to determine whether changes made to one variable indeed change another. This translates to high internal validity, which researchers for obvious reasons prefer.

The most important reason that not all studies are conducted in laboratory settings, using randomised control designs, is external validity. A researcher interested in performance anxiety can of course devise a challenging task, which the athletes then perform in the laboratory. If the level of challenge is manipulated, then it becomes possible to see whether more difficulty translates to more anxiety. The problem is that something studied in a laboratory, such as athletes' anxiety prior to or during a challenging task, is bound to differ compared to studying performance anxiety prior to or during a real world competition. It therefore becomes very difficult to generalise from the laboratory results to the field, and in validity terms, this means that the external validity is low.

Another factor besides the environment that also impacts external validity is the people involved; many studies in psychology are still conducted with undergraduate students as participants. Which makes sense from one perspective; they are easily approached if their teachers are also the researchers. Some departments and schools of psychology still require their students to participate in studies, in exchange for study credits, claiming also that the experience is beneficial to the students. A major problem exists if the researchers are interested in generalising their results to other populations than undergraduate students of psychology. Whereas the external validity may be high if the sample of students is used to draw conclusions about the population of undergraduate psychology students, it will most likely be very low to non-existent for other populations. Despite this, studies are still published where the people (cultures, etc.), situations (e.g. environment) and/or times (past/future) are not representative for the intended purpose and population; any conclusions reached by the researchers are consequently flawed. This is an increasing problem in science. One reason being that Honours and Master students are nowadays encouraged to not only write a thesis but also to publish their findings together with their supervisors in peer-reviewed journals. This trend is encouraged by a publishing culture in which academic staff needs to publish regularly to retain their continuing employment status (see Chaps. 5 and 6 for a more extensive discussion). When students collect their empirical data with the help of their fellow students, an increasing number of publications are inevitable based on young university students, while conclusions often are drawn outside of this rather limited population (e.g. results from university students being used to explain sedentary behaviour in the general population). The fact that external validity is threatened is rarely acknowledged.

Statistics

When data are analysed, the old saying 'garbage in produces garbage out' is worth remembering (Kass et al., 2016). That is exactly why operationalisation, reliability and validity are such important concepts to consider as soon as any form of measurement is involved. Regardless of how data is acquired, it needs to be of sufficiently high quality to be usable in statistical analyses. Because ultimately, the data is collected for one purpose only: to answer scientific questions (cf. Kass et al., 2016). In the next section, we will discuss psychometrics and cross-sectional questionnaire data, but first some additional statistical issues.

One such issue, albeit rarely discussed, is how sample size affect statistical results. This is exemplified in an article by Zhu (2012) entitled *Sadly, the earth is still round (p < 0.05)*. Zhu found that the correlation coefficient between 14 pairs was 0.178, with a p-value of 0.544. Zhu then copied this dataset, and pasted it into one data file, adding it 8 times ($n = 126$). He then calculated the correlation coefficient again and found it to remain the same (0.178). The p-value, however, decreased to 0.047 and thereby suddenly became statistically significant (i.e. $p <$ .05). This simple example shows that numbers matter, and that more observations make it easier to find significant correlations (or differences, if other statistical tests are used). The recommendation from Zhu is therefore to 'NEVER draw a conclusion merely based on a p value' and to always when possible report effect sizes (p. 10). This statement receives support from the Board of Directors of the American Statistical Association (2016):

> Good statistical practice, as an essential component of good scientific practise, emphasizes principles of good study design and conduct, a variety of numerical and graphical summaries of data, understanding of the phenomenon under study, interpretation of results in context, complete reporting and proper logical and quantitative understanding of what data summaries mean. No single index should substitute for scientific reasoning.

Despite repeated calls to abandon psychology's dirty little secret (Bakan, 1966), the belief prevails that the p-value is an accurate reflection of the risk that the result obtained is due to chance (Lambdin, 2012). The more advanced the statistical toolbox becomes, the easier it is to also forget that everything originates somewhere; a self-report questionnaire is always a self-report questionnaire regardless of whether the differences observed are subjected to simple t-tests or advanced multidimensional analyses.

At the same time, why should researchers change a winning concept? Science has been doing just fine for a long time, right? This may explain the stubbornness that prevails in science to continue using and reusing the same methods, designs, procedures and instruments, because we know what we have but not what may come if we change. There are numerous examples in sport and exercise psychology where theories that once were fresh and innovative are now still defended and promoted as valid, and the methods to 'prove' their continuing validity are more tailored to the theory than to the underlying question, see also Chap. 6. Self-report questionnaires are often used in sport and exercise psychology research, and the responses given on Likert-type scales, that subsequently are subjected to statistical analyses—this is not an uncontroversial practice.

Likert-Type Scales

These scales, named after their inventor the American organisational psychologist Rensis Likert, can at best be regarded to generate interval data—although statisticians more often consider them merely to produce ordinal data. The number of steps can vary from three upward; five- and seven-step scales are probably the most used ones. A common property is the uneven number, with the middle one often labelled 'Neither agree nor disagree' (= 3 on a five-point scale) and with lower numbers anchored with labels such as 'Strongly disagree' (=1) and 'Disagree' (=2), and higher numbers with 'Agree' (=4) and 'Strongly agree' (=5), respectively

Likert-type scales are often used to help quantify how much there is 'of something'. For example, an exercise psychologist who is interested in measuring how motivated people are to perform regular physical activity creates a number of items that hopefully taps into this construct (a validity issue). The respondents are asked how much they agree with the item-statements using a five-step Likert-type scale. While our exercise psychologist may think about scale levels, maybe even questioning whether equal distances exist between steps (is the difference between 1 and 2 the same as between 4 and 5?), praxis within the field nevertheless seems to treat this type of scale as possessing interval scale qualities. The reasoning behind this—conveniently disregarding the lack of equal intervals—is often similar to the one offered by Graziano and Raulin (2010): 'Most test scores are not true interval scales, but by convention, we treat them as interval scales, because they are closer to being interval scales than ordinal scales' (p. 73). A statistician would probably also highlight the lack of a true zero and the need because of this to use non-parametric statistical methods when evaluating differences obtained on this scale that in reality only qualify as an ordinal scale.

Our exercise psychology researcher does not agree, supported by the majority of researchers who considers Likert-type scales to 'approximate interval scales'; our researcher is therefore happy to use parametric statistical methods. The lack of a true zero is less of a problem than the lack of equal intervals between scores on the scale, at least from a purely statistical sense. This is an example of a pragmatic approach to research, as was discussed in Chap. 5.

Psychometrics and Cross-Sectional Questionnaire Data

The increasingly recognised (over) reliance on psychometric questionnaires, often deployed in simple cross sectional studies, has become widely accepted as normal practice in sport and exercise psychology. Ostensibly, there are a number of reasons why this approach is popular. The following section will explore some of these reasons and discuss whether self-report questionnaires truly are the most appropriate, and whether they deserve such a large proportion of journal space and research effort. To begin with the positives: (a) as the name implies, psychometric questionnaires generate numbers, and further still, these numbers can be used to calculate types of 'reliability' and 'validity'—albeit referenced against accepted norms in a statistics book, and not always something a coach or athlete would consider 'valid'. The provision of numeric ratio data, decimal places and all, and indications of reliability/validity serve an important psychological purpose (for the researchers) in alleviating the 'crisis of legitimation' (Martens, 1987; Smith & Sparkes, 2009). One could question, of course, whether modelling abstract linear functions in multidimensional imaginary space is the ideal way of doing science, but for many this has become the accepted norm; (b) questionnaires are incredibly convenient ways of gathering data, especially about psychological and social psychological phenomena. Even before the advent of the Internet, one could simply post a large number of questionnaires together with pre-paid envelopes and get a large number returned—sufficient to run a basic statistical analysis on. And better still—for those researchers who teach at universities—it was possible to simply stroll into a lecture theatre full of undergraduate students and ask them to complete the survey before the lecture begins. Boom: $n = 200$ straight away! When it became possible to post questionnaires on websites, it became even cheaper and easier, and one could simply email invitations to people for free. Most researchers are busy in their academic roles, with a large proportion of their time devoted to teaching, meetings, committees, administration and more. Hence, if questionnaires can be easily distributed and returned with 'reliable' and 'valid' data while you do other work, why would you do anything else? (c) Everyone else is doing it—or at least it can seem that way sometimes. Andersen, McCullagh and Wilson (2007) reviewed the publications in the three leading sport psychology journals during 2005, finding 85 papers of which 49 relied on 'arbitrary psychometrics' (25 used only these 'arbitrary' measures, and a further 24 combining psychometrics with objectively observed data). A further four papers reported on the development of new questionnaires. Thus, on one side of the argument, there is safety in numbers: reassurance from being part of the current trend; feeling at the forefront; and likely receiving peer reviews from others who are using the same methods. Another way of looking at it is this: if you are not benefitting from the quantitative numerical data and speed/convenience of psychometric questionnaires, you will be left behind by your peers who are pursuing this line of research. They will publish more papers than you, cite each other (lots) and receive tenure, contracts, grants and accolades, while you will be either (a) an unemployed academic or (b) an employed non-academic. At this moment in the development of sport and exercise psychology, if a researcher is not—at least occasionally—deploying psychometric questionnaires in their research... well... how can we say this? *They may find themselves under significant pressure to do so.*

So what is the harm in that? What is wrong with doing what everyone else does, forming a little club, and all mutually agreeing to support each other in this venture? It turns out, researchers in psychology have been criticising this measurement tradition for some time. Michell (2000: p. 639) argued simply that: 'psychometrics is a pathology of science'. Noticing the same 'safety in numbers' argument detailed above, he also opened with the following quote 'There is no safety in numbers, or in anything else' (Thurber, 1939). In arguing the case, Michell reasoned that: 'in a pathology of science not only is some hypothesis accepted within the mainstream of a discipline without a serious attempt to test it, but that fact is not acknowledged or, in extreme cases, is disguised (p. 641)... in psychometrics we have a situation in which: (a) a basic, empirical hypothesis (namely the hypothesis that psychological attributes are quantitative) is accepted as true without it ever having been seriously tested for its empirical adequacy, and (b) the fact that this hypothesis has never been satisfactorily tested is disguised' (p. 650). By disguised here, Michell is arguably implying that potential problems with psychometrics are not acknowledged or spoken about and—quite the opposite— that psychometrics is presented as the gold standard: excellent, valid and inherently robust. For Michell, this critique largely starts and ends with the difficulty of determining whether psychometric measures can ever really reflect complex phenomena such as intellectual abilities, personality traits and social attitudes. Ostensibly, he argued that no, they cannot, but he also railed against the failure of psychology as a field to seriously test this foundational assumption.

The criticism of attempting to ascribe quantitative numerical representations to psychological constructs that cannot be directly observed has a long history dating back to at least 1946 (Stevens, 1946, 1951, 1958). Criticisms of psychometric measurement become more recognised from the mid-1990s and have been consistent, forceful and—overall—persuasive (Andersen et al., 2007; Barrett, 2003; Borsboom & Mellenbergh, 2004; Michell, 1990, 1996, 1997a, 1997b, 1999, 2000; Narens & Luce, 1986). Fundamentally, these critiques consistently demonstrate that psychological and social phenomena do not fit with the assumptions of quantitative measurement. A score of 4 is not double a score of 2; 0 does not—in fact—mean 0 on many questionnaires; and there is no clear way of comparing 2 measurements made using difference scales (when compared to say, converting km to miles or feet to m). To those brave enough to pursue this issue further, Barrett (2003), Michell (1990) and Narens and Luce (1986) are some of the more accessible, readable deconstructions. Andersen et al. (2007) also made a similar case, specific to sport psychology. The arguments against generating arbitrary numbers to represent complex psychological phenomena are quite compelling, albeit depressing to those of us who do rely on psychometrics from time to time. Andersen et al. (2007: p. 664), for example, stated that: 'Sport and exercise psychology researchers use numbers extensively. Some of those numbers are directly related to overt real-world behaviors such as how high an athlete jumps or how far some object is thrown, but many of those measures do not have such intimate connections to real-world performance or behavior. They often involve self-reports on inventories or surveys that are measuring (or attempting to measure) some psychological, underlying, or latent variables such as task and ego orientation or competitive state anxiety. What those scores on self-report inventories mean may be somewhat of a mystery if they are not related back to overt behaviors'.

In contrast, the argument that has been most widely recognised as the strongest attempt to defend psychometrics, and reject Michell's thesis, was published by Lovie (1997: p. 393):

> There are no absolute, ahistorical mathematical truths or methods, only locally developed and locally maintained collective commitments and practices; what the ethno-methodologist Eric Livingston has termed the 'lived work' of the practising mathematician.

Lovie argued that measurement in psychometrics is different from measurement elsewhere and governed by implicit consent, trends and norms. 'We are different, and we do it our way.' It is the most fundamentally Kuhnian defence imaginable. Barrett (2003: p. 11, *emphasis added*) summarised that position as follows:

> When confronted with this [the unsuitability of psychometric measurement], many psychologists retort that psychological measurement "is different from" measurement in the natural sciences. When pressed to explain

the new axiomatic basis (or specific conditions) for this special measurement in psychology, there is complete silence. The issue here for many in psychology is not so much that Michell may be wrong in his exposition of the theory of measurement and continuous quantity, but whether what he states is in any way relevant to psychological and psychometric measurement. However, this "relevance" question is itself based upon a false premise. That is, that there exist different kinds of quantitative measurement which are relevant to particular domains of enquiry. There are not. *The axioms defining quantity and the theory of continuous quantity that underlines quantitative relations and structures are not "optional".*

It is further possible to argue that the problem exists at two levels, both measurement and analysis. Most statistical analysis models contain, within them, assumptions about the nature of the reality being studied. Looking outside of the current trends in sport and exercise psychology, analytic techniques such as agent-based modelling, neural networks and machine learning (Farmer & Foley, 2009; Macal & North, 2010) actually develop their underlying assumptions alongside the analysis of data (or they can, at least). Such a model—once built and tested—contains within it assumptions that reflect the behaviour of the system. In contrast, the assumptions of linear modelling—that we use for correlations, regressions, structural equation modelling and the like—are effectively fixed, as set out in the textbook (e.g. Field, 2002, 2013). Adopting assumptions beforehand may be influencing: (a) what we look for, (b) how we analyse it and (c) what we find. The assumptions of linear modelling are: that all variables have normal distributions (multivariate normality) and similar variances (homoscedasticity); that all relationships are linear, not curved in any way (linearity); that key independent variables are truly independent of each other (no multicollinearity); and that variables are not correlated with themselves over time (no autocorrelation—[See also 'Likert Scales', above]). These are (almost) always the assumptions of linear modelling, yet each of these assumptions can be queried in relation to studying psychological phenomena. For example, on many measures of perceived competence, people rarely rate themselves as below average—so everybody tend to be 'above average' (which is impossible—the Dunning-Kruger Effect, cf. Dunning, 2011; Kruger & Dunning, 1999).

This may lead to a non-normal curve (Schlösser, Dunning, Johnson, & Kruger, 2013). Likewise, homoscedasticity is tricky, as the moment-to-moment variation in say, affect, is much greater than the variation in personality traits (which should, by definition, be quite consistent—but this would conflict with the no autocorrelation rule). Perhaps most difficult to test: are all these relationships linear? Or are there likely to be non-linear interactions, such as stepped functions, exponential curves or hyperbolic functions? Imagine the impact of negative affect from a coach who clearly cares for her players and is passionate and energetic—the result might be an inverted-U relationship to positive affect in the players. Some negative emotion may be viewed as 'wearing her heart on her sleeve', but any more is disconcerting. Alternatively, if the negative emotions were accompanied by conveying strong ego/performance goals or perfectionism, they might be viewed as almost always unpleasant—perhaps producing an exponential decaying function. Neither would be linear, and it could change as a function of context. We do not know if this is the case because we rarely test it, and assumptions of linearity would not permit us to look for such a pattern.

Some papers do report testing the assumptions of linear modelling before performing statistical analysis based on linear modelling. Of course, if our measurement tools are forcibly creating imaginary multidimensional linear functions for us (as per the previous paragraphs on psychometric measurement), the resulting data may pass such a test more readily. Nevertheless, *neither* the psychometric measurement used *nor* the linear modelling analysis approach have been shown to ideally fit the psychological 'things' being measured. In the vast majority of cases, the only demonstrable compatibility is between the (arguably inappropriate) measurement instrument and the (potentially inappropriate) analysis technique: those two things fit together perfectly once we ignore the complex and non-linear nature of the things we are actually studying. In this way, the use of linear modelling techniques to analyse psychometric data can start to look like a 'house of cards', with its own seemingly robust and reliable internal logic, but almost no reference to the reality of the thing it refers to. It is, perhaps, the perfect Kuhnian paradigm: a club to which many of us belong; presented as robust, valid and ideal, and which none of us can legitimately question without immediately becoming either a 'failure' or an 'outsider'. Yet as many of the authors cited above have demonstrated, the 'validity' of this popular approach is actually derived from internal logic and—viewed more objectively—often appears inappropriate for the scientific study of complex psychological phenomena. If we go back and look at the strengths of psychometric measurement, as detailed at the start of this section, they may look quite different now. *They generate numbers. They are incredibly convenient. Everyone else is doing it.*

The only telling counterargument to the criticisms made by Michell and colleagues, regarding psychometrics, is as follows: What's the alternative? What's your solution? It needs to be clear that this argument does not invalidate the criticisms. Recognising that something is problematic and detailing why is a completely different task to developing and refining new approaches—which typically takes enormous time and effort. If we had to have a perfect and ideal replacement approach before we were allowed to criticise something, nothing would ever be criticised. It is a defence frequently deployed by politicians as a reason for persisting with damaging or unpopular policies: what's your suggestion? With the implication being that if you haven't got one, shut up and go away. This argument is reflected in the (rather strongly worded) quote of Brandolini (2013—http://bit.ly/1TZwL9w): 'The amount of energy needed to refute bullshit is an order of magnitude bigger than to produce it.' In simple terms, the two tasks are completely separate: (a) identify a problem, describe it, assess its impact and consequences; (b) develop and test solutions to that problem, which may require the formulation of many potential solutions, and extensive trial and error. Task (a) clearly informs Task (b), but they do not come as an inseparable pair. Lack of completion of (b) does not invalidate (a). Clearly we should devote energy to Task (b), developing and refining new approaches, as opposed to clinging to an approach that is demonstrably problematic. The best we can say of psychometric measurement and correlation—using linear models—is that such an approach can occasionally be appropriate but that it is currently over-represented in the sport and exercise psychology literature. The references to validity and reliability are internally defined, and bear little relation to any objective reality of cognitive and social phenomena. In that knowledge, to persist with relaying almost exclusively on such a technique is a deliberate deception—of the self and others. It might get published, it might get cited, it might lead to income from grants or people licensing the instruments developed—but is it moving us closer to a better understanding of psychology? Do we in fact overvalue the method but undervalue the knowledge?

Methodolatry

The clash and struggle between paradigms, the resultant discussion whether qualitative or quantitative methods are 'the best', or whether one statistical method is better than another may explain why researchers such as Chamberlain (2000) voiced concerns about methodolatry: 'an overenhanced valuing of methodology' (p. 287). That is, when the tools used become more important than the question, they are supposed to help answer. This call for caution has been made before, for example, by Romanyshyn (1971) and again by Koch (1981) and Danziger (1990); the latter two warning that 'method fetishism' needs to be watched as meaning may be lost when the tool becomes more important than the topic investigated. Even Tukey (1962, the creator of 'Tukey's honest significant difference test') was seriously concerned about the risk that statistical tests may draw the attention away from the empirical data. There certainly needs to be a healthy and critical discussion of the methods researchers chooses to use; methodolatry is the opposite, an unhealthy struggle to defend inferior methods and protect the legacy of using such methods in published research.

Although Chamberlain (2000) focused on qualitative methods used in health psychology, his message is equally applicable to quantitative methods used in sport and exercise psychology. And with the development of advanced statistical methods—such as Latent Growth Curve Modelling, Structural Equation Modelling, and Rasch Modelling—some researchers seem more keen on discussing various forms of factorial invariance, fit indices and longitudinal trajectories than what the data actually tells them about their original research question. Of course, discussing the method(s) is to some extent always warranted—we are not arguing against spelling out the pros and cons—but when a researcher crosses the line between a relevant and focused discussion of the tool's merits, clearly forgetting the original question and solely focusing on the tool, then a word of caution is warranted.

Methodolatry is not the same as what Sparkes (2013) refers to as methodological fundamentalism—although it is easy to envision a researcher who is both a methodological fundamentalist (or fetishist) and a methodolatrist. This could be a researcher convinced that the only true way to conduct research is the experimental approach in a well-controlled laboratory environment, which by this (imaginary) researcher's definition always includes random allocation to treatment groups, manipulation of the independent variable(s) and quantifying the dependent variable(s) with a maximum of control to reduce error variance. The above steps would have been taken in order to securely pave the way for cause and effect conclusions using the most advanced statistical methods possible. The results are for this researcher secondary to the intricacies of the statistical analyses; in fact, the initial research question is barely given any space in the concluding discussion. Although this example was voiced from a quantitative perspective, Chamberlain (2000) described how the qualitative researcher may become preoccupied with obtaining and analysing data, extensively discussing its trustworthiness, saturation, and recurrent patterning, and ultimately forgetting the phenomenon under investigation.

This trend towards over-emphasising the method—whether it be quantitative/statistical or qualitative—is supported by the increasing number of textbooks devoted to single research methods. These textbooks often describe in a step-by-step fashion exactly how a certain method should (should, not could) be applied and the data subsequently analysed. If consensus existed among researchers, these prescriptions would be less of a problem. But since several textbooks focusing on the same method often exist, with descriptions (prescriptions) that differ to some extent, it is not surprising that this can create confusion and problems. For example, when a researcher submits a manuscript to a scientific journal, there is a risk that the editor and/or peer reviewers will not fully appreciate or approve of the chosen method. They may instead subscribe to a slightly different approach, thereby rejecting a manuscript because it does not conform to '*the only* right way'. Whether the topic studied and questions posed are relevant and appropriately answered becomes less of a priority because the chosen tool is not used in the exact way a 'true believer' would. If a reviewer of a manuscript—who is fervently opposed to one school of thought—is not transparent when the suggestion is made to the editor to reject a manuscript, then high-quality manuscripts may be rejected on the wrong grounds. Not for their lack of quality or stringency, merely for the failure of the submitting researcher/s to believe that there is only one correct way of using a particular method.

Maybe editors and peer reviewers alike should listen more closely to two experienced qualitative researchers. Smith and Sparkes (2012) conclude their chapter, entitled 'Making sense of words and stories in qualitative research', by supporting pluralism: 'It is much more preferable to open up our analytical possibilities, consider certain purposes using different types of analysis, and, when appropriate, shift our analytical visions. That is, we should consider using a variety of analyses in order to understand our data in different ways' (p. 129). This call for a more open pluralistic approach to qualitative research does not, however, imply that methods should be without structure or stringency, only that the topic is more important than any one method chosen to analyse words and stories. There are still better or worse ways of analysing data, but many tools exist that can be used to come as close as possible to the inherent meaning. Believing in the 'only right way' may seem fine as long as it does not hinder progress or knowledge build-up. Allowing dogma or method-fascism is nevertheless a threat to everything science and research is meant to stand for; consequently, everyone involved needs to be aware of these risks and open to alternative solutions.

In criticising such an approach, Chamberlain (2000) argued: 'Methodolatry is characteristic of most psychology, and psychology has been overly concerned with methodology almost since its beginnings. Historical reasons for this relate to the dominance of behaviourism, a strong emphasis on being objective and the pre-eminence of measurement' (p. 286). That measurement has been a significant part of sport and exercise psychology from its conception has been discussed in previous chapters. Whatever we may think about quantitative research and whether measurements are a blessing or evil in sport and exercise psychology research, they will remain an important part in the foreseeable future. To know both strengths and weaknesses thereby seems appropriate for everyone involved in doing research (Kass et al., 2016).

This statement brings us back to our earlier acquaintance Stevens (1951), the psychophysicist, who defined measurement as 'assigning numbers to objects according to agreed-upon rules'. Stevens (1946,

1957) further classified variables into four levels or scales of measurement: nominal (names, e.g. men, women), ordinal (order, first, second third, etc., but without equal intervals), interval (order and equal intervals) and ratio (order, equal intervals and a true zero point). From a purely statistical viewpoint, ratio scales with a true zero point are superior to the other three levels of measurement. In real life there are many measures that are less than ideal for being subjected to statistical analyses. For example, few variables are perfectly normally distributed (bell shaped); instead we accept 'approximately' normally distributed variables. Most statistical methods are fairly robust towards violations of normality, but when a multivariable dataset is analysed, many 'approximations' may add up to severe violations, and the need to abandon parametric and instead use non-parametric statistical methods (parametric meaning that they assume that variables, among other things, are approximately normally distributed around the mean). The preceding discussion has in parts been rather abstract, so we therefore continue with three concrete examples.

Some Examples

The following section will delve deeper into three constructs from sport and exercise psychology—burnout, mood and achievement goals—and explore how these have been operationalised in order to measure them. All three instruments have subscales and their intended target audience differ widely, at least from when they were conceived (people in helping professions; psychiatric outpatients; athletes and exercisers). Nowadays, they are all frequently used in sport and with athletes, exercisers and coaches as respondents.

Burnout

First burnout; originally made measurable by Christina Maslach through the Maslach Burnout Inventory (Maslach & Jackson, 1981). Burnout was then described as a syndrome with three dimensions: emotional exhaustion, depersonalisation and lack of personal accomplishment.

Maslach and colleagues assumed that the relationships between provider and recipients in healthcare settings (e.g. health professionals vs. patients) and educational settings (teachers vs. students) could cause burnout. The primary burnout dimension was labelled emotional exhaustion, which with mounting levels may in turn lead to an effort by the provider to distance her-/himself from recipients (i.e. depersonalisation) as a way of coping when demands exceed available resources. For some this may also cause feelings of diminished personal accomplishment, although this third dimension is frequently not highly correlated with the other two (Lee & Ashforth, 1996; Shirom, 2005). A later version was developed to offer a context-free alternative; the construct was also broadened somewhat and the second and third dimension as a consequence renamed cynicism and professional efficiency, respectively (Schaufeli, Leiter, Maslach, & Jackson, 1996).

What is interesting with the burnout construct is that it has basically remained unchanged over the years since its conception (Lundkvist, Stenling, Gustafsson, & Hassmén, 2014); it is still predominantly measured by three dimensions, such as in the original MBI (Maslach & Jackson, 1981) or in slightly altered forms when used in sport and exercise settings in the form of the Athletic Burnout Questionnaire (ABQ) and Coach Burnout Questionnaire (CBQ; see Raedeke & Smith, 2001). Alternatively, with two (of the three original) dimensions: (a) emotional and physical exhaustion and (b) disengagement, which is similar to cynicism (OLBI: Oldenburg Burnout Inventory; Demerouti, Bakker, Vardakou, & Kantas, 2003).

Given that burnout—when studied using qualitative methods—frequently is described as a much more multi-faceted and complex syndrome (e.g. Lundkvist, Gustafsson, Hjälm, & Hassmén, 2012), the lack of newer and more comprehensive instruments may initially seem somewhat surprising. One reason is probably the tendency by peer-reviewed journals and their editors to be more likely to accept a study using an established inventory rather than a new and less used one. The reasoning seems to be that an instrument used extensively over a long period of time must produce scores that are both valid and reliable. An alternative answer is of course that peer reviewers, although being experts in their respective fields, may have a lot to lose if a newer and better instrument replaces the one they have used for many years in their own research and maybe even to a large extent built their academic career on. While peer reviewers are supposed to assure that only good quality research is published, they are only humans that may also be inclined to ensure that only research that fits their own preferences is accepted. Thereby acting as a conservative defence force instead of contributing to extending the knowledgebase and making sure that novel and creative research is rewarded by being accepted for publication.

The above can also be discussed in terms of 'construct underrepresentation' (Standards for Educational and Psychological Testing, 2014, p. 12). That is, when an instrument fails to capture the full (or a significant proportion) of the construct and only captures a narrow part of it. This is unfortunately not uncommon as many instruments either are too narrow in their conceptualisation of the construct or miss it altogether. Before we sound too critical, consider the following statement in the *Standards*:

> Nearly all tests leave out elements that some potential users believe should be measured and include some elements that some potential users consider inappropriate. Validation involves careful attention to possible distortions in meaning arising from inadequate representation of the construct and also to aspects of measurement, such as test format, administration, conditions, or language level, that may materially limit or qualify the interpretation of test scores for various groups of test takers. (p. 13)

That the three dimensions described above only partly capture Burnout is not a particularly bold statement. Yet few efforts have been made to develop new instruments that not are inspired by the original conceptualisation by Maslach and colleagues.

Mood States

Another anomaly in the sport and exercise psychology literature, namely the use (and abuse) of an otherwise reliable and valid instrument, the Profile of Mood States (POMS). It was originally developed for assessing transient, fluctuating affective states in people undergoing counselling or psychotherapy (McNair et al., 1971/1992). The 65-item 5-point (0–4) adjective rating scales comprise 6 mood or affective states: Tension-Anxiety, Depression-Dejection, Anger-Hostility, Vigour-Activity, Fatigue-Inertia and Confusion-Bewilderment. Psychometrically its quality was deemed satisfactory, at least for its intended target population: Psychiatric outpatients (McNair et al., 1992). The POMS first appeared in 1971 and has since then also been used to answer sport and exercise psychology related questions. Not the least by Morgan who based his mental health model partly on the POMS, with the specific aim 'to introduce a mental health model for use in predicting and understanding maximal physical performance in sport settings' (Morgan, 1985, p. 70). Morgan admits that the model is narrow, incomplete and conservative:

> It is narrow because it is restricted to selected psychological states and traits; it is incomplete because it does not incorporate potentially relevant variables of a physiological, biomechanical, and medical nature; and it is conservative because any predictive ability generated with the model will underestimate the actual potential to predict maximal physical performance. (p. 70)

Despite these shortcomings, Morgan (1985) reported eight separate studies including various athlete populations, such as elite wrestlers, elite and university rowers, distance runners and college athletes including swimmers; it was also with this book chapter that the 'iceberg profile' started to get traction. That is, high scores on Vigour and low scores on the other five subscales; the 'iceberg' becomes visible by graphically displaying Vigour as the fourth of the six subscales. Interestingly—but not surprisingly—small and non-significant differences were detected between athletes. A later meta-analysis based on 33 POMS studies concluded that a slight difference possibly could be detected between successful and less successful athletes, but that the variance explained was less than 1 % (Rowley, Landers, Kyllo, & Etnier, 1995)—a startlingly low proportion. It seems Morgan was right when he already in his original 1985 chapter concluded by stating:

> The basic thesis underlying the mental health model described here may not seem very provocative since it merely specifies that athletes characterized as anxious, depressed, hysterical, neurotic, introverted, withdrawn,

confused, fatigued, and/or schizoid would be less likely to succeed in a given sport than would an athlete who had positive mental health. In other words, the model possesses a common sense or intuitive appeal. (p. 78)

Indeed, this seems to be common sense. But nevertheless an interesting example when an instrument intended for psychiatric outpatients, such as the POMS, is applied in a completely different setting, in this case, even used to predict sport performance. That only 1 % of the variance could be explained in Rowley's meta-analysis and 99 % were explained by other factors is a sobering thought and an example of construct irrelevance (or construct contamination) as described in the *Standards* (p. 12).

There are many other examples when POMS has been used in an effort to answer research questions that given the instruments strengths and limitations simply cannot be answered. Consider, for example, the researcher interested in the link between physical exercise and depression: does exercise reduce depression? The answer can be 'yes', provided that the participants present with elevated scores on the POMS-depression subscale. A completely different answer will be reached if the participants are not presenting with elevated scores, simply because the POMS was created to measure five negative mood states (and one positive: Vigour). If participants at the pre-test are not scoring much above 0 (Not at all, on the five-point Likert-type scale) on Anxiety, Confusion, Depression, Fatigue and Tension, then no intervention regardless of how effective it is will cause scores to decrease because they are already as low as they can get (Hassmén & Koivula, 1997; Leunes & Burger, 2000).

On the other hand, if the aim is to detect increasing negative mood states, the POMS may be the best instrument available. For example, when elite athletes are training hard and approaching an overreached state, negative mood states tend to increase as well. So for non-depressed exercisers, POMS is not a very good alternative, but for athletes approaching an overreached state, it may help them or their coaches to decide when more recovery is needed instead of more training, thereby reducing the risk for developing an underrecovery syndrome (Kenttä & Hassmén, 2002). The takeaway message from these examples is that a valid and reliable instrument—such as the POMS—can provide valid and reliable answers in one setting, while proving of little value in other settings.

This turns our attention to the fact that validity and reliability can be discussed from at least four different angles: the test developers', test distributors', test users' and test takers', respectively. When the POMS test originally was developed, the target group was clearly specified (psychiatric outpatients). Even with restricted access and sometimes steep costs, it is difficult for a test developer to prevent that a test distributor sells the test to any buyer deemed legitimate; it is practically impossible for a test developer to control in what context the test will be used, for what purpose, and who will be asked to complete it. This means that the person administering the test must ensure that all prerequisites are fulfilled so that validity and reliability are not compromised by non-intended use. Something that is not always the case in sport and exercise psychology where both students and researchers sometimes assemble a collection of tests that may or may not be suitable for the research questions they are trying to answer. Finally, in this section, there is the example of achievement goal theory (Nicholls, 1984, 1989), which offers a qualitatively different set of challenges and issues to consider.

Achievement Goals

It is difficult to imagine someone being motivated towards everything, all of the time. For most people, motivation is directed towards some type of goal and thereby also fluctuates in intensity and over time. One type of goal is achievement-motivated; Nicholls (1984, 1989) described how children in an educational setting either evaluated their competence (goal achievement) in relation to their own past performances, or in relation to the performance of others. The former has become known as mastery or task goals, and the latter as performance or ego goals. See the previous chapter for an extensive discussion of achievement goal theory; we will in this chapter focus only on issues relating to measuring achievement goals.

Two instruments were more or less simultaneously developed, one of these being the Perception of Success Questionnaire (POSQ; Roberts & Balague, 1989; Roberts, Treasure, & Balague, 1998). The second named the Task and Ego Orientation in Sport Questionnaire (TEOSQ; Duda & Nicholls, 1992). Whereas the POSQ measure task and ego orientation with 6 items for each subscale, the TEOSQ does it by 7 and 6 items, respectively. Wordings and content are, however, very similar, which is not surprising given that Nicholls and/or collaborators to him developed both inventories. Among them Roberts, who in the third edition of *Advances in Motivation in Sport and Exercise* (Roberts & Treasure, 2012) states that: 'Although other scales exist, the POSQ and the TEOSQ are the scales that best meet the conceptual criteria of measuring orthogonal [i.e., independent] achievement goals in sport' (p. 13). Roberts further suggests that even if other scales are developed in the future, '...the constructs identified must be conceptually coherent with achievement goal theory' (p. 13). Do you remember the statement made by Razon et al. (2012, p. 356) that appear earlier in this chapter? Reiterating the cautionary words of Noble and Noble (1998):

> Emphasis should be placed on understanding perception, not on studying the results of the Borg scale. Until that is done, the study of perceptual response during physical activity will reflect only what the Borg scale measures.

It is tempting to exchange some words to make this statement applicable also to the study of achievement goals:

> Emphasis should be placed on understanding *achievement goals*, not on studying the results of the *POSQ/TEOSQ*. Until that is done, the study of *goal achievement in sport and exercise* will reflect only what the *POSQ/TEOSQ* measure.

Our previous conclusion that such statements can be applied to most inventories—because the definition we make and how we chose to operationalise a construct will always be challenged and contested—thereby seems to hold true. And Roberts and colleagues have indeed been challenged, not the least in respect to whether task and ego goals are the only achievement goals worth contemplating, or if there are more facets to achievement goals than these two, see Chap. 6. From this follows that also the scales created to measure task and ego goals can be challenged, although if the most important criterion is that any new scale 'must be coherent with achievement goal theory' (Roberts, 2012, p. 13)—which in this case arguably means 'coherent with a very narrow view of one version of achievement goal theory'. If that pessimistic viewpoint were to be the case, then it seems highly unlikely that we will see any major breakthrough, either regarding the theory, or how the construct is operationalised and measured.

Concluding Remarks

Measurements in sport and exercise psychology research are here to stay, but the postpositivistic dominance is broken with the increasing focus on constructivism and qualitative methods—the toolbox is becoming more complete and researchers may finally realise that the questions they are trying to answer are more important than the tools at their disposal. This statement is not saying that statistical tools are unimportant, rather that even advanced analyses rely on the quality of the data. If a cross-sectional questionnaire with questionable reliability and validity is used, then not even the most advanced statistical analyses can help the researcher present trustworthy results. Some may even use advanced statistical tests to cover up the shortcomings of the data; Andreski (1972) called this 'quantification as camouflage'. It seems pertinent to be aware of this risk with the advent of ever more advanced statistical tests. As such, textbooks helping sport and exercise psychology researchers to analyse and interpret their data better and more appropriately are needed, see, for example, Ntoumanis and Myers (2015). Likewise such messages need to be taken seriously, and taught earnestly. Just remember that advanced statistical methods can never compensate for inferior instruments or scales, the questionable practice of treating ordinal scales as something they are not, and devising new and even more advanced statistical analyses without acknowledging—and remedying—the shortcomings of the available data.

8

Research and Practice in Applied Sport and Exercise Psychology

At the 2015 FEPSAC Conference, keynote speaker Chris Harwood reflected on the 'gap' between: (a) the way we teach sport psychology at university and (b) what practitioners will need to know when they begin supervised practice (and thereafter) (Fédération Européenne de Psychologie des Sports et des Activités Corporelles [FEPSAC]—Harwood, 2015). Effectively, this difference reflects the 'research-practice gap': wherein what is researched, written about and read—and thus accepted by most graduates—can be relatively unhelpful when it comes to sitting down opposite an athlete seeking psychological support. Harwood used the metaphor of a ravine that has to be crossed by those brave enough to 'make the leap' into applied practice. The research-practice 'gap' is a common problem across all of science, and not-at-all unique to sport and exercise psychology. One might argue that the 'gap' is perhaps more pronounced in sport and exercise psychology, or more current, or more persistent. After all, in 1979, Martens reflected: 'I am disturbed by the gulf between those who do sport psychology research and those who interpret the sport psychology research to practitioners' (cited in Smith & Bar-Eli, 2007; p. 37). Twenty-seven years later, Vealey still referred to this 'schism' (Vealey, 2006; p. 144). Thirty-six years after Martens, Keegan (2015) was imploring practitioners:

© The Author(s) 2016
P. Hassmén et al., *Rethinking Sport and Exercise Psychology Research*,
DOI 10.1057/978-1-137-48338-6_8

(a) to make better use of research evidence, (b) to demand higher-quality evidence from researchers and (c) to open up the processes of applied practice to be researched. Of these, Vealey's summary is perhaps most succinct: 'Research is viewed as incomprehensible, pointless and boring, while practice is viewed as pseudoscientific and ineffective. [We should be] asking real world questions, with an eye on the person in context, aiming for practical theory... not theoretical practice' (Vealey, 2006; p. 148).

Case Example: 'The Scales Fell from My Eyes'

By: Richard Keegan

The following experience may be a familiar one for many readers. A conversation with the coach of an elite rugby team once left my fledgling world-view in tatters. After 4 years of training in sport and exercise psychology, I had just started my PhD, and at the time, I considered myself an achievement goals researcher. When asked about what I was studying, I explained that some athletes were naturally very competitive (i.e. ego oriented), and some focussed on performance, development and process (i.e. task oriented). I explained that research showed elite athletes tended to score high on both. 'Yeah I know', he said, 'that's obvious'.

'Ah but the cool special thing I'm interested in is that you can either have athletes worried about failing and trying to avoid it – which is generally bad – or focussed on doing well and succeeding – which is generally good.' Same answer. 'But Im studying the motivational climate', I said, 'that's the thing that the coach can control'.

'Well, now you're talking', said the coach, 'tell me what I can do to improve the motivation of my athletes'.

'Well. It turns out that when athletes feel the climate around them is highly competitive, that has very mixed outcomes. The ones who like that, and are generally winning, quite like it but the rest may not enjoy it: and may start to lose motivation. When athletes feel the climate around them promotes effort, improvement and collaboration, most of them will enjoy it more, and stay motivated.'

'Again, I could have told you that. Any of us could. Is this research with elite athletes?'

'Erm, no mainly school children and university athletes.'

'Right. Ok. Um. So what can I do to make the athletes feel that way?'

'Actually, our questionnaires don't tend to ask that, they just ask how the athlete feels generally. "On this team".'

'That doesn't help me very much. Is there anything I, as the coach, can do to improve the motivation of my athletes?'

'Actually maybe not. Athletes with the same coach seem to develop wildly different perceptions of their motivational climate.'

'Last chance Richard. Is there anything I, as the coach, can do to motivate my athlete more?'

'Um. Oh yeah. The TARGET framework. You can use that. Tasks, Authority, Recognition, Grouping, Evaluation, and Timings. Each of those can be either "task" or "ego". There.'

'And has that been tested in elite sport, and proven to work?'

'Erm. Not really. In fact, some aspects don't seem to work so well. It's mainly gone out of fashion.'

The coach had been very patient with me. I was young, and desperately keen to help (and to prove myself!). But this conversation had been awkward. To make matters worse, my PhD data—based on interviewing athletes at different ages and levels—consistently failed to match specific coach behaviours with specific motivational outcomes. For me, the rope snapped during a focus group with eight-year-old children: children who theoretically should not be able to differentiate between normative comparisons (ego goals) and effort improvement (task goals). Firstly, they could clearly differentiate. Second, they would consistently disagree about the effects of any specific coach behaviour. One would say he likes praise from a coach. The girl next to him would say: 'But only if he means it, not if it's fake'. Hmm. Another child would say he dislikes criticism from a coach. The boy next to him would say: 'No I need that to improve. And it shows that she cares about my improvement'. Eight-year-old children. This culminated in what I call the 'Oh shit' moment, when I was trying to explain the problem to my PhD supervisors. After I had made several awkward, embarrassed attempts to explain the lack of consistent links between coach behaviour and the impact on motivation, one supervisor summarised: 'So what you're saying is…. It's like…. Well… Shit.'

I had a choice between falling into line and continuing to obey the 'rules' of my paradigm, or following the data. The above experiences had made a big impression on me. I had to question the theory I had 'grown up with' and consider that it might be wrong (or at least, inadequate to inform applied practice).

What Is the 'Research-Practice Gap'?

To fully understand the research-practice gap, we need to understand the different aims and activities of each, and the different skill sets required in each domain. As it becomes clear that each of these skill sets can be quite advanced, requiring extensive training and practice, then the reason for a gap becomes clear: very few people have the time or inclination to accumulate *both* these very different skill sets. These two very 'hard-earned' skill sets, with very different languages, aims and methods, can become quite difficult to reconcile. Once a professional has finally 'made it' within one or the other domain—research or practice—very few people seem willing to learn the language, aims, skill sets and assumptions/expectations of the other side. Thus, the researchers 'get on with' research, and the practitioners 'get on with' practice, solving different problems using different methods and approaches, with little requirement to communicate. In this way, a significant opportunity to advance both research and practice is lost—in sport psychology, exercise psychology and performance psychology (as well as many other fields). Of course, this doesn't preclude the two groups from interacting and talking to each other, but for reasons explored below, that also doesn't seem to happen.

Why don't researchers and practitioners speak to each other? Paraphrasing Norman (2010): in most typical research, there are clear links between hypotheses, tests or evidence and conclusions. But in applied practice, these links are tenuous (at best). Instead, there is much reliance upon 'best practice', where 'best' is often agreed via unofficial consensus, using short-term measurement of variables that are easy to measure—as opposed to those that are of most significance. Long-term measures are seldom taken (arguably, this observation regarding measurement applies equally to both practice and research in sport and exercise psychology). Further, methods are seldom compared in applied practice. Note that in most cases, it is not-at-all easy to find ways of understanding and comparing different instances of applied practice. Research usually prefers carefully controlled conditions, forming abstract characterisations of the phenomena under consideration and studying them in a controlled research environment. Similarly, the theories within research are often simplified and abstracted to a pristine form—and this is argued to be necessary in order to facilitate their testing. Of course, this can mean the deletion or exclusion of 'outliers', even though most elite athletes are, by definition, outliers. Focussing on the 'parsimony' principle, most people find the conclusions of research are easiest to understand, and most compelling, when all the variables are simple, comprehensible and controlled. The real world of applied practice is complex and messy, with uncontrolled and poorly defined variables; often behaving in ways that contradict the neat, logical assumptions of the researcher. In this way, the researchers attempting to study applied practice see a messy and complex world with no control and rigour. By contrast, the practitioners attempting to engage with research see a world of stale, abstract and irrelevant findings that would never survive contact with the complexities of the real world. Each is repulsed by the other, and the result is a 'gap'.

What Are the Consequences of Allowing a 'Research-Practice Gap'?

There are a number of 'impacts' that emerge from permitting a research-practice gap, and these are often of increasing magnitude, in proportion to the size of the 'gap'. The simple overview would be that: (a) research is not used for its intended purpose—or at least its moral purpose—of informing practice and generating improved outcomes in the real world; and (b) practice is not sufficiently 'evidence based', sometimes to the extent that people start redefining 'evidence' as their own opinions and experiences—which is not how evidence-based practice is intended to be used (Chambless, 1999, 2006; Chambless & Ollendick, 2001; Crits-Christoph, Chambless, & Markell, 2014; Gardner & Moore, 2005). There are additional concerns, however. First, perceiving a disconnect between 'scientific' research and applied practice can undermine the confidence of those seeking psychological support. Athletes, coaches, governing bodies and the like may all either shy away from seeking applied services, or perhaps simply be seduced by 'alternatives' that seem equally 'scientific' (i.e. not very). For every tightly regulated practitioner who undergoes many years of training and adheres to strict ethical standards, there are many more who are not regulated, not scientific and not 'constrained' by ethical considerations. In many ways, unregulated providers of psychological support—the mind coaches and excellence practitioners—can actually outcompete the tightly regulated and qualified practitioners: partly because they can (and do) use former clients as advertising, and partly because those who underwent significant and expensive training to attain registration as a psychologist simply are unable/unwilling to 'sell' the benefits of being scientific and evidence based. Remember, most ethical codes for psychologists demand that practitioners be evidence based (cf. Keegan, 2015), whereas unregulated practitioners are not constrained by this rule and can choose whether to adopt it or not. So imagine the debate between the different camps (let's imagine just two, for simplicity). Unregulated service providers: 'We promise awesome results, using the latest techniques – techniques that are so new they're untested by those boring scientists… and we have already worked for all these famous athletes…. and those regulated practitioners aren't even evidence-based anyway; they barely even talk to the researchers!' To which the regulated and registered psychologists can only reply: 'We would never promise awesome results, that's unethical. And we cannot use previous clients as advertising; that's unethical too. We do try to use theories and techniques that have been tested, but many have not been tested well enough… some of them are not very applicable, and actually… yeah most of the research isn't so helpful to applied practitioners – so it's very hard to be evidence-based.' *Who would you give your money to?* The disconnect between research and practice does more than simply deny quality evidence to applied practitioners, it also undermines the selling and marketing of applied psychology. There are further consequences, however, because if-and-when clients receive a non-optimal service from a non-regulated practitioner, their opinion about *all* applied psychology will be affected. Very few such clients will emerge from a bad experience and think 'I will make sure I use a regulated practitioner next time'. By way of adding a little balance to this coverage, it is also quite possible that the regulated and evidence-based practitioners—when deprived of suitable evidence by the research-practice gap—can also generate poor outcomes for clients (perhaps more ethically, but still ultimately leaving potential unmet, or offering support that is viewed as ineffective).

The research-practice gap also makes it much more difficult to train future practitioners, as there is no consistent vocabulary, no strong models of practice, and thus no way of understanding what practitioners do, or why. This can reduce training in applied practice to an 'art' or 'craft', wherein important rules and principles are not understood or conveyed. In fact, regarding the 'science-versus-art' debate within sport and exercise psychology, we arguably know more about the differences between Rembrandt and Escher than we do about the differences between consulting styles and philosophies. This lack of vocabulary and understanding can lead practitioners to make vital decisions about philosophy or delivery style quite arbitrarily—that is, 'choose one you like' (which is how some trainee practitioners seem to interpret Poczwardowski, Aoyagi, Shapiro, & Van Raalte, 2014)—as opposed to this being a carefully reasoned and transparent decision. If the gap between research and practice were closed, perhaps this would be a decision where we could, for example, analyse the consequences and effects of adopting each style in different situations. This situation can undermine our understanding of philosophy-of-science in applied practice, and delivery style, such that there is no way of defining, comparing or evaluating different approaches. Right now, how would we tell which approach suits a client best: cognitive-behavioural therapy, humanistic counselling, rational-emotive therapy or perhaps just whatever approach is espoused in the latest self-help book? It quickly becomes possible for practitioners to claim the 'eclectic' label, but not in a good way where they are able to adopt different styles depending on the needs of the client. Increasingly, 'eclectic' becomes an excuse to do whatever felt right at the time, for any (or no) reason, and then retrofit one's actions to one of many frameworks that might legitimise them (as discussed by Keegan, 2015). Practitioners can quickly end up adopting incoherent and incompatible methods, goalposts can be easily moved, claims for effectiveness can be overblown; and clients eventually pick up on this. They don't like it. As such, echoing the above point, the research-practice gap can undermine training and reporting processes, ultimately undermining the quality of applied psychological practice. A good relationship between research and practice would create a shared language for describing, analysing and evaluating applied practice—scientifically. Yes, different epistemologies will accept different types of evidence, and we can explore what that means one day...but right now we aren't even having this debate—researchers and practitioners don't talk (enough) and it leaves applied practitioners 'flying blind' to a greater extent than we'd find acceptable (if, e.g. we researched it).

From the research side of the divide, most researchers arguably start their careers with the aim of informing—perhaps even revolutionising—applied practice in their field. Very few PhD students begin their journey with an ambition of achieving a high h-index. Unfortunately, in order to participate in the game of science, researchers are usually expected to adopt the: (a) assumptions; (b) theories; (c) methods; and (d) measurement instruments that are considered acceptable in their field. In Martens' time, these were (a) strong positivist assumptions; (b) parsimonious theories, often borrowed from social psychology; (c) experimental methods, often conducted in labs away from where the real action occurred; and (d) behavioural observations, and questionnaires. In modern times, we tend to see research that promotes (a) postpositivist assumptions, often reduced to naïvely positivist assumptions (e.g. generalisability, strong inference, etc.); (b) parsimonious theories, sometimes developed within sport and exercise psychology, but often adopted from elsewhere; (c) social-cognitive methods depending heavily on questionnaires and survey data—leading to extensive use of correlations and correlational models; (d) parsimonious (and so quite abstract), internally consistent, cross-sectional deployment of questionnaires.

Described this way, it is difficult to see much advancement since Martens' impassioned plea for researchers to abandon the lab and get out in the field. Why? Because in both scenarios—historical and modern—applied practitioners, athletes and coaches arguably find the outcomes of research equally irrelevant. Research done in a sterile lab, away from all the noise of the real world: irrelevant. Research depending on linking subjectively rated feelings with other subjectively rated feelings, *saying little-to-nothing about the environment that caused them*: irrelevant. But the problem for the researchers is this: there is too much risk and effort involved in breaking the paradigm to make it worthwhile. Trying to deliver research that would be extremely relevant to practitioners would involve using different assumptions, theories, methods and measurement instruments. Firstly, such an approach would risk being cast out as unscientific. Second, such an approach would receive little or no support in terms of supervision and existing literature (where the theories, methods and measures would be drawn from). One would be forging a new path, with no clear foundations on which to build and no guarantee that other researchers will approve. At the very beginning of one's research career, this doesn't seem like an appealing option. In itself, this can be quite a disincentive; however, the problem gets worse. What is incentivised in research settings is also quite unhelpful to applied practice. Researchers are judged on the number of papers they produce, the popularity of the journals they publish in and the number of times other researchers 'cite' their work (Callaway, 2016). These core values can then be combined into measures of impact such as the h-index: the number of papers with a citation number of $\leq$ h. For example, if someone has 40 papers published, but only 6 that have received 6 or more citations, their h-index is 6. This number is frequently referred to by review committees, tenure committees and grant funding panels. Hence, in that context, researchers have to do work based on what has gone before them, and create work that has a very good chance of being cited. At present, applied practitioners rarely ever write journal articles—so there is no chance of being cited by applied practitioners. Hence, there is no point in doing work of relevance to applied practitioners. Instead, researchers are incentivised to produce papers that—for the main part—extend and propagate the same assumptions, theories, methods and measurement instruments. The most famous and successful researchers will broadly have been cited a lot by other researchers—boosting their h-index—not by applied practitioners, boosting their real-world impact. Hence, unless we can (a) encourage new researchers and research projects that directly focus on applied practice, (b) persuade applied practitioners to start writing in journals and citing the most relevant and helpful research papers and (c) create systems that facilitate and reinforce/reward highly applicable research—perhaps something very different to the current citations and h-index system—then the research-practice gap will remain. It may even widen. Hence, not only do researchers find that their work fails to make much of an impact on applied practice, this problem seems to worsen and be reinforced as researchers progress 'up the chain'.

As a beginning on the journey to closing the research-practice gap, and reducing or avoiding the problems outlined in this section, the following passages will explore three broad 'strategies': practical theories; theories-of-practice; and theoretical practice. Only two of these approaches are presented as solutions to the research-practice gap, but all three need to be explored and understood. Chapter 10 will subsequently explore the 'post-revolution' world where—among other issues—the research-practice gap can be closed and a thriving culture of evidence-based sport and exercise psychology can grow.

Practical Theories and Theories of Practice

Picking up from Martens' (1979) critique of the way he believed was sport psychology evolving, he specified that we should seek practical theories, not theoretical practice. This might be equated to the idea that 'there is nothing more practical than a good theory' (Lewin, 1952, p. 169). Many philosophers of science (e.g. Popper, Lakatos, etc.) as well as many well-known scientists (e.g. Hawking, Einstein) have argued that theories should be developed to help solve practical, real-world problems. 'Well of course!' one might retort, but note these arguments were developed in response to a plethora of very popular theories that were, in fact, not useful and not (ultimately) scientific. The research-practice gap, however, works two ways—and so we must consider both practical theories (bridging from the researcher's side) and theories of practice (bridging from the practitioners' side). Note that neither of these options requires 'theoretical practice'—wherein favourite theories presumably drive all key decisions in applied practice, and/or practitioners are expected to adopt a favoured theory and use it throughout all of their practice. The following section will define, explore and critically examine each of these approaches, with a view to understanding their place in addressing the research-practice 'gap' (as noted above, this can also become the gap between teaching/ training and applied practice).

Theoretical Practice

In a world where theories and paradigms dominate how research is done (e.g. Chap. 5), and we expect practitioners to base their applied work on the literature that this generates (see 'scientist-practitioner model', below), theory-driven practice is the result. In some ways, given that we rarely attempt to test our theories to destruction, or seek to 'gold standard' evidence that a theory really does withstand scrutiny, theory-driven practice is a fair description of the outcome. A theory—good or bad, and with key claims often untested—can be used to tell a practitioner what to do with clients. So long as a practitioner is prepared to simplify an athlete's uniquely personal and complex needs into one of our very simple theories, that is, *untested*, or insufficiently tested, and *highly simplified* (i.e. parsimonious). To clarify here, many theories in sport and exercise psychology contain two or three categories into which behaviours/emotions/ strategies can be classified. Some more but still relatively few categories are the 'parsimonious' preference. And much of the research in sport and exercise psychology is, quite famously, either based in labs away from actual performance settings (cf. Martens, 1979, 1987) or based on cross-sectional survey data and correlational analysis (cf. Vealey, 2006; Keegan, 2015)—that is, insufficient evidence to know a theory is 'true'.

Let's think of an extreme (intentionally silly) example, but one that might resonate with those who are familiar with applied psychological practice. After several hours speaking with a psychologist, exploring life history and many important moments in their life, an athlete is told by the practitioner: 'It is clear to me that you are thinking like a fish, and you need to think more like a robot'. Confused, the athlete seeks clarification. 'Well you see, fish have very small brains, which really only focus on self-preservation and making snap judgements to avoid being eaten. They are reactive, not proactive. Robots are much more analytical and rational. They plan and execute. By following your first instinct all the time, you are letting your inner fish dominate your life. We need to cultivate your inner robot.' Being based at a university, the athlete asks if the advice has been supported by research. 'The model we use is *based on* science, inspired by science, but not actually used by researchers. It is more "real world".' The theory being used by this practitioner is both insufficiently tested, and a gross simplification. We can go further and imagine a coach with a team, trying to create the optimal social atmosphere. In some ways this makes the example more forceful. The same practitioner might advise: 'You need to create a less fishy atmosphere, and promote robot-ness instead'. The coach may protest that she feels she is already doing that. 'Ah but the players are giving very high fish scores in their Perceives Fish-Robot Climate Questionnaires [PFRCQ].' The coach might ask what she can do to remedy the situation. 'Well actually it depends on the individual athlete, but you could do things in a less fishy manner, and try to help them use robotty language and goals.' The coach might ask if that advice has been tested scientifically. 'The model we use is based on the latest quantum neuroscience. We have lots of studies proving that fish and robots are different; but using that information to inform practice? That's very contemporary right now: much too new to have been tested yet by those slow boring researchers.' The coach might seek clarification that there are only fishy and robotty social environments. 'Yes, every single behaviour you exhibit promotes either fishiness or robot-ness, and we need to create more of the robot-ness.

There are no other 'Nesses' in the complex social environment of a team.' Exhausted, the coach might even inquire as to what a 'Ness' is: fishiness or robottiness. 'Ah it's a complex network of neural quantum magnetic ion activations, that occurs either in the fish brain or the robot brain.'

Now. Paraphrasing the comedian Stewart Lee, (fortunately) *neither of the above stories are true*. But what they tell us about the research-practice gap may well be true (or rather, reflect the lived reality in sport and exercise psychology—i.e. be true). If there is a sufficient gap between the researchers and practitioners, neither paying attention to the others nor checking/evaluating each other's work, then one side of the divide may end being rather unscientific. In the above examples it is the applied practice side, but in fact both sides of the divide may ultimately be 'unscientific', in different ways. Researchers working away furiously on theories that might never have been intended to support real-world application could also be viewed as a poor manifestation of science. Yet many regulatory bodies actually expect applied practitioners to use theories and research, even if it does not actually help them in applied settings. The reason for this is the scientist-practitioner model; or rather, the way we interpret and implement the scientist-practitioner model.

The Scientist-Practitioner Model in Sport and Exercise Psychology

Following its foundation at the Boulder Conference in 1949 (Benjamin & Baker, 2000; Raimy, 1950), the scientist-practitioner (SP) model has gained prominence in many other areas of psychology, and is currently receiving increased attention in sport and exercise psychology, following Weinberg's (1989) influential paper. For example, consecutive conferences of AASP have emphasised a requirement for papers to support/facilitate an SP perspective, requiring: '…clarification of the integration and reciprocal relationships among theory, research, and interventions/practice' (AASP Conference Speaker Guidelines, 2013).

The increased formal regulation of applied sport and exercise psychology has meant that practitioners are increasingly held accountable for their practice—with annual registration, mandatory record keeping and obligatory continued professional development. Within these processes, there is an increasing demand for the integration of scientific principles into the practice of psychology (Chwalisz, 2003; Hayes, Barlow, & Nelson-Gray, 1999). Consequently, the 'scientific process' is presented as extremely relevant to applied practitioners—who may frequently be asked to defend their consulting processes and the quality of their decision-making (Acierno, Hersen, & Van Hasselt, 1996).

The core of the scientist-practitioner model is most succinctly explained by Shapiro (2002, p. 234): adapted here for sport and exercise psychology. A scientist-practitioner should: (a) deliver psychological assessment/testing and psychological intervention procedures in accordance with scientifically based protocols; (b) access and integrate scientific findings to inform consulting decisions; (c) frame and test hypotheses that inform consulting decisions; (d) build and maintain effective teamwork with other relevant professionals that support the delivery of scientist-practitioner contributions (e.g. coaches, trainers, physiotherapists, other sport scientists, team managers, etc.); (e) provide research-based training and support to other relevant professionals in the delivery of sport psychology (examples as per d); and (f) contribute to practice-based research and development to improve the quality and effectiveness of sport psychology consulting, i.e. researching one's own practice and disseminating the findings. Notably, those who are well versed in the philosophy-of-science will already have noticed that criteria a–c contain a number of assumptions about the nature of how science should be conducted, and this observation arguably captures the conflict at the heart of the scientist-practitioner model: a conflict which has previously been argued to have *undermined the proper implantation of the scientist-practitioner model*—its 'fatal flaw' (Albee, 2000, p. 247). Authors such as Eysenck (1949) and Shapiro (1955) argued that the scientist-practitioner model should only reflect positivist assumptions. However, many others have argued *both* that a positivist philosophy underpins the scientist-practitioner model *and* that this is inappropriate: deepening the divide between researchers and practitioners, and suppressing other highly relevant, legitimate and useful philosophical stances (Breen & Darlaston-Jones, 2008; Corrie & Callahan, 2000; Goedeke, 2007; Kanfer, 1990; O'Gorman, 2001; Page, 1996).

The primary goal of the scientist-practitioner model is to equip psychology practitioners with skills to apply basic scientific principles (APA Committee on Training in Clinical Psychology, 1947); basing professional activities on scientific foundations. The model aims to produce psychologists that are able to both provide successful services and capable of contributing to the research literature during their professional career (Belar & Perry, 1992; Drabick & Goldfried, 2000; Milne & Paxton, 1998; Stoner & Green, 1992). The scientist-practitioner model was conceived to integrate science and practice, such that 'each must continually inform the other' (Belar & Perry, 1992, p. 72). However, so long as sport psychologists equate the scientist-practitioner model and 'being scientific' with ideas of positivism, then there may remain significant resistance to the adoption of the scientist-practitioner model in sport and exercise psychology. Practitioners adopting different philosophical paradigms will simply reject the scientist-practitioner model, even if it means being thought of as 'unscientific' (Albee, 2000; Belar, 2000; Chwalisz, 2003; Drabick & Goldfried, 2000; Gaudiano & Statler, 2001; Stoltenberg et al., 2000; Stricker, 1997, 2000). Thus, if our regulatory regimes promote a scientist practitioner model, but our interpretation of the scientist-practitioner model is based on naïve positivist assumptions, then the 'gap' between researcher and practitioners will widen.

Reclaiming 'Theoretical Practice'

It is arguably appropriate to expect our applied practitioners to be scientific: psychology is a science after all. It is inarguably inappropriate, however, to expect all applied practitioners to embody the assumptions of naïve positivism—an approach disproved as long ago as Hume (1738) and clinically dissected by Popper (1959, 1969). Further, as explained elsewhere in this book, while positivism often suffices as a philosophy in the physical sciences, it fails comprehensively when addressing complex mental and social phenomena. Martens (1979, 1987) made these points very eloquently, but even when we agree with his arguments, our research and applied practice has remained broadly the same (cf. Vealey, 2006).

If sport and exercise psychology is to achieve a strong alignment between research and practice, as required by the scientist-practitioner model, then we must accept a wider variety of ontological and epistemo-logical stances as being 'scientific'. That is not to say that researchers and/or practitioners should make it up as they go along (unscientifically), but rather we should recognise, adhere to and transparently report coherent philosophical stances. We should be accountable regarding philosophy. If a researcher or practitioner claims to be adopting a phenomenological approach, we should hold them to that and not approve of 'switching' to other stances for no reason (the 'bad' type of eclecticism noted earlier). But first, we must recognise, talk about, understand, implement and evaluate different approaches: in both research and practice. In this way, it may one day be possible to achieve a type of theoretical practice that works. It may be hypothetically possible to develop theories that are a little more nuanced and contextualised, not dogmatically parsimonious and generalising across all sports/levels/cultures. It may be possible to develop ways of practitioners being closely involved in the generation and 'testing' of theories, within their practice, rather than waiting to see what evidence the researchers can offer up. As such, there may be a future in which 'theoretical practice' might become workable. Nonetheless, as long as our theories remain highly abstract, generalised, parsimonious and relatively untested: that is, not tested 'to destruction' but rather 'applied' to different problems—so long as this remains the case, then theoretical practice will be rightly decried as inappropriate and unworkable.

Practical Theories

As alluded to earlier, many authors have argued that theories, themselves, are not particularly important (i.e. not worth defending or protecting too ferociously). Rather they are merely tools to assist in the solving of important problems. Martens' was arguing that, in his view, theories had become the dominant driving force in sport psychology; that we had become a profession driven by our tools and gadgets as opposed to providing efficient solutions to meaningful problems. Martens (and many others since) argued that the theories driving sport psychology research were not 'fit-for-purpose' when it comes to applied practice. Such a situation is extremely problematic, because—put simply—one would expect leading theories in sport psychology to be useful in real-world sport psychology. But ostensibly, they aren't. The following is a short list of criticisms of leading sport psychology theories, generated by undergraduate students who were three weeks into a second-year class. The responses were produced following two seminars in which the students had been asked to propose theory-based interventions (e.g. Felde, Pensgaard, Lemyre & Abrahamsen, 2010) for hypothetical athletes requiring support (taken from Keegan, 2015; p. 247–253):

- There are multiple theories for each topic—anxiety, motivation, confidence and so on—even discounting the really old ones…they can't all be right. Which one should we choose, and why?
- The core tenets of each theory could be applied to almost any athlete, any time, anywhere. Surely they're supposed to help this specific athlete, or problem?
- The theories are usually very simplistic, with perhaps 2–6 core considerations. The real people in our examples are much more complex than this. Do we just have to simplify and 'shoe-horn' them into these frameworks?
- The theories tell us exactly what to look for and measure—often even having accompanying measurement tools/questionnaires that are specific to that theory. What might we be missing by adopting these theories and only looking for what they tell us to?
- Most of the popular and most heavily researched theories do not differentiate between ages, competitive levels, contexts, personal backgrounds, ethnicity and culture…how are we supposed to apply one to this specific athlete?
- Once we do apply one theory to the athlete, it seems to suggest a large number of possible interventions. Which one is right, or how could we tell?

It was interesting how quickly undergraduate students were able to express these concerns—once they had been 'given permission'. Students quickly realised that basing applied interventions purely on 'textbook' theories would be highly problematic, and probably ineffective. Of course, one must also consider the weight of evidence testing theories and interventions, as well as one's hard-earned professional judgement during such a decision, but does this cancel out the damage done by the relative paucity of relevant, highly applied, theories?

Perhaps we need to reconsider what a theory is, or should be. A popular and well-argued explanation was given by Stephen Hawking in his book *A Brief History of Time* (1988; p. 11—italics and parentheses added):

> In order to talk about the nature of the universe [or the mind]... *you have to be clear about what a scientific theory is.* I shall take the simpleminded view that a theory is just a model... and a set of rules that relate quantities in the model to observations that we make. *It exists only in our mind and does not have any other reality.* A theory is a good theory if it satisfies *two requirements*: [1] It must accurately describe a large class of observations on the basis of a model that contains only a few arbitrary elements, and [2] it must make definite predictions about the result of future observations. For example, Aristotle's theory that everything was made out of four elements, earth, air, fire and water, was simple enough... *but it did not make any definite predictions.* On the other hand, Newton's theory of gravity was based on an even simpler model, in which bodies attracted each other with a force that was proportional to a quantity called their mass and inversely proportional to the square of the distance between them. Yet it predicts the motions of the sun, the moon, and the planets to a high degree of accuracy.

Two conditions: a theory must explain the existing observations and it must make testable predictions about future events. Without meeting these two conditions, then the rules specified by the theory could just as well be the rules of a game or a sport. There is also a theme that the theory should, ideally, be as simple as practically possible and I would add that, if it is to serve our purposes, the theory must be communicable such that someone other than the 'holder' can understand it too. But that's it.

We can go on to consider what makes a good theory, as opposed to a bad one, but the theoretical 'working model' used by practitioners in applied practice can be discussed in these terms. This chapter is arguing that these theories often fail this basic test—as well as being insufficiently tested—making them not fit for purpose, and thus contributing to the research-practice gap.

Hawking's definition is consistent with that of Popper (discussed in Chap. 1). In his attempts to delineate scientific theories from either non-scientific or pseudo-scientific theories, Popper offered a range of criteria for a 'good' theory. Firstly, a good theory should be 'bold' in that it should rule out, or prohibit a range of events or possibilities. One key criticism of many theories, raised by the students above, is that they often permit numerous and even contradictory possibilities. The following passage illustrates the problem as Popper saw it, in relation to psychotherapy (1963; p. 368—italics added):

> I may illustrate this by two very different examples of human behaviour: that of a man who pushes a child into the water with the intention of drowning it; and that of a man who sacrifices his life in an attempt to save the child. Each of these two cases can be explained with equal ease in Freudian and in Adlerian terms. According to Freud the first man suffered from repression (say, of some component of his Oedipus complex), while the second man had achieved sublimation. According to Adler the first man suffered from feelings of inferiority (producing perhaps the need to prove to himself that he dared to commit some crime), and so did the second man (whose need was to prove to himself that he dared to rescue the child). *I could not think of any human behaviour which could not be interpreted in terms of either theory.* It was precisely this fact—that they always fitted, that they were always *confirmed*—which in the eyes of their admirers constituted the strongest argument in favour of these theories. *It began to dawn on me that this apparent strength was in fact their weakness.*

So by prohibiting certain eventualities, a theory exposes itself to being false, and Popper viewed this as a strength. As such, practitioners should not be swayed by theories that appear unfalsifiable, or perhaps able to explain any and all circumstances. This may even mean the theory/model is not scientific in any formal sense—because there is no way to ever test it and falsify it. The more possibilities a theory rules out, the better. Pragmatically—as noted by the undergraduate students earlier—this is actually very useful, as we need our working model to identify specific courses of action and preferably not to permit/allow any 'treatment'.

Further to the above, if a theory rules out possibilities that we might ordinarily expect (or makes unusual/unexpected predictions), and these predictions are then tested but remain unfalsified, then the theory is a good one. Successfully predicting things, which other theories failed to, is clearly a strength: especially if it can be done with as few rules and qualifiers as possible. This latter idea of simplicity originates from the trend that many existing and popular theories tend to 'sprout' additional qualifiers and 'get-out clauses' when faced with problematic observations—the so-called Duhem-Quine principle (Gillies, 1998).

So from the above, it is clear that good scientific theories should be helpful to applied practitioners when contemplating their 'case formulation'. The theory or model should explain any data gathered during the intake and aspects of the relationship, and make concrete predictions about what will be helpful. As such, the theory is a useful *tool* to be used for the benefit of the client: it is expendable. When a tool is not right for the job, a tradesperson would use a different tool, and the same should arguably apply to the practicing psychologist. However, in the 'free market' of tools for tradespeople, sellers care deeply about how useful their tools are, and conduct market research exploring what the practitioners want in a tool, on order to win their custom. Those sellers know that their customers, the tradespeople, have choices and could simply choose another more useful (or useable) tool. In contrast, many theories in sport and exercise psychology do not appear to have been designed, or at least evolved, with practitioners in mind. In many cases, the theories have evolved in such a way as to facilitate measurement (using questionnaires) and research (using correlational methods)—both of which use weight of numbers, naïve positivist assumptions and assumptions of parsimony to forcibly simplify real-life complexity.

Now. A particularly talented or rich tradesperson, who found the available tools unacceptable, could either build or commission the perfect tool for the job. There is a free market for this and a clear mechanism for the tradesperson to perform such a task. There is even likely to be a tidy profit in it if other people want to buy the new tool she created. In contrast, applied practitioners are rarely given an opportunity to participate in the creation and testing of sport and exercise psychology theories. In the current system, practitioners are cast as passive recipients or customers, receiving whatever theories and evidence researchers decide to offer them. It is difficult to imagine the mechanism through which a practitioner could take a new theory 'to market', for others to view, evaluate and perhaps adopt. Further, there is little or no reward to the applied practitioner for taking such an approach. Practitioners don't benefit particularly from citations and h-indexes. In fact, offering one's best ideas to others might be seen as entrepreneurial suicide. Hence, there is no mechanism nor any incentive to attract the ideas, feedback or creative contributions of applied practitioners in sport and exercise psychology.

Imagine, though, what might be the benefits of obtaining feedback, ideas, theories and research data from applied practitioners. Imagine how many of the above problems might be addressed, or at least tractable. We might be able to create an avenue for generating better theories, better research, better outcomes for clients, a better reputation for sport and exercise psychology…and more. If only we could find ways of creating theories that were focused on being practically useful, as opposed to theories that lend themselves to whatever methodologies and trends happen to dominate research at the time. The first step in evaluating each theory should be to apply to criteria from Hawking and Popper, above: explanation, falsifiability, clear predictions, easily expressed/ conveyed (and so, effectively, transparent and 'accountable') and ultimately *solving an important applied problem*, not an abstract, unimportant problem (on this point, 82% of humanities papers are never cited, and 32% of social science papers [Remler, 2014]: areas that sport and exercise psychology arguably occupy). So, for example, when we receive papers claiming to explain fractionally more variance in some subjectively rated concept that seems several steps removed from real-life… we should arguably be rejecting those from the outset and discouraging people from doing that research. We should be asking practitioner what types of theories we need to build, and what problems they perceive in existing ones—and then using that information both in the commissioning of research and in its evaluation. The first priority of 'practical theories' should be to support real-world athletes, coaches, practitioners, parents and governing bodies; one of the lower (lowest?) priorities should be advancing researchers' citations and impact factors. Sport and exercise psychology needs practical theories, but at the moment, we seem to have it all back to front.

Theories of Practice

As an additional consideration, not explicitly put forward in Martens' dichotomy of 'theoretical practice' versus 'practical theory', there is also an option for research to examine the 'art' of applied practice. Like any phenomenon, the processes of applied practice can be studied, described, modelled (or theorised) and evaluated. Recent work by Poczwardowski et al. (2014) and Keegan (2015) has started to describe the processes followed by practitioners. Keegan's model specifically suggests linkages between key processes followed by practitioners, and testable predictions. For example, the model could be used to predict that 'the quality of the needs analysis will contribute significantly to the quality of the outcomes'; or 'practitioners who maintain a consistent philosophical approach with each individual client will likely produce improved client experiences and outcomes'. Notwithstanding these very recent developments, sport and exercise psychology currently generates relatively little research examining the processes and mechanisms of applied practice. The following is a quote from a magazine article in computer design, with the word 'design' replaced by 'applied sport and exercise psychology'. The resulting passage is equally applicable to sport and exercise psychology, but it demonstrates once again that the problem is not unique to our own field: 'We know surprisingly little about how to do applied sport and exercise psychology. *There is no science of the practice*…. Applied sport and exercise psychology is still an art, taught by apprenticeship, with many myths and strong beliefs, but incredibly little evidence. We do not know the best way to do applied sport and exercise psychology. The real problem is that we believe we do. Beliefs are based more on faith than on data' (Norman, 2010—*italics* added).

As noted earlier, there is a strong tendency in sport and exercise psychology—and many fields—to cast applied practice as an art or craft: mythical and magical processes not open to the scrutiny of researchers. On the one hand, this is understandable given the profound differences in assumptions and methods between researchers (positivist, reductionist, lab-based and quantitative) versus practitioners (for whom almost all of those assumptions are inappropriate and ineffective). On the other hand, such a shroud of mysticism undermines the credibility and transparency of any discipline it affects: almost in direct proportion to the (figurative) magnitude of the research-practice gap.

What might be the barriers to researching the processes of applied practice? Well it is difficult. The methods and assumptions used by researchers would struggle to capture the process at all. It is also possible that researchers believe the size of their potential audience is limited. How many practitioners out there are likely to read, and more importantly cite, research that examines the processes and mechanisms of applied psychological practice? At present, if we compare to the number of other researchers, combined with all the students being force-fed the very same abstract and highly simplified theories, and the likelihood of receiving citations from those people—there is no contest. This is another reason why practitioners need to engage in writing, for formal journals and textbooks: writing that has traditionally been dominated by 'researchers' and 'academics'. Encouragingly, the 'outlets' for such writing are beginning to appear. There is the '*Journal of Sport Psychology in Action*' (AASP); the '*Journal of Applied Case Studies in Sport and Exercise Sciences*' (Taylor and Francis) and the journal '*Case-studies in Applied Sport and Exercise Psychology*' (Human Kinetics). At the time of writing, however, a review of the submissions, and outputs, of these journals reveals very few applied practitioners writing about the processes of applied practice…and rather too many academic researchers writing about the applications of their research.

What would be the benefits of researching applied practice? This should be a simple answer by this stage: (a) we would understand the processes of applied practice better; (b) we could therefore give our applied practitioners increased ability to deliver positive outcomes (and avoid negative outcomes) when they work with clients; (c) the very theories and research generated by researchers would be immediately used by practitioners in the real world, not simply remaining in journals where they may or may not be picked up by other researchers: actual 'impact'; (d) we could improve the training of applied practitioners and reduce the unreliability of simply letting trainees work it out for themselves in an 'apprenticeship' style of post-university training; (e) we could also, therefore, improve the accountability and transparency of applied practitioners and facilitate informed and meaningful reviews of practice and case studies; (f) thus, ultimately, we could increase the credibility of the field of sport and exercise psychology. Overall, therefore, it goes without saying that there is incredible value yet to be realised in proactively researching the processes, assumptions and mechanisms of applied practice.

Additional Approaches to Bridging the Research-Practice Gap

The preceding sections offer several options for bridging the research-practice gap, but a simple framework (Stokes, 1997) also offers additional cues as to where we might find additional opportunities. The framework offers two dimensions: (a) 'quest for fundamental understanding' and (b) 'consideration of use'. Each of these dimensions can simply be divided into 'high' versus 'low', and so classic academic research would typically score high on 'quest for fundamental understanding' ('pure science') but low on 'consideration for use' (that's somebody else's problem). In contrast, most practitioners would typically be very focused on how science is being used, and much less concerned with generating 'fundamental understanding'. Transitioning from 'typically' to 'ideally', we might seek to generate fundamental knowledge about the processes of applied practice (theories of practice), and to ensure that practice is informed by the most up-to-date and relevant research (practice theories and evidence-based practice). There are other options, however.

Stokes' framework is perhaps best remembered for its reference to 'Pasteur's quadrant', wherein many influential ideas (particularly those of Louis Pasteur) appear to have originated from the quadrant that is *both* highly concerned for producing new knowledge *and* its practical application. This high: high quadrant is often thought of as the most innovative aspects of Stokes' approach. Pasteur, as Stokes noted, never undertook a study that was not immediately applicable, or inspired by an applied problem. Pasteur's fundamental contributions to science, however, instigated the entire field of microbiology and revolutionised the way we view the cause and prevention of disease. The consideration of Pasteur's quadrant illuminates a path where applied practice is not inherently antagonistic to scientific rigour. Understanding, and being open to, this usage-inspired basic research enables us to move away from the either/or logic of research versus practice and encourages us to look for research questions that can contribute to both. Choosing an applied and interesting/relevant phenomenon, and uncovering the basic science underlying it, can set the stage for generating research that is recognised both by researchers and practitioners as highly meaningful and important. Hence, if we were able to create, encourage and recognise researchers who care deeply about applied practice, or practitioners who are interested in generating new knowledge, we may be creating the Louis Pasteurs of sport and exercise psychology. This might be achieved through training new recruits, upskilling and reskilling existing contributors and ensuring that the systems we create actually reinforces such skill sets (as an example, most academic contracts place almost no value whatsoever on applied practice and professional registration. Likewise, as noted earlier, there is little or no value for practitioners in publishing in many national regulation frameworks).

There remains, within Stokes' framework, a fourth quadrant: the low: low quadrant. Such individuals, groups or projects/activities would have little interest in generating new knowledge or ensuring that applied practice is supported and optimised. What sort of people or activities would be so disinterested in either of those aims? In short, it is arguably the consumers. People who receive the outputs of the scientific research and/ or the services offered by practitioners. When we think about what proportion of the population are either researchers or practitioners in sport and exercise psychology (or both!), we are, in fact, left with a very big group indeed. Thus, even if this large group is more passive, and consumes rather than produces, they must still contribute enormously to how sport and exercise psychology is understood, interpreted and valued.

So let's review, briefly, who and what might constitute this fourth quadrant. Stokes (1997) was clear that this group would be concerned with neither the creation nor the use of knowledge, but may still explore and interact with the topic area. Using the example of ornithology informing the (at the time) popular hobby of birdwatching, he cited Peterson, the well-known author of birdwatching guides. Moreover, Reeves (2006) suggested that research in this quadrant targets the instrumental and educational developments that are preliminary to the activities in Bohr's and Edison's quadrants. Thinking about that for a moment, the importance of the 'fourth quadrant' becomes clearer. Almost everyone entering or interacting with the other three quadrants will originate from this 'fourth quadrant'. All of their expectations, understanding, biases and critical faculties will have been developed within this fourth quadrant. What people ask of a science, expect from a science, and think of as science will be determined by the knowledge and activities within the fourth quadrant. That sounds important. Anybody becoming a researcher in sport and exercise psychology will have started out in the Fourth Quadrant. Anybody becoming a practitioner in sport and exercise psychology will have started out in the Fourth Quadrant. Any athlete, coach or parent receiving applied sport psychology support will likely be in this fourth quadrant, and anybody hearing about sport psychology on TV or through media reports of research findings will inhabit the fourth quadrant. Yet what are the contents of this quadrant? What do people typically expect of sport and exercise psychology, and how close is that to what researchers and/or practitioners deliver? Does anybody really know, and if not, shouldn't we be studying this? Further, we might need to explore how to engage better with the people in that fourth quadrant. In this way, we might be able to create better 'default' understanding of sport and exercise psychology, more realistic expectations of our research and practice, and ultimately better implementation of the knowledge and understanding generated by practitioners and researchers.

Conclusion

In summary, this chapter has reviewed the wider debate regarding the research-practice 'gap'—occurring throughout most areas of science—and illustrated how it may apply to sport and exercise psychology. Even in our specialist field, there is a long history of such a gap being explicitly acknowledged, criticised and, unfortunately, causing problems. Options for reducing the 'gap' in sport and exercise were also reviewed, and there is reason for optimism after all. Sport and exercise psychology is—by nature—a highly applied discipline, with most of the content intended to be used by practitioners, coaches, athletes and parents on a daily basis. Contrast this to some disciplines where the scientific content is so specialised that only a very few people can understand or apply it: sport and exercise psychology are happening all around us every day. The potential population of the 'fourth quadrant' is enormous, but we are currently paying those people little or no attention. Thus, when they engage with either practitioners or researchers their expectations can be wayward, and this can undermine the effectiveness of those exchanges. Likewise, practitioners and researchers appear to be quite disengaged, for the reasons discussed at the beginning of the chapter. The consequences of these 'disconnects' are ostensibly quite severe, and warrant serious consideration. This chapter has built the case that we can address this problem by: (a) reconsidering the meaning of 'theoretical practice'; (b) building practical theories with the 'end users' in mind, and being clear that the end users are not simply other researchers; (c) considering theories of practice, not merely theories limited to concepts and abstract ideas; (d) increasing the frequency and clarity of discourse between practitioners and researchers; (e) creating more people who can inhabit 'Pasteurs Quadrant' and speak the language of both research and application, jointly considering both sides of each issue; and (f) improve the knowledge, language and discourse in the 'fourth quadrant' by deliberately and frequently engaging with the wider public and 'consumers' of sport and exercise psychology. In this way we might change the nature of the exchange from a product that consumers can 'take or leave' into a co-development, conversation and relationship. As an additional benefit, this may lead to the redirection of people's attention from other sources—media, social media, blogs and so on—to the scientific researchers and highly qualified practitioners we really want people to listen to. But unless we start that conversation, why would people listen to us? There are plenty of other protagonists competing for their attention, and we need to engage more widely, as well as clearly demonstrating the value of our own 'product'. If that involves simultaneously improving the very nature of our sport and exercise psychology 'product', great!

9

Developments to Enable Progress

Nailing the Colours

The primary purpose of this chapter is to provide the intellectual foundation for the final chapter, where we attempt to describe what a post-revolutionary world of sport and exercise psychology research might look like in some detail. Thus far, we have diagnosed various problems in the field, described research practice in both functional and dysfunctional forms, and made some piecemeal recommendations for future practice. The lenses through which we have viewed the field—or used to determine what is 'functional' or 'dysfunctional' —have been explicit, for the most part, but we have yet to fully 'nail our colours to the mast' where a normative theory of research is concerned. What philosophical theory of research do we endorse in the final analysis? What sort of principles should guide research practice? How could these principles be implemented both by individual researchers, groups and institutions? It is the goal of this chapter to answer such questions.

The chapter begins with a positive and in-depth exploration of Popper's mature theory of science, as reconstructed following the various criticisms of Kuhn, Lakatos and Feyerabend (amongst others). We choose a specific

© The Author(s) 2016
P. Hassmén et al., *Rethinking Sport and Exercise Psychology Research*,
DOI 10.1057/978-1-137-48338-6_9

essay as the focus as it provides the most explicit and coherent arguments *against* the relativism in Kuhn and Feyerabend, while maintaining a clear vision of what good research practice *should* involve if we are to achieve progress. We go on to highlight cases from earlier chapters where we believe this attitude and method has already been demonstrated in sport and exercise psychology, to help illustrate the point.

As we pointed out in Chap. 1, Popper was a logician, so the argument is logical rather than sociological (or psychological) in nature. This therefore raises the old issue of the possible versus the actual. Or as Lakatos put it: 'from a logical point of view, it is quite possible to play the game of science according to Popper's rules... the only problem is that it has never happened in this way' (Lakatos, in Motterlini, 1999: p. 98). Even if this is true, it does not rule out the possibility that it *could* happen this way, so we conclude by offering a realistic assessment of the social conditions conducive to establishing a critical rationalist 'constitution' and outline a possible professional ethical code (of sorts) for sport and exercise psychology researchers.

The Myth of the Framework

The subtitle is the title essay of the final book published by Popper in the year of his death (Popper, 1994). Given that the essay was originally prepared in 1965—the year of the Bedford College conference—it contains arguments clearly levelled at Kuhn's view of science and all forms of intellectual relativism (e.g. Quine, Feyerabend). It is Popper's clearest and arguably most emotive attempt to rally against what he saw as a mistaken and highly dangerous set of views about science. It takes in his studies of pre-Socratic philosophy (Popper, 2001), some of his early autobiographical accounts (Popper, 1978) and also his political philosophy as detailed in his 'war effort': *The Open Society and Its Enemies* (Popper, 1945). It is therefore perhaps the best single account of Popper's unified theory of science, expressed in passionate and unambiguous terms. In the following passages, we trace Popper's argument as closely as possible as the basis of a constitution (of sorts) for research, which is transformed and applied into a code of professional ethics in the final section of the chapter.

Popper's argument in *The Myth of the Framework* is composed of 16 parts, numbered in roman numerals. We summarise each step in turn below.

I. Popper establishes the nature of the Myth he will criticise. It is the myth of relativism that says truth is relative to our intellectual background and of the impossibility of mutual understanding between different cultures and generations.

II. He establishes his general intellectual (and moral) stance: that *'orthodoxy is the death of knowledge since the growth of knowledge depends on disagreement'*, and argues that the greatest step towards a better and more peaceful world was taken when the 'war of swords was replaced by the war of words' (p. 34).

III. Popper defines the Myth specifically in the following terms:

> A rational and fruitful discussion is impossible unless the participants share a common framework of basic assumptions or, at least, unless they have agreed upon such a framework for the purpose of discussion. (pp. 34–35)

He goes on to argue that the extent to which a discussion is fruitful is inversely related to difficulty (see Fig. 9.1). That is, discussion between participants who share a common framework is pleasant but rarely fruitful; whereas discussion between people holding different frameworks, though often difficult, leads to the valuable extension of intellectual horizons.

IV. Popper uses a historical example to show that agreement is an unrealistic goal of a discussion ('we must not expect too much') and that even where common assumptions are absent, common problems are often sufficient to yield fruitful outcomes (e.g. the production of new and interesting arguments), even if arguments are inconclusive.

V. He asserts that the Greek enlightenment (and human rationality) was born of 'culture clash', where people with different frameworks came together and chose to engage in critical discussion rather than cultural transmission (or conquering).

VI. Human rationality is made up of two components: (a) poetic inventiveness (myth-making or storytelling) and (b) criticism and critical discussion (criticising and improving on cosmological myths). Popper argues that (a) is universal and as old as human language, whereas (b) is relatively recent and was invented only once, by the Ionian School of philosophy led by Thales (followed by Anaximander). Popper goes on:

> The critical tradition was founded by the adoption of the method of criticising a received story or explanation and then proceeding to a new, improved, imaginative story which is in turn submitted to criticism. This method, I suggest, is the method of science. (p. 42)

VII.   Popper repeats the idea that critical discussion of this sort is rare and difficult, requiring ingenuity (in criticising and creating theories) and, above all, a recalibration of expectations. The natural instinct of

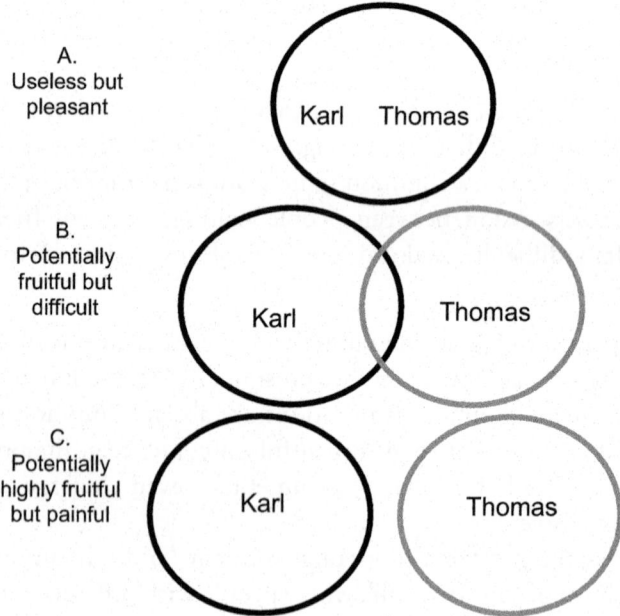

A.
Useless but pleasant

B.
Potentially fruitful but difficult

C.
Potentially highly fruitful but painful

Fig. 9.1 Possibilities for constructive discussion and growth in knowledge

participants in a debate is to win. Rational discussion, by contrast, does not aim at conversion: 'it is enough if we feel that we can see things in a new light or that we have got even a little nearer to the truth' (p. 44).

VIII. One of the main tendencies that supports the Myth is cultural relativism: the view that truth is relative to a specific cultural background. This is true in trivial cases of local laws and customs (e.g. driving on the left or right side of the road) but dangerous when applied to important moral and ethical matters (e.g. the freedom of citizens, the punishment and reform of criminals, etc.)

IX. Relativism is attractive because people confuse it with fallibilism (the true insight that all humans are prone to be biased). Popper argues that the doctrine of human fallibility cannot be used to support relativism because:

> There exists a very different attitude towards absolute truth [between fallibilism and relativism]... To the fallibilist, the notion of truth, and that of falling short of the truth, may represent absolute standards – even though we can never be certain that we are living up to them. But since they may serve as a kind of steering compass, they may be of decisive help in critical discussions. (p. 48)

X. Another form of relativism is attacked here, namely, 'ontological relativism' made popular by Quine who argued that different languages contain different assumptions about the structural characteristics of the world, embedded in their very grammar. Popper agrees that translation may make discussion difficult, but not impossible.

XI. In direct opposition to cultural and ontological relativism, Popper points out that culture clash is diminished if one or other of the opposing parties regards itself as superior (or inferior) to the other. The former case leads to a reluctance to change views on the part of the superior party; the latter case leads to a kind of blind acceptance or conversion on the part of the inferior party. He accepts that frameworks of various kinds act as 'intellectual prisons' but that we can become aware of them through culture clash. As awareness grows, we may break out of prisons into new, larger and wider prisons. Breaking out of an intellectual prison, however, is not a matter of routine and 'can only be the result of a critical and creative effort' (p. 52).

XII. Popper explicitly applies these ideas to the philosophy of science, drawing on his experiences as a young man where he noticed that every argument against Freudian and Adlerian[1] frameworks, for example, was interpreted by them so as to fit into the framework: 'criticism against Freudian ideas was due to repression; against Adlerian ideas as due to the desire to prove your superiority, thereby compensating for feelings of inferiority'. He concluded that the need for theories is immense, but that we must avoid getting *addicted* to a theory. Breaking out of our intellectual prisons is a twofold process: (a) we must formulate our beliefs so they can become a target of criticism; (b) we must demand that theories can be compared to others, which is made possible where they offer solutions to the same or similar problems. Discussions that follow are always possible and fruitful.

XIII. Popper targets Kuhn's view of science specifically, arguing against his 'incommensurability' thesis, describing in detail a number of counterexamples (mainly in physics) where the struggle *between* proponents of different frameworks *did* occur *and* led to fruitful results. He is willing to concede to Kuhn that 'there are irrational conversions', that 'there are scientists who follow the lead of others…accepting a new faith because the authorities have accepted it' and, regretfully, that 'there are fashions in science and there is social pressure'. He even accepts that normal science may one day come to dominate a field of enquiry, but that this would signal 'the end of science as we know it' (p. 57).

XIV. Having conceded ground to Kuhn, Popper reasserts his basic positive argument for fruitful critical discussion between frameworks.

XV. He mentions as an aside another special form of the Myth that says we must 'define our terms' before a discussion is possible (an implicit nod to Wittgenstein and his followers). Popper points out that such argument leads to an infinite regress.

---

[1] Popper spent time with Adler in the 1920s, working in social guidance clinics with working-class children in Vienna as he studied for his PhD in psychology.

XVI. The final section contains a 'logical diagnosis' of the Myth, where it is likened to the doctrine that it is impossible to discuss fundamental principles (or axioms). This view is mistaken since it rests on the assumption that rational discussion must have the character of a proof: a logical derivation from admitted premises. Popper therefore defines two methods of criticising: one correct, one mistaken. The *mistaken* method starts from the question: how can we justify this thesis from this theory? Whereas the *correct* method asks: what are the consequences of this theory? Are they acceptable to us? A potential criticism of the *correct* method is that 'preferable consequences' are judged as such by reference to our framework, leaving a model of self-justification. Popper counters by arguing that:

> We can *choose* to set ourselves standards of explanation, and methodological rules, which will help us achieve our goal and which it is *not* easy for any theory or framework to satisfy. Of course, we may chose not to do this: we may decide to make our ideas self-reinforcing.... But if we choose to do this... we will be turning our backs upon that tradition of critical thought (stemming from the Greeks and from culture clash) which has made us what we are, and which offers us the hope of further self-emancipation through knowledge. (p. 61)

What emerges then from Popper's essay is a strong logical and historical argument for the possibility and value of critical discussion between different frameworks (III); an appeal for the recalibration of expectations for critical discussion (IV, VII); and a passionate argument for the necessity of difficult and effortful culture clash for the growth of knowledge (V, VI). Yet in the final reckoning, Popper asks us to accept these arguments as a matter of *faith* (XVI). This argument—that taking a critical rationalist approach to science rests on a *choice*, or in the *belief* in Popper's specific definition of rationality—has struck some as insufficient to challenge the various forms of relativism that endanger science (cf. Bartley, III, 1962). However, if viewed as a sort of 'constitution' for research, which is itself always open to criticism and 'amendment'—critical rationalism applied to itself—it is possible to put this stance on more defensible footings (cf.

Bartley III, 1990; Munz, 1985). Box 9.1 outlines a set of critical rationalist rules and standards that might form the basis of a constitution for a
scholarly society (i.e. those informing conferences, journals and education programmes, such as the accreditation of qualifications).

Box 9.1 A Critical Rationalist Constitution for Research

1. The *goal* of critical discussion is the growth of knowledge (or simply
   clarifying a problem), *not* for one side to be declared the 'winners'.
2. Researchers holding different frameworks should be encouraged
   to debate as a stimulus for fruitful culture clash.
3. Critical discussions must be kept free of the influence of status
   (beyond blind peer review); the *quality* of argument is all important, *not* who is making it.
4. Protect against the onset of normal science (or 'theory addiction') through regular checks and facilitated culture clash (see 2).
5. The clear and unambiguous statement of research problems is a
   necessary condition for critical discussion.
6. Beliefs and theories should be formulated so that they can be
   criticised (i.e. state the conditions under which criticism would
   be accepted) (also helped by 5).
7. The primary goal of research education should be developing
   ingenuity in creating and criticising theories.
8. All of the rules and standards noted above (1–7) are open to
   improvement.

The attitude, if not the method, of critical rationalism has already been
glimpsed at points throughout this book. In Chap. 1 we encountered
Martens' (1987) attempt to outline (albeit mistakenly) opposing frameworks in sport psychology, with a view to initiating a critical discussion
that has undoubtedly been fruitful. The quote from John Nicholls in
Chap. 2 beautifully captures the Popperian spirit of constructive culture
clash, even if his theory has occasionally been defended in a staunchly
anti-Popperian spirit since his death (see Chap. 6). And in Chap. 8, we saw
what a critical rationalist approach might mean for the research-practice

gap and for applied practitioners in general. Between the glimpses, however, much of what we have reported and critically analysed has been decidedly anti-Popperian (or Kuhnian) in nature. We therefore turn to a conjectural sociological explanation for the current state of affairs, bringing together threads of arguments that have appeared in the previous eight chapters, in order to expose the workings of a system that, we argue, stymies progress in sport and exercise psychology.

A Sociological Fly in the Philosophical Ointment

Returning briefly to Chap. 1, we saw that powerful criticism has been levelled at critical rationalism, not least by Popper's former student, Paul Feyerabend. Feyerabend's most compelling objections were: (a) that the philosophical rules and standards offered by the Popperians must themselves be open to criticism and reform and (b) methodological prescriptions must be understood against the social and psychological realities of scientific life to be of any value. We quote again the relevant passage in full:

> Methodology, it is said, deals with what should be done and cannot be criticised by reference to what is. But we must make sure that the application of prescriptions leads to desirable results; and that we consider historical, sociological and psychological *tendencies* which tell us what is possible under given circumstances, thus separating feasible prescriptions from dead ends. (Feyerabend, 1975: p. 149)

Before we get carried away with methodology and 'what should be done', then, it seems appropriate to consider what is possible (psychologically and sociologically) and the circumstances under which subsequent prescriptions might be feasible. We have already encountered Kuhn's sociological view of science, of course, but this relatively benign account may be sharpened by reflecting on a more critical interpretation. One of the most prominent sociologists among the group of critical theorists was Pierre Bourdieu, who eventually directed his considerable conceptual arsenal at his own kind: academics. As he put it himself: 'every sociologist is a good sociologist of his rivals' (Bourdieu, 1975: p. 40).

Although there are similarities in Bourdieu's and Kuhn's accounts of science—both see it as a highly conservative practice—Bourdieu's version (1975, 1991) is more granular, in that he sees academics engaged fundamentally in a complex struggle for power and domination. First, Bourdieu argues that science is an autonomous social 'field', insulated from society, containing its own distinct rules and resources. A field is not a benign site for the practice of normal science, but a site of continuous *struggle* for recognition, which is achieved through the accumulation of various forms of 'capital' (Bourdieu, 1975).

Capital is a finite resource in any field: if one scientist has more, another must have less. In the case of 'social capital'—the extent and importance of one's professional networks—those in the higher echelons of power tend to hang together to the exclusion of others. It is not uncommon, for example, to see the same names on the editorial boards of journals in sport and exercise psychology, or the same groups of people congregating at conferences (see Chap. 6). Indeed, in our survey of four of the main editorial boards in the field (first reported in Chap. 4), 73 % of the respondents had been invited to the board by people they knew. Similarly, in the case of 'cultural capital'—for example, qualifications, knowledge of theories, academic writing skills and so on—PhD bursaries are limited in number; there is limited space in a handful of recognised journals; and only a few who can be recognised as experts (e.g. delivering keynote lectures at conferences, holding positions on journal editorial boards). Capital may also be converted from one form to another (Bourdieu, 1975). A student with rich parents (economic capital) may, for example, approach a world-class institution or leading expert to self-fund a PhD. They would thereby access the right kind of networks (social capital) and gain qualifications, knowledge and skills (cultural capital) that are valued in the field (e.g. knowledge of SDT and how to administer questionnaires and perform regression analysis—see Chap. 4). Their rise through the ranks of sport and exercise psychologists would presumably be swift, though hardly radical.

With the accumulation of valued forms of capital, a scientist eventually accrues what Bourdieu called 'symbolic capital', and with it the power to determine the 'official fiction' of the field (Bourdieu, 1975: p. 24). That is to say, 'they try to impose the definition of science that best conforms to their specific interest... the one best suited to preserving or increasing their specific capital' (Bourdieu, 1991: p. 13). This 'logic of practice' produces a structure, or order, that consists of objects (tools, textbooks, institutions) and a specific scientific habitus (dispositions, language) produced by education, all of which serve to perpetuate the interests of the powerful. This is most clearly seen in scholarly journals, which, 'by selecting articles in terms of dominant criteria, consecrate productions faithful to the principles of the official stance... whilst censoring heretical productions' (Bourdieu, 1975: p. 30). Qualifying Kuhn, then, revolution is the business of those richest in scientific capital. And as Fischman (2014) has noted, since there are no checks and balances to mitigate the power of journal editors, we place a great deal of trust in the hands of so few who are the ultimate arbiters of what counts as progress, what theories and methodologies are considered acceptable or unacceptable.

New entrants to a field, according to Bourdieu (1975, 1991), have two strategies open to them: (a) 'succession', which is risk-free and comes with a guaranteed but predictable career, or (b) 'subversion', which is infinitely more costly and hazardous and brings no profits unless complete redefinition of the dominant order is achieved. Succession is naturally the most popular strategy and involves a 'tacit adherence to the rules of the game' implying an investment and inclination to play the game. Such a path also leads to the 'training of selected legitimate scholars to take control over the instruments of research and publication' (Bourdieu, 1991). As we noted in previous chapters, this appears to have been the case in our field both historically (Chap. 2) and more recently (Chap. 5 and Chap. 6), with clear lineages from 'founding fathers' to current journal editors visible in many cases. Subversion does occur, however, but Bourdieu claims that this is only possible in rare cases where researchers high in symbolic scientific capital choose to leave 'socially superior fields' in order to develop new areas of study and thus 'realise themselves' (he uses Fechner and Freud as examples).

The outcome of this 'logic of practice' in the social sciences, according to Bourdieu (1975, 1991), has been the widespread adoption of positivism as 'the most legitimate form of science', with its criteria of individual objectivity and unproblematic truth. This, we recall, was Martens' point about sport psychology back in the late 1980s (see Chap. 1) though for Bourdieu such an outcome is entirely logical, given the success of natural scientific explanations in the twentieth century. We also noted this residual tendency for positivist criteria and standards in Chap. 4 with respect to the growing popularity of grounded theory and also pointed out how this may have partially caused a research-practice gap in Chap. 8. Hence, following Bourdieu's line of argument, in this 'space of competition, where agents and institutions work at valorising their own forms of capital' (Bourdieu, 1991: p. 7), the perpetuation of dominant ideologies and practices is inevitable—a kind of cultural determinism. In summary, then, Bourdieu suggests that most scientists are stuck in the game, struggling for recognition, where the rules and goals of the game are determined by a few powerful individuals—those rich in symbolic, scientific capital—with the aim of promoting their own interests. Given the data cited in Chap. 6, it is also worth pointing out that dominant 'de facto insider group' (Merton, 1975) in our field appears to be still very much white, Western and male.

Assuming we accept Bourdieu's account (which has a similar outcome to Kuhn's), we return then to Feyerabend's question from the beginning of this section and ask: to what extent is it possible to break (or subvert) this 'logic of practice'? How feasible is the application of a critical rationalist approach in sport and exercise psychology? At first glance, Bourdieu's rather deterministic account would suggest that it is not very feasible at all. However, going back to Marx, critical sociologists have found it difficult to account for change, especially positive change inspired by individual action. This has meant that their politics often stand in conflict with their sociology (Popper, 1945)[2]. Bourdieu allows for change through individual agency only in very special cases where specific individuals are endowed with symbolic capital (e.g. Fechner—see Chap. 2). They have the power to determine the 'habitus' and 'doxa' of the field: to set new norms and standards, new goals and new tacit rules for behaviour. Yet he also suggests that such moves would be illogical in most cases since the

---

[2] Marx offered an economic determinist sociology, the logic of which held that two classes would emerge and were bound to fight one another until the inevitable revolution. His political exhortations in publications such as *The Communist Manifesto*—for example, 'workers of the world, unite'—therefore make little sense if the revolution is inevitable (Popper, 1945).

powerful are most likely to have reached their position through championing the very ideas and behaviour that constitute the status quo. One potential but unlikely route to change, then, is for 'subverters' to accumulate sufficient symbolic capital to alter the norms of the field.

Bourdieu and others have, however, argued that the power of the 'ruling class' may be mitigated by exposing the mechanisms through which power operates. In the context of masculine domination in society, Bourdieu labelled one of those mechanisms 'symbolic violence' and noted that:

> The transformative action [of symbolic violence] is all the more powerful because it is for the most part exerted invisibly and insidiously through insensible familiarisation with a symbolically structured physical world and early, prolonged experience of interactions informed by the structures of domination. (Bourdieu, 2001: pp. 37–38)

In other words, symbolic violence is effective because it is naturalised, taken for granted and assumed to be part of the structure of things (recall the point in Chap. 6 on 'that's just the way things are'). Other critical sociologists with an interest in the mechanisms of power have reinforced this inverse relationship between power and visibility. Bourdieu's famous contemporary, Michel Foucault, for example, pointed out that 'power is tolerable only on the condition that it mask a substantial part of itself; its success is proportional to its ability to hide its own mechanisms' (Foucault, 1978: p. 86). Similarly, the political theorist Steven Lukes noted that 'the effectiveness of power is enhanced by being disguised or rendered invisible, by 'naturalisation' (i.e. through acceptance of conventions), and by 'misrecognition' of its sources and modes of operation' (Lukes, 2005: p. 141). The conclusion we might draw from this insight seems to be this: if power is exercised most effectively when it is *least* visible (to the dominated), its effectiveness will be diminished if it is made *more* visible.

We have attempted already in a number of the preceding chapters to undertake such a task. We have shown how researchers applying Self-Determination Theory 'save' the theory from criticism and how advocates of Grounded Theory attempt to close down debate about its central tenets

(Chap. 4). We have described the operation of 'old boys clubs' and the dominance of white, Western males in the upper echelons of power and anatomised anti-scientific practices used by some proponents of Achievement Goal Theory (Chap. 6). We have pointed out the ways in which measurement tools are perpetuated despite fatal flaws in the reasoning behind them (Chap. 7). And we have suggested that the goals of this academic game (e.g. improving your 'h-index') may be doing harm to the relationship between research and practitioners (Chap. 8). We have tried, in short, to explore the ways in which dominant ideas in sport and exercise psychology research have been established and continue to be perpetuated. But this is not enough. We need to go further than the critical sociologists and offer a positive vision and guidelines for the future based on normative models of science.

In this chapter we have thus far built an argument for a positive critical rationalist approach to research and we have noted the potential mechanisms that may prevent it from being realised. We have done so, in the spirit of the critical sociologists, so that readers may make better-informed *choices* about how they conduct themselves—as researchers, supervisors, teachers, students, reviewers, journal editors—in the future. There is no doubt that this is a difficult undertaking, with multiple forces acting in the opposite direction. Tenure systems in North America and Australia and the Research Excellence Framework (REF) in the UK certainly exert pressures on academics that support a Kuhnian or Bourdieusian approach to research. The critical rationalist approach also appears inconsistent with some of our natural cognitive biases—e.g. confirmation bias, bandwagon effect, congruence bias (Kahneman, 2012)—that may restrict our ability to really look for errors in our ideas, to break with the status quo or to truly test theories and give them up with effective criticism. Yet Popper himself was not blind to the sociological processes at work in science (see section XIII of the Myth); and he understood too well that personal psychological beliefs and biases can be overcome and superseded by strengthening 'institutional attitudes' (e.g. 'I have a personal preference for my theory, but as a scientist I am duty bound to give it up in light of convincing criticism') (Popper, 1978). Indeed, it is the goal of the final section of the chapter to further strengthen this positive argument and provide illustrations of how such ideas might manifest themselves in the field of sport and exercise psychology.

A Professional Ethics for Sport and Exercise Psychology Researchers

Having considered and resolved, to a degree, the main objections of the sociologists to the possible prescription of critical rationalism to sport and exercise psychology research, we return to an attempt to outline the theory in purely positive, constructive terms. We have already offered normative guidance for institutions (Box 9.1), which contained implications for individuals but did not specify guidance for individual behaviour. Such a task was undertaken, however, by McIntyre and Popper (1983) in the context of the medical profession. Based on a critical analysis of existing professional ethics derived from nineteenth-century medical acts—underpinned by positivist ideas of certainty, accumulation and authoritative expertise—McIntyre and Popper (1983) propose a new medical ethics composed of ten theses. We conflate the ten theses into six more general propositions as a basis for a conjectural critical rationalist professional ethics for sport and exercise psychology. Some of the ideas are familiar, of course, and overlap with Box 9.1, but the prescriptions have a more individual and applied connotation.

Statements 1 and 2 represent claims about the limits of human knowledge and therefore authority. McIntyre and Popper (1983) believed

---

Box 9.2 A Critical Rationalist Professional Ethics for Sport and Exercise Psychology

1. Our knowledge far transcends what any individual can know and changes quickly. Therefore, there can be no authorities. There can be better and worse scientists, and the better scientist is aware of their limitations.

We are not authorities

2. We are fallible and it is impossible for anybody to avoid making mistakes. The idea that we must avoid mistakes has to be revised.

   We are liable to make mistakes

3. Errors may lurk in even our best tested theories. It is the responsibility of the professional to search for these errors, a task that is helped by the proposal of new theories.

   Search for errors

4. Our attitude towards mistakes must change. Hiding and forgetting mistakes must be regarded as a deadly sin. Rather, we must search for mistakes and investigate them fully.

   Do not hide mistakes—investigate them

5. We must train ourselves to be self-critical, but also accept that criticism from others is necessary and especially valuable if they approach problems from different backgrounds or frameworks.

   Be self-critical and invite criticism from others (especially outsiders)

6. Rational criticism should be directed to clearly defined mistakes and be expressed in a form that allows its refutation. It should be inspired by the aim of getting nearer to the truth and should therefore be impersonal.

   Offer clearly defined, impersonal criticism (and invite it back)

that inclinations towards authority and omniscience were at the heart of much that was wrong (even dangerous) in the medical profession—covering up mistakes to avoid recrimination may even lead to avoidable deaths—and therefore based their alternate code on fallibilist footings. Statements 3–6 represent the consequences of accepting

1 and 2: they are behavioural prescriptions for conduct in research (and may also be applied to practitioners). Since we have tried to be as clear and pithy as possible in our adaptation of this professional ethics, some examples of the potential practical implications for both researchers and journal editors and reviewers are offered here for illustration (Table 9.1). A full discussion of the implications is reserved for the final chapter.

Some of the proposals in Box 9.2 should be self-evident and self-explanatory, based on what has already been said; others require some explanation. Proposal 4b, for example, makes reference to Sparkes' (2002) call for researchers to write in the style of 'confessional tales', or accounts that problematise research, revealing the truth of the process rather than covering it up with impersonal retro-sanitised accounts. The notion that scientific papers are written in a deliberately misleading manner is not new. As far back as 1963, the Popperian biologist Sir Peter Medawar asked 'is the scientific paper a fraud?' and gave a clear and affirmative answer. For Medawar (1963), reports of scientific studies were presented in a positivist fashion, following an inductive logic and presenting discoveries as indisputable facts. Such an approach also demands the editing out of mistakes and errors, for they would surely burst the bubble of certainty. Although, following Medawar, it is now a broadly Popperian convention that underpins many natural scientific papers, there remains a systematic 'editing out' of mistakes and false starts that continues to misrepresent the actual practice of science. As Howitt and Wilson (2014) conclude: 'Doing science and communicating science are quite different things; in the 50 years since Peter Medawar expressed his concern about the scientific paper, little has changed' (p. 484).

The confessional approach, then, is far more consistent with critical rationalism since it would: (a) highlight errors and allow other researchers to make better critical appraisals and (b) allow more of the community, especially students, to learn from the mistakes of others. Yet a very brief literature search of the field of sport and exercise psychology revealed only three papers that have thus far taken an explicitly confessional approach (e.g. Schinke et al., 2012). It may be that confessional tales still represent too radical a break from the established norms (see Chap. 6 and earlier in

Table 9.1 Proposals for bringing a critical rationalist professional ethics to life

Proposition	Researcher behaviour	Reviewer/editor behaviour
(3) Search for errors	(a) Undertake methodological approaches that are most likely to reveal errors in a theory (i.e. avoid soft but convenient 'tests' such as correlation/regression)	(a) Invite critical reviews or meta-analytical studies that focus on exploring anomalous data in bodies of popular research (e.g. SDT research). Encourage authors to comment on 'progressive' or 'degenerating' shifts
(4) Do not hide mistakes—investigate them	a) Search for anomalous data, especially with well-tested theories (e.g. AGT), and treat this data seriously. Interpret data with reference to multiple competing theories where possible (or invent new theories)	(a) Inspect a study's results closely and challenge instances where anomalous data is explained away (especially with the use or creation of ad hoc hypotheses)
	(b) Write papers in the style of a 'confessional tale' (Sparkes, 2002), admitting errors and allowing others to learn from mistakes	(b) Be tolerant of alternative writing styles and of the publication of unavoidable mistakes that the research community may learn from
	(c) Conduct and report on case studies of applied practice, especially where experience problematises received theory and practices (also see Chap. 8)	(c) Make space in journals for the publication of honest, 'warts and all' case studies
(5) Be self-critical and invite criticism from others (especially outsiders)	(a) See 4b (above) (b) Seek out and attend conferences arranged by rivals and deliver papers inviting the harshest form of critical discussion	(a) See 4b (above) (b) Arrange conferences and symposia with the explicit aim of facilitating culture clash (with the goal of learning from the discussion, rather than declaring a winner)
	(c) Seek reviews from researchers outside of your immediate social and professional circles	(c) Seek out reviewers for papers who come from very different subdisciplinary backgrounds as the author(s)

(continued)

Table 9.1 (continued)

Proposition	Researcher behaviour	Reviewer/editor behaviour
(6) Offer clearly defined, impersonal criticism (and invite it back)	(a) When offering theories or explanations, define the conditions under which criticism would be accepted	(a) Offer clear guidelines for authors and reviewers concerning the way theories and arguments should be presented and how they should be criticised
	(b) Ensure that criticism of others is rooted in an explicit philosophical stance and directed at the argument rather than the individual(s)	(b) Consider publishing the account of peer-review process in journals, allowing others to benefit

this chapter), though it is slightly more common to see researchers writing 'reflexive accounts' (we found approximately 40 papers), which may be natural precursors to the emergence of full confessional tales (Sparkes & Smith 2013).

Proposals 6a and 6b are also difficult and therefore deserve further explanation. With respect to 6a, we have already made piecemeal recommendations as to the ways in which, for example, SDT and AGT could be made better targets for criticism (Chap. 4 and Chap. 6, respectively). That is to say, while it is possible to derive clearly testable hypotheses from these theories (they are technically 'scientific', under a Popperian definition), researchers have largely chosen not to act in a scientific manner (but for understandable reasons, as we have seen). Popper's deceptively simple but intellectually challenging principle for promoting scientific behaviour was to require all researchers to specify the conditions under which theories would fail. This, we recall, is what Einstein did, but what Freud and Adler could not.

In his personal account of working under Popper, Agassi (2008) described how this principle informed the famous Tuesday afternoon seminars at the LSE, where speakers were asked to present an interesting problem *and* a solution, before being pressed for the conditions under which it would fail. For Agassi, these seminars were the most intellectually stimulating and invigorating experiences one could imagine but 'unreasonably demanding' for most (Agassi, 2008). Popper's behaviour, it seems, did not live up to his own heady principles (Agassi, 2008), but this does not mean the principle cannot be converted into guidance for authors and reviews in journals. Knudson, Morrow and Thomas (2014) have recently noted the absence of clear evaluation standards in a range of kinesiology journals, yet their recommendations for improving such standards are not informed by a particular view of progress in science. It is instances such as these, then, that an explicit critical rationalist ethics can be useful. Not only does it define processes and standards for progress (see below), but by taking an explicit and informed stance about publication standards allows for more effective critical discussion of the same standards. That is to say, if a journal were to publish a generic list of criteria (e.g. like that offered by Knudson et al., 2014), someone may accept or reject them. But if criteria are derived from a well-developed logical philosophy of science, a critic has to engage explicitly with the underlying view in order to criticise the criteria. And this would surely lead to a better quality debate, and therefore likely improvements in the evaluation criteria.

The final proposal (6b)—formalising the depersonalisation of criticism—is highly contentious. It certainly has a whiff of positivism about it, and those of a relativist or constructivist persuasion are likely to remind us of the myth of individual objectivity. Indeed, there are few who can claim to have done more damage to positivism than Popper (Magee, 1973), yet he also championed a form of 'objective knowledge'. For Popper (1994), however, the objectivity of knowledge is derived from 'intersubjective criticism', *not* from some personal quality of the researcher. Once written and published, a theory becomes an object in what Popper called world 3: the world of human-made cultural artefacts, as distinct from the world of physical objects (world 1) and the world of the human mind (world 2). Once in world 3, a theory becomes objective from its originator insofar as it is subject to the interpretations and criticisms of the broader community. As a theory undergoes criticism from the community, its weaknesses are exposed and it is revised and reformulated, or dies altogether. What emerges from this process of intersubjective criticism, then, is more corroborated, more truth-like, more trustworthy product. In short, more objective knowledge.

Of course, the academic community already has some mechanisms for promoting the depersonalisation of criticism. As we saw in Chap. 3, this is arguably the primary purpose of a double-blind peer-review system. However, we have also seen that the peer-review system has come in for sharp criticism in recent times, and we would argue that it is ripe for 'rethinking'. Following the critical rationalist professional ethics, journals may consider widening or extending the peer-review process, publishing papers along with reports of the review process, allowing more of the community to learn from, and engage in, the discussion. Some journals in related fields (e.g. *International Journal of Sports Science and Coaching*) regularly feature articles followed by multiple critical responses, before allowing the authors of the original article a 'reply to their critics'. Opening up peer review in this way—for peer review does not imply that the process ends at the point of publication—will surely establish new norms for critical discussion of the big ideas in our field. And, if researchers ensure that criticism is aimed at the idea or argument rather than the researcher, and if this principle is protected via published guidelines (Cf. Knudson et al., 2014), criticism is likely to be more effective. Such a move is fundamental under a critical rationalist ethics since 'the growth of knowledge depends on disagreement' (Popper, 1994: p. 34).

Conclusion: Defining and Enabling 'Progress'

We began this chapter with a positive and constructive argument for taking a critical rationalist approach to research and explained how it could become manifest in various dimensions of research practice. We then considered Feyerabend's question concerning the extent to which this may be possible in the given social environment. We therefore counterposed Popper's views in the *Myth*, with Bourdieu's rather conservative vision of science, which leaves little room for changing the status quo. Nevertheless, Bourdieu, like Kuhn, *does* leave room in 'extraordinary' (or 'subversive') cases, and the broader critical sociological approach suggests that dysfunctional power-plays of the kind Bourdieu describes are mitigated by rendering the mechanisms of the 'logic of practice' more visible. In this space we offered a tentative professional ethics for researchers and described a few concrete proposals for progress.

Back in Chap. 1 we discussed the various definitions of progress implicit (and sometimes explicit) in the four main philosophical views of science. Given the title and purpose of this chapter, it is necessary to conclude with a brief reflection on the nature of progress. We summarise the four views below:

Popper—Theories become increasingly truth-like (i.e. they explain more facts) and better corroborated (i.e. they survive more and harsher criticism).

Kuhn—The range of the paradigm is extended and deepened (i.e. the paradigm achieves intellectual monopoly) and more precision measurement tools are created.

Lakatos—More scientists work on progressive research programmes, or creating progressive shifts in degenerating programmes.

Feyerabend—There is an increase in the invention and proliferation of new alternative theories and new standards for research (sometimes including the revival of defunct theories and research programmes).

At an individual level, we have argued for a Popperian definition of progress, and occasionally for a Lakatosian definition at the group or institutional level. Much of the critique featured in previous chapters has been aimed at research practices that seem to lack such a compass, or which draws implicitly on a Kuhnian compass. And while we acknowledge, with Kuhn and Bourdieu, that a critical rationalist vision may run counter to current (and historical) trends, or even be contrary to natural human social and psychological tendencies (or biases), we have tried to argue that the adoption of the kinds of proposals illustrated in Table 9.1 *are* possible, with considerable effort, *and* that they will lead to progress, so defined. With such progress, it is argued, comes the growth of knowledge and with it the increased likelihood of solving important practical problems in our field (cf. Popper, 1945) and thus, a closing of the gap between research and practice. We do not expect full agreement with this view, but by making the position clear and transparent, we hope to at least improve the quality of the critical discussion that may follow.

10

Planning a Post-revolutionary World

Introduction

The purpose of this final chapter is to offer positive and constructive options for the future of sport and exercise psychology. Over the course of this book, much ground has been covered, from philosophies of science to contemporary sport and exercise psychology research. Much of it makes for a less-than-optimistic prognosis if our field continues unabated on its current course. Problems and challenges have been identified and discussed, with the implications weighed. It is now time to offer some concrete suggestions for a (currently imaginary) 'post-revolutionary world' of sport and exercise psychology research. The preceding chapters have made the case that in sport and exercise psychology the current approaches taken—by researchers and, to a lesser extent, practitioners—are often problematic. Not because all research performed so far is intrinsically or intentionally bad; there has certainly been much interesting and innovative research published over the years. Rather, our field faces a choice. One option would be to continue with business-as-usual, hoping that any weaknesses will 'naturally' fix themselves in good time, if our science is simply permitted to follow its course. There is little or no evidence that such self-correcting or natural/inherent correctness follows from simply allowing researchers to research as they see

© The Author(s) 2016   **243**
P. Hassmén et al., *Rethinking Sport and Exercise Psychology Research*,
DOI 10.1057/978-1-137-48338-6_10

fit: the history and sociology of science present clear evidence to the contrary. An alternative—one that appears to be necessary based on the preceding chapters—is to explicitly and deliberately rethink research in sport and exercise psychology: to revise some aspects, persist with those that genuinely withstand critical scrutiny and, overall, make a conscious effort to ensure that our science 'advances'. Where historians and those who research the scientific process have detailed the strategies and attitudes that contribute to genuine scientific progress (see the end of Chap. 9), we must deliberately apply those to our own work: both individually and collectively. Such an approach will, we argue, speed up progress and help to prevent some of the (unnecessary) pitfalls. Although as cautioned by Vealey (2006):

> ...we can be critical of the 'box' used at various points in history, it is hypocritical to criticize previous research traditions as ineffective. All our research traditions were effective in showing us the way, similar to working through a maze where at times backtracking and rethinking is required (pp. 147–8).

Another reason for a serious rethink is time alone: the first scientific journal in sport and exercise psychology was published nearly 50 years ago—half a century. Academics 50 years ago inhabited a very different world compared to today: personal computers did not exist, the Internet was not something we could effectively carry around in our pockets, and academic freedom was not hampered by a thriving audit culture emphasising metrics, citations and grant income.

Likewise, elite sport nowadays is different from 50 years ago: money rules, wins and losses are instantly communicated worldwide, and more athletes and coaches than ever before seem to struggle with stress and mental health issues. At the same time, lack of regular physical activity has resulted in a society battling obesity and numerous mental health problems; children today present with illnesses previously only found in the elderly. Many explanations focus on a sedentary lifestyle that prevails from infancy to late adulthood. Some do too much, many too little: research continues to enquire as to why (among many, many other research questions). To understand the impact of all previous, present and future changes, sport and exercise psychology researchers need to adapt their tools and scrutinise their theories in order to study and understand what happens, and to offer insights that can benefit those studied, as well as society at large. Such a review and rescoping might also be argued to represent (or at least necessitate) a rethink. However, a rethink should never occur without considering the story so far (cf. Vealey, 2006); history has clearly shaped the present and will—to the extent it is allowed—continue to affect how sport and exercise psychology research is performed. Hence, it is necessary to quickly summarise the story that lays the basis for any potential rethink and/or 'post-revolutionary world'.

The Story So Far

The impact of Popper, Kuhn, Lakatos and Feyerabend is (or should be) indisputable, both on the history of science and the way we have approached writing this book. Although we do not go 'all the way' with Feyerabend to the conclusion that 'anything goes', it is important to consider his anarchist desire to disrupt the status quo, encourage creative thinking and bring a philosophically versed pluralistic scientist out of the closet. Free debate, pluralism and challenging standards were Feyerabend's solution, and it is eminently possible to apply these strategies when we (collectively) rethink sport and exercise psychology research.

History is at times a heavy burden, and the impact of Wundt, Fechner and the early drive towards measurement still affect our field. The many cross-sectional studies using standardised inventories still contribute to the knowledge base even though some merely seem to reiterate what is already known (and yet, many others that don't 'work' are never even submitted for publication). We do acknowledge, of course, that interpretivism and social constructivism have changed and expanded the traditionally individual-focused and nomothetic approach to sport and exercise psychology research, to also include a social (even sociological) perspective. With the increasing use of qualitative methods and idiographic approaches, the trend towards mixed-methods research is strong, and groups of mixed-discipline researchers joining forces to solve real-world problems proliferate: much has changed for the positive as a result of rethinking the dominating paradigms and ways of conducting and organising research. The advent of open access outlets has revolutionised how research is disseminated; mostly for the better but also creating some new challenges in the form of predatory journals.

So our recent history contains both progressive and regressive/conservative forces, but is it really necessary to fundamentally rethink how sport and exercise psychology research is performed? This book has constructed the case—one at least worthy of consideration—that researchers *should* rethink what is known, how it came to be known and if the road ahead of us requires different tools and strategies to those that brought us here. As argued herein, dominant theories such as achievement goal theory and self-determination theory, or methods for theory generation such as grounded theory, are rarely challenged. And when they are, there are invariably at least some proponents who are quick to defend and dismiss any criticisms—sometimes (notably) in the very same journal issue in which the criticism/challenge occurred, and sometimes actively labelling their counterargument a 'refutation' (which technically would be very final and objective). Such an approach displays all the hallmarks of the 'dogmatism' criticised by Popper. Such an aggressive defensive strategy is ostensibly supported by the audit culture and methodological fundamentalism we have discussed; sometimes further supported by the advantage that biomedical models of research have held over the humanistic and social sciences. Put simply, in order to dominate citations and grants, one must be a proponent of the dominant paradigm (preferably one of the originators, in fact), as citations and grant income are limited and finite. Thus, anything that questions the main paradigm—either by threatening it or simply offering an alternative—must be quashed proactively, not simply ignored. However, these sometimes fierce discussions are not necessarily signs of progress, if the main purpose is either to kill off competitors or vigorously defend existing views, theories and methods.

Even where examples have been provided in this book quoting specific papers and researchers, we are not arguing that such behaviour takes place in isolation; there is a context. It cannot be viewed as the fault (or a character flaw) of any specific individual. All the issues we have described in this book take place within a wider system, and we are all part of 'the system', as researchers, authors, reviewers, editors and as members of editorial boards and research councils. Sport and exercise psychology is a microcosm of the wider world of science: we still appear to play similar games, with similar rules, and adopting similar tactics. As such, the following section involves a wide-ranging discussion including many of the key protagonists in our scientific system: every researcher, every undergraduate and postgraduate student, editors and reviewers for scientific journals, members of editorial boards and research councils, chancellors and vice-chancellors. Even politicians and decision makers at the highest level of government. Society has changed so much that there is a need to rethink the overall purpose of science, the goals of research as a whole, and what society can and should expect to gain from it.

While the language of a 'revolution' can imply combat and chaos, we would recommend a more sensible and peaceful transition into the post-revolutionary world, for sport and exercise psychology research. Not all progress is linear or incremental, as our account of the history of science has shown. Yet, to a large extent, the history of sport and exercise psychology seems to lack comprehensive overhauls and total changes in how we approach our science. The knowledge-base has grown bit by bit, often expanding in applicability, often offering findings that (almost exclusively) claim to support a small number of favoured theories, and often using very similar methods. Thus, the contents of journals in sport and exercise psychology do not appear to be markedly different today compared to 10, 20 or even 30 years ago. What has changed, admittedly, over the past decades are the statistical methods that can be used to analyse data, driven forward by the computer-revolution. The addition of constructivism as a belief system, complementing (and challenging) those that historically have dominated sport and exercise psychology research, has also helped to move the field forward. Yet, there is still a long way to go until the full potential is realised. The following sections outline some reflections and speculations about how the field of sport and exercise psychology would proceed in a post-revolutionary world. If our readers have followed the argument of the preceding chapters, there is nothing particularly scary or revolutionary here. When viewed rationally, in the cold light of day, perhaps these proposals could one day become the new 'business-as-usual'.

Imagining Post-revolutionary Research

How would research be conducted after a hypothetical revolution in sport and exercise psychology? How would we identify, formulate and then test research questions? What research methods might emerge, and how will data be interpreted? Further still, which philosophical standpoints will be adopted, and how will researchers behave as a collective group? Chapter 1 described the current trends in the philosophy underlying sport and exercise psychology, as well as the sociological processes driving these trends: it seems inevitable that these would be quite different following a 'revolution' in this field. Chapter 1 also offered insights into how future research practice would be different: it could be 'Popperian', 'Lakatosian' or 'Feyerabendian'. In contrast, while it might be unfair to characterise his historical account as something he advocated for, we are explicitly recommending a movement away from 'Kuhnian' approaches to research, or at least the approach he termed 'normal science'. Note though, that there were occasions when Kuhn crossed the line from describing how he felt science was done, historically, to arguing that this approach—paradigms, puzzle-solving and the dogmatic protection of favoured ideas—must be effective, or correct, because it is what happens. This arguably conflates observation with justification, in the same way as observing crime or discrimination does not—in fact—mean that those things are right-and-proper. In fact, given how Kuhnian paradigms appear to so neatly encapsulate so many aspects of sport and exercise psychology research, there may be a transitionary step that each researcher may go through on the way to 'revolutionising' research in this area: 'anti-Kuhnian'. For example, if one feels the emotional tug to 'do what everyone else is doing'; to adopt 'widely accepted' methods to the extent that it may even require amending or changing your research question; or designing research studies that simply 'demonstrate' or 'apply' a favoured theory—researchers must first resist these temptations. It may not be necessary to have a replacement strategy immediately ready to hand. In fact, as argued elsewhere in this book, identifying a problem is orders of magnitude easier than offering a solution, but absence of a solution does not invalidate the criticism, or concern. So as a first step, researchers in sport and exercise psychology might simply resist falling into old habits, in easy patterns and 'smooth' approaches—because by choosing the relative comfort and safety of working within paradigms, we are arguably doing more harm than good. Step 1: resist. Step 2: develop and justify the alternative.

A classical paradigm contains clear instructions for each of the following, and in that way may be seen as undermining the potential for true progress in scientific understanding: (a) what is to be observed and scrutinised; (b) the kind of questions that are supposed to be asked and probed for answers in relation to this subject; (c) how these questions are to be structured; (d) what predictions made by the primary theory; (e) how the results of scientific investigations should be interpreted; (f) how is an experiment to be conducted, and what equipment is available to conduct the experiment. If each of the above issues is tightly constrained—either tacitly or explicitly—then what possible option is there to discover something 'new'? This book has argued throughout that such restrictive paradigms are common in sport and exercise psychology, with examples, and that where they are dominant, or unquestioned, then the options for scientific progress are significantly reduced.

The three 'templates' offered as alternatives to Kuhnian paradigms are Popperian, Lakatosian and Feyerabendian—although this may not be an exhaustive list. Fundamentally, Popper's approach would involve the switch from seeking to extend and support theories to attempting to falsify them: testing them to destruction. Popper generally argued that we learn more from how theories break than from seeking to support them. Sometimes, a theory can be repaired, other times it must be replaced. But if each new theory is an attempt to resolve the problems and weaknesses of its predecessors, then progress is arguably occurring. We are not becoming 'more certain' of a specific theory, but rather each theoretical solution to a problem is tentative, and we actually assume it will eventually be proven wrong—even if we don't know how just yet. Further to this, Popper argued that we should seek to research problems that are practically meaningful, even if they are difficult and even if other researchers are not studying them. Hence, for example, in motivational climate research (as detailed in Chap. 6), the most practically meaningful problems regard the specific ways that key social agents—coaches, parents, teammates—can actually influence motivation. Yet for the main part, research in this area has focussed on what happens after any 'motivationally relevant' behaviours have been perceived and interpreted by the athlete, and limited to a relatively general impression (e.g. a dichotomous or trichotomous distinction). Once we know, for example, that athletes perceive the same coach very differently, or even the same behaviour by the same coach very differently, it is sorely tempting to short-circuit this process by gather all our data from one or the other (usually the athlete's perceptions, occasionally the coaches). That way, there is no need to reconcile the complex interactions between intentions, behaviours, perceptions, interpretations and impact. Following such a proposed 'revolution', researchers would be less inclined to 'do what everyone else does' by handing out relatively simplistic questionnaires, usually at one single time point. Instead, while acknowledging that it will be very difficult, researchers might seek to tease out relationships between each of the above steps, including how they differ and are inconsistent. Instead of seeking to minimise and obscure such inconsistencies, we might seek to understand when and why they occur, and how to manage them. Popper would arguably reason that a small contribution to overcoming this difficult problem is infinitely more valuable than any study that adopts the same workaround as many others to circumvent that problem but deliver data that may—ultimately—become worthless if-and-when somebody else solves the 'hard' problems. Thus, Popper's two main contributions to a post-revolutionary world would be: (a) to seek to falsify our theories—expressing them in falsifiable terms and then attempting to do so—such that scientific understanding can improve as one theory replaces another; and (b) seeking to address meaningful and important problems with practical value to real-world application. Practical and applied does not have to conflict with scientific (as also discussed in Chap. 8).

Lakatos, as noted in Chap. 1, was a student of Popper and broadly agreed with the logic offered by Popper. He also acknowledged the claims of Kuhn that, regardless of the apparent rationality and logic offered by Popper, it is simply not how science is actually done by scientists. Popper described what should happen, in a perfect world, whereas Kuhn described what often tends to happen. There was convergence, for example, what Popper argued should be 'normal' or 'best practice' was described by Kuhn, but rather as 'extraordinary'. In both cases, significant change and overhaul of scientific understanding were possible. One argued we should conduct all science like this, the other that—for some reason—such strategies are 'extraordinary' and not normal. Lakatos tried to position his approach as the ideal compromise between these positions: attempting to describe when and why groups of scientists studying a particular topic should shift from normal (or 'degenerative') strategies to extraordinary (or 'progressive') strategies.

A simplified way of thinking about the difference is to consider a hypothetical 'theory numbering system'. Under Kuhn, there is only 'Theory 1', which is not particularly open to change or modification. Under Popper, each falsified theory might be considered cast aside, especially if a promising replacement is available. Hence, for Popper, progress might be viewed as 'Theory 1' becomes 'Theory 2' becomes 'Theory 3'; even if Theory 3 contains many similar attributes to Theory 2, it might be considered as new and different. Lakatos' solution to the tension between Kuhn (little or no progression) and Popper (fast, sweeping progression) was to try and specify that while the hard core of a theory may remain unchanged, its 'auxilliary' aspects may be updated in the face of falsification. Hence, Lakatos would offer: Theory 1.0, becomes Theory 1.1, then Theory 1.2 and so on, until it became clear that Theory 1 was unable to compete with Theory 2. At such a point, Theory 2.0 would be developed to Theory 2.1 then 2.2, in each case retaining the 'hard core' but changing the 'auxilliary' hypotheses or mechanisms. Take, for example, the various versions of achievement goal theory, if we draw from sport and educational settings. Nicholls' version might be thought of as Version 1.0, and the 'trichotomous' version put forwards by Elliot (1999) and Church, Elliot and Gable (2001) might be viewed as version 2.0. The 2 × 2 model of achievement goals put forwards by Elliot and McGregor (2001) could be Version 3.0 and so on (further new versions continue to be proposed). Within each, refinements are often made, but often not explicitly, leading to all sorts of confusion while proponents of one theory conspicuously attack and criticism versions of a competing theory that may be out-of-date. Hence, with Lakatos, Popper's focus on falsification was largely retained, but instead of being euthanised, a falsified theory would be required to evolve and adapt (and given every chance to do so). In this approach, therefore, researchers are certainly not naively following the canons of their prevailing paradigm, but neither could they be viewed as the 'wasteful' with regard to treasured theories and methods—a criticism levelled at Popper. Instead, a Lakatosian post-revolution researcher might keep careful records of a theory's 'hard core' and evolving 'auxilliaries', noting when certain auxiliaries were failing and—ultimately if no auxiliaries could be derived to protect the 'hard core' of the theory—then noting the precise nature of the damage to, and revisions required in, the core of the theory. This is an important difference to Kuhn's normal science, wherein any possibly auxiliary would be adopted, sometimes even post-hoc and sometimes without ever being tested, and viewed as further evidence in support of the core theory/model. Both Popperian and Lakatosian approaches, therefore, remain fundamentally different to what Kuhn considered to be normal science. In these approaches, 'progress' requires modifying, updating or replacing the existing favoured theoretical framework, or at least attempting to find reasons to do so (attempting falsification). In Kuhn's normal science, progress involves somehow gaining confidence in one's favoured theory, and applying it in more circumstances. Both Popper and Lakatos denied that there was any meaningful progress in such an approach, and this book has largely made the same argument.

Finally, there is another, often overlooked template for how to conduct research: the 'epistemological anarchism' of Paul Feyerabend. This was not, necessarily, a hopeless regress to simply declaring that the answer to any question is 'fish', or accepting that all scientific observations can only be explained as the will of a supreme overlord. Instead, Feyerabend could be interpreted as arguing that science becomes stronger when it contains more diverse ideas: more diverse theories and more diverse methodological approaches—the same argument that was made about ethnic, geographic and gender diversity in Chap. 6. In this respect, Feyerabend rejected both the normative ordering, leading to convention and consistency, as well as rejecting the possibility that any rational formula or process could ensure 'progress' within science. In fact, Feyerabend effectively argued that the only way we can evaluate a single theory is by comparison to many others, thus we need as many theories as possible in order to be able to compare and evaluate. There is no objective standard of good or bad theories (or methods), but the existence of many standards allows the comparison of relative strengths and weaknesses. Going full circle, this might explain why it is in the interest of the first (or very early) theories on a topic to suppress the development of any others, because the existence of other theories would create a comparison and expose weaknesses in the dominant theory. Thus, a scientist conducting research in a Feyerabendian spirit would be unconstrained by discipline area, showing no loyalty to one or another theory, or any particular method, and unconcerned by 'widely accepted' norms or practices. Whatever problem appeared interesting could be investigated in whatever manner seemed most appropriate. If the importance of the problem could be explained and the manner of attempting to address that problem seemed coherent, there is no problem. No need to address the same problems as other people, using the same theories, methods or assumptions. The data is generated and simply left bobbing in a sea of other competing 'pieces of knowledge' where—effectively—the cream might rise to the top. The more heterogeneous the mix of ideas, the more scope there is for separation, presumably, but even then it depends what sort of problem is being considered, and one person's problem is another's opportunity. No firm ground.

Notably, neither a Popperian, Lakatosian or Feyerabendian template for how to conduct science would be constrained to 'fitting in' with the prevailing preferences for theories, methods or assumptions. There is no deference to authority, no insistence on citing certain 'founding fathers' (as an aside, this is a patently sexist term). No 'clustering' around certain theories or certain methods—trends in sport and exercise psychology that have been critically analysed throughout this book. The protection of pet theories and fiercely favouring certain methodologies are both rejected by all three 'post-revolution' approaches to science. Two approaches, Popper and Lakatos, suggest that progress is cumulative and largely rational, achieved through finding flaws in existing knowledge and then improving it, whereas Feyerabend argued that progress is relative. The pattern that Kuhn described as normal science, and which we have criticised as necessitating a 'revolution' in sport and exercise psychology, either denies progress ('no new ideas') or defines progress as simply 'increasing confidence in the only theory/method we use'.

Two further—relatively simple—suggestions leap to mind that would be very different to current practice (revolutionary?), but which are actually very easy to implement. First, following the previous discussion of 'parsimony' in Chap. 6, it is clear that there is no law or requirement to pursue parsimony above truth—in sport and exercise psychology or in any field of science. In particular, if we are studying a complex 'thing'—which the psychology of sport and exercise arguably is—then adopting assumptions, theories or methods that are extremely simplistic (or parsimonious) could be a huge error. Just as viewing all colours in the most parsimonious way possible (say a dichotomy of dark vs. light) would be a gross over simplification, so is the case in sport and exercise psychology. Not only that, such simplicity might be preventing us from pursuing a deeper understanding of the deeper mechanisms and processes by which a rich diversity of colours is generated in nature and perceived by humans. Of course, it may be slightly more difficult for researchers to acknowledge and recognise—rather than simply blotting out—complexity in their subject matter. But is it better? Our story suggests that both historically and logically, insisting on parsimony can cause more problems than it solves. There are, in contrast, philosophical assumptions, theories and methodologies that explicitly acknowledge complexity and manage it in ways that do not attempt to minimise, dismiss or ignore it.

Second, in a discipline where discussing philosophy-of-science has become almost frowned upon, perhaps the exact opposite would be better. Where consistently failing to declare philosophical assumptions has been the norm for many decades, perhaps researchers should be required to declare this in every paper. After all, findings can only really be interpreted in relation to their underlying philosophical assumptions, so if they are missing from a paper, how should we interpret the findings? Further, failing to declare philosophical standpoints permits 'switching', or a type of 'eclecticism' that—rather than being inclusive and flexible—becomes mercenary and anti-scientific (cf. Keegan, 2015). One example, characterised by Keegan (2015), is the recommendation that 'This technique works for any athletes, you should all do it'. Such a statement would clearly be based on strong positivist assumptions of generalisability and a 'reality' that is concrete enough to allow such a claim (i.e. all people are basically the same). If an athlete returns to their psychologist saying 'But it didn't work' (which happens often enough to be a worry), what would a typical response be? The most common 'knee-jerk' response would be 'Oh well, everyone is different, try this other thing instead'. Now, one way or another 'everyone is different' emerges from totally different philosophical assumptions to positivism—be they interpretivism or constructivism. So such a response would be a fundamental switch of underlying philosophy, but if no-one ever declared their underlying assumptions, how would we know? It would take a very sharp mind to spot, and even then probably long after the offending scientist has departed the scene of the crime. Instead, imagine if all researchers and research papers explicitly declared their philosophical stance from the outset. First, it would prevent a lot of people reading papers if they fundamentally disagreed with the philosophy adopted. Second, it would provide strong and sound 'foundations' upon which theories, methods, findings and interpretations all necessarily stand. Without clear philosophy underpinning them, those things are simply floating in a meaningless void. Philosophy lends meaning to findings, determines our attitude to theories and provides clear anchor points for methodology: how on earth can we proceed in science without clearly identifying the underlying philosophy-of-science? That we appear to at all is extremely impressive, but arguably more a matter of luck than judgement. In a post-revolutionary world, researchers would be required to explicitly declare philosophical assumptions in any research paper, and that (of course) would require understanding the philosophy-of-science too (which would also be quite revolutionary).

Imagining the Post-revolutionary Journal

Given their central roles in stimulating, evaluating, selecting and showcasing research, journals would inevitably operate very differently in a post-revolutionary world. The papers they contain might be very different—in their content, presentation and tone. The way that papers are promoted, evaluated and recognised would be different. The way that papers are read and understood would be different. The criteria of evaluation for papers, and the approach to reviewing may change significantly. Reviewers and editorial boards may be recruited, trained and instructed differently, and editors would—almost unavoidably—have different priorities, attitudes and approaches. It may even be the case that the things we value—and therefore our metrics for evaluating journals—must fundamentally change in order to facilitate a revolution in sport and exercise psychology. But what might we expect to see in a world where theories, methods, knowledge and application were all understood differently? Following the critiques offered in the previous chapters of how research is guided, conducted, presented and interpreted, the following text offers a (necessarily speculative) overview of how journals could contribute to, and support, a more progressive world for sport and exercise psychology.

Starting from the very top of the hierarchy and working downwards, we could begin with the way governments (and therefore universities, publishers and ultimately academics) actually evaluate research. So long as the scientific value of a research article is judged in terms of citations, in the form of impact factors, h-indexes and the like, then potential problems abound. The h-index has known biases (especially regarding age/longevity); citation indices value quantity over quality; peer review and 'impact' (or uptake by other researchers) are both resistant to new or controversial ideas; and 'originality' is a beauty that is in the eye of the beholder. Most importantly, those using it to judge research, takes no account for topic area. At the broad level of fields of research, this is widely recognised, but even within an area as specific as sport and exercise psychology, one would receive many fewer citations if one studied a new topic or niche area—so it is better to simply follow the crowd. Such a situation would lead to paradigms and regressive science, which is precisely the situation this book is trying to avoid. Impact factor contains many of the same issues. Based on the assumption that impact factor reflects scientific quality, it produces a widespread impression of prestige and reputation, though no experimental data support this hypothesis (Brembs & Munafò, 2013). Neither impact factor nor h-index is in any way reliable indicators of the substantive quality of research: of a research paper, a particular researcher or a particular journal. In particular, both are highly likely to propagate Kuhnian paradigms by encouraging a 'clustering' of research efforts around particular ideas, theories and methodologies.

One commonly suggested solution is simply to 'decouple' government funding of universities and researchers (and also university rankings) from impact factors and citations (and other similarly meaningless metrics). For example, if universities can demonstrate that they are employing research-active staff and generating research, then they should be funded more for demonstrating the 'process' than the 'outcome'. This would be a huge step in permitting researchers to study any topic they liked, question any theory they like, invent new theories and more. At present, the wrong choice of topic, or stepping outside the accepted norms of your peers are effectively 'career suicide'. Remember the earlier analysis we presented, showing research currently clusters around a very small number of theories and methodologies. How can we possibly find anything new if we use the same guiding principles, methods and interpreting frameworks as everyone else? Following such a change, universities should also desist from using such metrics in selection, retention and promotion decisions, and instead devote due care and attention to the practices, strategies and integrity of their researchers. Imagine being evaluated on the genuine merit, ingenuity and potential of one's idea—rather than being told that's 'too hard' and so quality has simply been redefined as a number: a number that really requires you to 'play the game' of citations, h-indexes and impact factors (there are better metrics available, e.g. m-index allows for career duration, and relative weighted citation index indicates citations relative to others in the same field of research, but ultimately as scientists, we should know better than to trust too much in any system reducing complex phenomena to a single number).

By consequence, the contents of journals would likely become much more diverse, daring and interesting. At present—in the pre-revolutionary world—some brave journals and editors already encourage more diverse content. As examples, PlosOne and the BioMed Central series clearly specify that papers which are methodologically sound will be published regardless of whether the theories are popular, or whether the findings are considered 'interesting' or 'plausible' by reviewers. In pursuit of this aim, such journals also strongly encourage their authors to include their original data and ethical approvals, and they publish these online as supplementary material. Even in a world where governments and universities still base important decisions on indexation data widely recognised to be unreliable, journals could assist the cause by roundly ignoring such metrics. Unfortunately, at present, most journals announce their impact factor on their homepage and gleefully broadcast any increase in it each year. Publishers and journals have come under criticism for this but generally ignore it. If anything, it is generally accepted (e.g. Moustafa, 2014) that journals proactively pursue increased impact factors by: (a) favouring papers that sit in the middle of established 'citation networks' (i.e. at the centre of the paradigm); (b) favouring papers that cite their own journal; (c) rejecting perfectly good papers in order to reduce the 'denominator' in the calculation of impact factor—papers such as replications, new or unpopular topic areas and papers that may question the core paradigm; (d) favouring review papers (even when those reviews are simply summarising [sometimes re-summarising] a series of modest and uninteresting papers); and in some instances (e) becoming 'invitation only' journals, inviting papers from already well-established 'big names', never early- or mid-career researchers, and not even considering papers submitted freely, regardless of quality. The reliance on metrics such as these shifts the emphasis from advancing science and contributing to the world onto simply 'playing the game'. Faced with the constraints of metrics, trends and paradigms, it is far too easy to simply say 'well, that's reality'—without realising that by doing so, we create and propagate that reality.

Hence, there is enormous scope for post-'revolution' journals to be incredibly different—at least in terms of how they are managed and administered. Journals and publishers could, quite easily, reject the claimed importance of impact factors, h-indexes, rankings and comparisons. Key strategic decisions could be made with completely different goals in mind. We could replace 'what will increase our impact factor?' with 'what will contribute meaningfully to knowledge and/or debate in this topic area?' Now, that is not to tar all journal editors in sport and exercise psychology with the same brush: these issues are widely recognised across all scientific publishing (van Wesel, 2016). Furthermore, against a backdrop of relatively heavy reliance on such metrics by many key funding bodies and scientists, reflecting that in one's editing strategy may even seem quite a rational way to proceed. But imagine a different way. What if more papers were published in journals that attempted to replicate famous findings? If a key finding is supported, great. If not, that's even more interesting: leading to questions as to why and opportunities to improve our understanding. Imagine if a greater variety of theories and methodologies were permitted in leading journals. Some people may argue the recent adoption of more qualitative papers is sufficient, but arguably quantitative papers have gravitated towards psychometrics and correlation, and qualitative papers have gravitated towards grounded theory (see Chap. 4). To the extent that this claim is true—judge for yourself—then the resulting literature can hardly be argued to be methodologically diverse. Likewise, if only a small number of theories are permitted to exist for each core topic in sport and exercise psychology, and they are rarely ever critically compared or developed, then where are the opportunities for progress in our science? All researchers could do is accrue more support for those theories—truly paradigmatic behaviour. But, of course, replication papers, unusual (but perfectly sound) methodologies and new theories may not be cited as much as seemingly 'new' findings, using widely accepted methodologies and widely accepted theories. To a very large extent, the emphasis in citations, left unquestioned and unchecked by those in power, is a significant contributor to the problems described in this book: the reasons a 'rethink' is required. Regardless of whether finding a slightly new combination of things to correlate is really new (or subtle variations of how to analyse such data), and regardless of whether 'widely accepted' is the same as 'good', to a large extent that is the diet we are currently served. Journals, their editors and their publishers could do a great deal to combat this, but a great many changes would need to be realised first.

For example, in sport and exercise psychology at the moment, it doesn't seem that any researchers are proactively critiquing existing theories, developing new ones or attempting new methodologies. They would not be published. Hence, few students would think to attempt to initiate such a project, and even fewer supervisors would want to spend time and effort supervising it. Hence, to initiate the process, journals may need to reconsider their scope, aims, instructions to authors and more—in order to proactively stimulate more diverse submissions. Submissions from non-English speaking researchers, who are often turned away due to minor errors in writing style or APA formatting (some journals now offer support for writing style and APA, which may significantly help authors from non-English speaking countries). Submissions from minority groups, offering important different perspectives, who may currently read our literature and think 'there is nothing for me in here'. Submissions containing new and novel ideas, theories, methodologies and so on that are currently not even being attempted, let alone written up as manuscripts. In sport and exercise psychology, it seems, such papers are rarely submitted and then turned away, but rather they have been so effectively discouraged that they are rarely ever even attempted. We would need to proactively stimulate the production of new and interesting papers, and then patiently wait. Of course, the other angle-of-attack would be to proactively discourage business-as-usual. Editors could steer the discipline, very effectively, towards progress and advancement by announcing that the 'balance' would change, with relatively disinteresting papers correlating a range of psychometric measures likely to be rejected unless they can clearly demonstrate a novel contribution. Or perhaps journals could keep a running list of theories that have been disproven, replaced, done to death or simply exhausted and clearly announce that further papers on that list would be rejected too—again unless they could demonstrate something important has been missed. What a change that would be, what a rethink. At present, certain theories and methodologies actually appear to be the only game in town, almost pre-requisites for publication, and would therefore be much more likely to be sent for review and/or published (this is a subjective judgement, nobody seems to be checking this as far as we know). But citation rates may well drop off without the creation of self-citing 'clubs', all working in the same manner on the same theory. The advancement of science, however, as defined by Popper, Lakatos and Feyerabend, would be greatly enhanced.

Further still, reviewers would need to be given clear instructions (cf. Knudson, Morrow, & Thomas, 2014), and perhaps even feedback on their reviews. Moreover, associate editors and editors should—more often than is currently the case—seriously read and reflect on reviews before passing them on to authors. Too many stories are told online and at conferences of completely contradictory or nonsensical reviews, and of course attempting to significantly change the review process so as to encourage diversity and advancement would either exacerbate this, be fighting against this (remembering that peer review is typically characterised as extremely conservative and regressive), or both. We would need to stimulate new and different submissions, and then we would need to shepherd them through review and ensure that the rejections are genuine, rather than 'too new', 'too different', 'implausible' or 'offensive'

Of course, we would still reject papers that were novel, but not solely for being novel. The instructions, options and feedback to reviewers would likely be very different in both producing and maintaining a 'revolution'. Furthermore, reviewers may be asked to reconsider certain points, or make them differently. Editors, or associate editors, may step in to clarify which changes are 'compulsory' versus 'advisory' versus 'for consideration'. Of course, there is also a recent trend to make reviewers more accountable, by including their names in the report to authors, and even on the final manuscript. This too has pros and cons, but it is—at least—different and shines a light on the potential problems caused by unaccountable, blind and unchecked reviews. Some journals even attempt to offer greater flexibility in the number of reviewers, and what can be done if/when an impasse or contradiction occurs—such as simply replacing a review (!) or inviting additional reviewers to both read the manuscript and the reviews and offer a resolution. At the moment, however, one bad review is death for a manuscript, and most new, divergent or progressive papers are almost guaranteed to always displease one reviewer. So they are rarely published. So new ideas are never born—or at least communicated.

There is another question that publishers, journals and editors could be asking—how can we ensure that our papers are read, by as many people as possible? Without doubt, the recent proliferation of open access publishing has vastly increased the potential for greater readership. If they want to, the public, policy-makers and practitioners—anyone with an Internet connection—can now find, download and read many scientific papers that used to be behind paywalls. *If they want to.* But what exactly are we doing to make scientific papers appealing to this wider audience? What would make an interested, non-academic, stranger want to read a scientific paper, written in dense jargonistic language, using theories and methods that seem both inaccessible and unrealistic? Why not simply read a newspaper, blog, or advert instead? Of course, this can have serious consequences, if every time a reader makes this choice they choose a less evidence-based, less scientifically informed source, and make decisions based on that, real harm could occur. This is, to a large extent, how the anti-vaccination movement became established and equally led a politician to the recent claim in an important referendum that 'the British people are sick of experts' (http://www.ft.com/cms/s/2/7c7f2dbe-3474-11e6-bda0-04585c31b153.html).

So long as we seek, publish and celebrate scientific papers based on the citations, this situation is likely to get worse. Why? Because citations only come from other scientists. Specifically, other scientists working on that topic, and more often-than-not, from other scientist who agree with and endorse what they read in the paper they are citing. So—again linked to the current emphasis on metrics of citations, impact factors and the like—we are simply creating and reinforcing a (relatively) small club of people to cite each other, and who cares if it's interesting or useful to practitioners, policy-makers or the public. Granted, some evaluation frameworks (not journals) now insist on 'impact' case studies of working with industry or similar, but this relatively independent of what journals choose to publish, or why. Imagine if journals, editors and publishers really prioritised achieving a wider readership than just 'other researchers in this topic'. You could even go further and ask what might be different if journals really valued being read in non-English speaking countries, or in places with limited (or no) Internet access. Would that be more valuable—scientifically and ethically—than achieving a high impact factor? Which would be more worthy of being advertised on the front page?

As noted in Chap. 9, there is—arguably—a significant disconnect between researchers and practitioners in sport and exercise psychology just as in almost every other field of scientific research. Assuming a key purpose of science is to be useful, then we must also prioritise its usefulness—to practitioners and policy-makers but also in general. The current emphasis on citations in deciding what is valuable may be limiting the usefulness of research to simply 'other researchers', and even then, only 'other researchers who tend to agree with this paper'. Occasionally, journals prioritise applied practice, for example, the *British Medical Journal* recently (and controversially) explained its lack of qualitative papers by claiming they felt the findings were less useful to medical practitioners. Many practitioners of sport and exercise psychology are quite explicit in their unhappiness with the academic literature we produce—it does not inform evidence-based applied practice (see Chap. 8). Once again, it could be possible for journals to explicitly encourage and promote this type of research, with calls for papers, special editions, clear subsections in each issue, promoting such papers to organisations that promote and regulate applied practice and of course making them open access. Once again though—especially in the early stages of such a strategy—citation rates would drop, because practitioners rarely ever write papers for journals. It is a great pity, as the study of how key ideas from theory and evidence are adopted, implemented and evaluated by practitioners would be extremely valuable.

As such, the journals representing sport and exercise psychology would be extremely different following a revolution. They would have little or no regard for unscientific and unreliable metrics such as impact factor and h-index. As such, they would be less concerned about citation rates of each paper, or the journal overall. From here, journals could focus on each paper's clarity, transparency, coherence (between methods, findings and claims) and potential for advancement. Journals could even go so far as to insist on breaking up the current 'citation rings', discouraging papers that simply fall into a paradigm and deliberately encouraging papers that seek to test theories (i.e. explicit attempts to falsify them), refine and reformulate theories, critique and replace theories and even develop new and tailor-made methodologies. The arguments presented in Chap. 7 clearly detailed how a heavy reliance on cross-sectional psychometric questionnaires and correlations is inappropriate for a subject matter that is complex, interactive and dynamic. What methods might be? At this point in time, very few people can contemplate this as their training did not address such options but they do exist in other areas of science. Journals could explicitly tailor their review processes to enable the changes being sought—from conservative and regressive to innovative and progressive—but this would require quite significant modifications to the peer-review process. Other areas of science have trialled this though. For example, many papers in particle physics are simply published 'pre-review' and then reviewed by those reading them—the so-called post-publication review—leading to changes and modifications before the paper is accepted and finalised. Change is possible. Finally, journals could seek to deliberately engage non-English speakers and minority groups, as well as practitioners, policy-makers and the public. These new priorities would involve different processes—for example, support in writing style (not rejecting papers outright for a few typos)—and different priorities. But when we contemplate the very purpose of science, and thus the very aims of sport and exercise psychology, it is clear that journals should be about much more than simply accruing citations.

Imagining the Post-revolutionary Conference

Along with textbooks and journals, scholarly and professional confer-ences are arguably the most important mechanism for the communica-tion (sometimes generation) of new knowledge in our field. International conferences organised by professional scholarly societies such as FEPSAC (in Europe), AASP (in the United States) and BPS (in the UK) repre-sent important annual events in the life of those in sport and exercise psychology. Yet, as described in the brief personal account in Chap. 6, they can often be sites for the expression of power by those in positions of authority; for the perpetuation and promotion of the status quo; and as mechanisms for the socialisation of young researchers into narrow paradigmatic conformity. How could organisations ensure that academic meetings live up to their often high-minded aspirations and avoid lapsing into petty bickering among warring cabals? What might an alternative post-revolutionary conference look like?

Before we elucidate a positive vision for conferences, it is worth point-ing out that very little evidence exists to support our assertions of their sometimes dysfunctional state. Beyond our own experiences and those of close colleagues (gossip), and occasional brief online conference reports, the actual reality and experience of conferences is largely undocumented. Unlike behaviour in academic publishing or research practice, which has been subjected to fairly extensive academic scrutiny, nobody to our knowledge has critically analysed the behaviour of researchers and prac-titioners at conferences. Notwithstanding this absence of research, we draw on our collective experience (over 50 conferences between us) and the theoretical accounts of Kuhn and Bourdieu (see Chaps. 1 and 9) to offer a brief characterisation of a 'typical' sport psychology conference. For the uninitiated, this 'pen portrait' may serve as an image that we aim to replace; for the seasoned conference delegate, it serves as a hypothesis for a critical discussion.

The typical conference opens with a keynote address, delivered by a well-known professor who is often charged with providing a high-level reflection on the 'state of the field'. The attitude of the delegates to such an address is meant to be reverential and deferential, though occasionally some bold individual may try to 'subvert' proceedings with an awkward question or two. Coffee and networking then punctuate a series of roughly themed (sometimes incoherently themed) parallel sessions typically consisting of a stream of 20-minute PowerPoint presentations which invariably overrun, leaving little time for discussion (AASP recently featured novel alternative approaches such as '5 slides in 5 minutes'). Where discussion does occur, social conventions dictate that questioning is polite and not too difficult. Only occasionally does a genuine critical discussion flare-up, the conclusion of which is normally determined by the power relationships of the interlocutors rather than the strength of argument. Interspersed between long uneventful parallel sessions are occasional symposia or roundtable discussions, typically featuring planned (or staged) discussion on more focussed topics or themes (the 2015 FEPSAC conference featured sessions on 'professional challenges working at the olympic level' and 'certification for sport psychology delivery'). Somewhere in the middle or second half of the conference will be a second keynote address with much the same character as the first. Again, the topic is usually large and important, such as 'the future of the discipline' (or the future of the paradigm). Awards ceremonies and gala dinners typically mark the end of the conference before delegates filter back to their universities and organisations, with much of the conference material and discussion lingering only briefly in their memory. Lucky delegates may have forged some useful new contacts (i.e. gained valuable social capital) to help them get ahead in the paradigm; others may have been subject to the kind of experience described in Chap. 6.

In contrast to this ideal type image, we outline our alternative positive post-revolutionary vision. In Chap. 9, we offered a critical rationalist constitution for research and a professional ethical code for researchers based on Popper's mature normative theory of science (Popper, 1994; McIntyre & Popper, 1983). The tentative principles we defined in Boxes 9.1 and 9.2—for shifting the goal of critical discussion, encouraging fruitful 'culture clash', protecting against 'theory addiction' (or normal science) and for the effective formulation of problems and theories to encourage criticism—may all be applied to the conduct of conferences. In the same way that we have advocated for clear guidance for reviewers and authors in the context of journals (above), such rules and principles would also be written down and made clear to all delegates. Box 10.1 sketches out a potential 'code of conduct' for a post-revolutionary conference.

Box 10.1 A Code of Conduct for Delegates at a Post-revolutionary Conference

1. Papers identifying errors and anomalies in well-established theories or research programmes are especially welcome.
2. Presentations should begin with a clear outline of the research problem and its history (i.e. the 'problem situation').
3. Where theories are presented, delegates are expected to specify the kinds of arguments and evidence they would accept as valid criticism of the theory.
4. Chairs must protect the allotted time for discussion.
5. Errors and mistakes should be pointed out by presenters, inviting criticism (i.e. 'confessional' style papers).
6. Critical questions should be addressed at arguments, not individuals.
7. Purely critical questions or arguments should be accompanied by alternative positive theories where possible.
8. A 'good' session is one that leads to growth in knowledge and understanding, or even just the clarification of a problem, which should be summarised by the chair.

To support the practical application of such a code, additional mechanisms and changes of structure would be required. As Steve Fuller argued after his keynote at the recent British Sociological Association meeting (Fuller, 2014), 'a conference is a distinct channel of academic communication; it is not a watered-down or zombie version of the academic print culture' (it is still common for researchers to literally 'read' papers at conferences). As such, and given the availability of Web 2.0 technologies, our post-revolutionary conference would feature the following structures and dissemination mechanisms (adapted from Fuller, 2014):

1. A conference website or blog site with fully enabled Web 2.0 capabilities (e.g. integrated social networking, delegate profiles, comment and reply sections, wikis) will provide an *interactive* online hub.
2. Instead of traditional abstracts, delegates will produce 2–3-minute video clips explaining what will be said in the paper, and how.
3. Screencast versions of PowerPoint presentations will be featured on the conference website, coupled with anonymous comment and reply features. Such presentations may also be screened in 'high-tech' poster sessions in a central lobby area.
4. By reducing the number of face-to-face presentations, more time and space will be made for symposia and roundtable discussion sessions, which will also be captured and made immediately available on the conference website. Online (potentially anonymous) feedback may then contribute to follow-up sessions where criticism is discussed.
5. Symposia and roundtable discussions will be organised that deliberately place researchers from opposing 'paradigms' in the same room, discussing common problems, with the aim of provoking fruitful 'culture clash' (see Chap. 9). To use an example from earlier in this chapter, proponents of the different versions of achievement goal theory (1.0, 2.0, 3.0) could be brought together to discuss, say, how to motivate children to engage in greater levels of physical activity.
6. A large hall should remain open throughout the conference for the spontaneous meetings of varied people around given topics attended by anyone with an interest (i.e. 'unconferences': https://en.wikipedia.org/wiki/Unconference). Physical and online notice boards (and wikis) may help such groups organise and record such meetings.
7. Funding for the conference should not be tied to the delivery of a formal presentation, but to the requirement to make one's presence visible through participation in the various online and offline activities (i.e. keeping more people engaged beyond the delivery of their own session).

This is not an exhaustive list and, clearly, none of these are new ideas. The technology required to support such practices is also well-established, with a proven impact in business circles (Tapscott & Williams, 2006) and freely available to anyone with an email address. However, with the exception of FEPSAC, who create non-interactive podcasts of keynotes and symposia, none of the big sport psychology conferences has yet to begin to take advantage of such opportunities.

One further qualifying point needs to be made with respect to points 4 and 5 (above) and the implementation of the code of conduct (Box 10.1). In short, how would discussions and symposia actually be conducted in this utopian Popperian fashion? Would they not be subverted by natural psychological biases and established power relationships? (see Chap. 9). Part of the answer to these questions lies simply in an appeal to individuals, first and foremost, to behave 'virtuously'—to adopt an institutional attitude that may run counter to their natural instincts—based on a clear and explicit argument for how and why such behaviour will lead to more favourable outcomes (Sassower, 2006: p. 25). This is a necessary but insufficient response, however, and is unlikely on its own to lead to mass behaviour change. For another part of the answer, we can look at a first-hand example of the conduct of a Popperian seminar, since Popper himself based his famous Tuesday afternoon seminars at the LSE on just such a code.

According to Agassi's (2008: p. 68) detailed account, Popper's seminars were 'a pioneering experiment of the first order' in that he allowed anyone attend and to speak, on any topic, so long as they spoke plainly and presented a clear and justified problem. Agassi also notes that, for the same reasons, the seminar was also plagued by procedural problems. The right of speakers to speak uninterrupted was seldom recognised, for example, and Popper would frequently demand of those offering theories to also present arguments that would make them admit that their speculations were false. Agassi points out that, while such conduct was terrific for those who could take it, for many it was too hard. Those who complained were chastised: 'we are trendsetters' Popper would argue, 'and it behooves us to demand of ourselves much more than the customary rules do' (Agassi, 2008: p. 69). Part of the problem here was that the 'rules' were often not made clear to speakers before they began. Popper, as chair, also clearly expected too much. Theories, for example, are hard to come by and are valuable even when they are untenable (Agassi, 2008). To push for expected refutations and alternative ideas is therefore unreasonable. The chairing of such sessions is therefore extremely important: the 'rules of engagement' need to be made clear to all in advance of a session and the chair needs to have the confidence and sensitivity to enforce the rules where speakers deviate, without expecting too much.

So, by following the suggestions made above, and with the production and promotion of a code of conduct like the one in Box 10.1 (but perhaps without Popper in the chair), we anticipate that the post-revolutionary sport and exercise psychology conference will bring about significant positive changes in the field. First, it would extend and deepen interaction in the conference. By making material available online, say, a month before the conference, delegates could begin to view and feedback on abstracts and presentations. Such feedback may even inform the conduct of symposia or debates during the conference itself. Better integration of social networking, 'unconferences' and wikis would also extend the discussion well beyond the end of the event. Second, by increasing the opportunities for critical discussion—through application of the code of conduct, convening interparadigmatic problem-based symposia and encouraging (anonymous) online comments and replies—the post-revolutionary conference would effectively institutionalise the principles of critical rationalism and thus expedite 'progress' in the field. Third, by subverting the conventional approaches to conferences, dissolving old authoritarian hierarchies and challenging paradigmatic monopoly, this new approach will help to mitigate the onset of 'normal science'. Finally, the post-revolutionary conference may also assist in bridging the research-practice gap (see Chap. 8), as academic material is made more accessible to a wider audience, who can watch videos and follow debates without having to wait until knowledge emerges from behind publishers' paywalls (assuming they can penetrate the academic language of the paper at all).

Imagining Post-revolutionary Research Education

At the foundation of good research, publishing and communication is philosophically informed and well-integrated research education. The post-revolutionary vision we have expounded thus far therefore hinges on the design and delivery of effective education programmes. If we are to counteract the conservative and idiosyncratic socialisation (even indoctrination) processes described by Kuhn (1962) and Bourdieu (1975), a carefully planned and skilfully delivered curriculum is necessary. Our vision is sketched in two parts: first, we consider the *content* of an education programme; second, we consider *how* such a curriculum might be successfully delivered.

A review of popular undergraduate curricula, and the contents pages of the research methods textbooks that inform them, typically reveals three problematic characteristics of current approaches to research education: (a) there is a heavy emphasis on the data collection and analysis aspects of research (especially statistics); (b) there is an artificial disconnect between the teaching of research and of substantive theory and practice; and (c) there is an almost complete absence of the philosophical principles informing research (typically a throwaway introductory chapter or lecture). Students experiencing such curricula are liable to develop only partial understanding of the subject, misplaced confidence in theories and an inability to think critically about the knowledge presented to them (see Chap. 3). With the help of Popperian ideas outlined in Chap. 9, our alternative vision aims to overcome these problems and facilitate the development of competent, confident, creative, self-aware (fallible), critical thinkers who can interpret, improve, design, deliver and apply high-quality research in sport and exercise psychology.

Critical rationalism, we recall, is both an attitude and method. The attitude may be summed up in a single sentence: 'I may be wrong and you may be right, and by an effort, we may get nearer to the truth' (Popper, 1994: p. xii). It is therefore an open, tolerant, optimistic yet critical and fallibilist attitude. The method or logic was expressed most simply in Popper's four-stage schema introduced in Chap. 1: $P_1 \rightarrow TS \rightarrow EE \rightarrow P_2$ (initial problem, tentative solution, error elimination, new problems) (in Magee, 1973: p. 65). Our first suggestion, then, is that an effective education programme be built on these two pillars. Students must be taught not only methods but also attitudes and fundamental philosophical ideas.

More specifically, at the attitude level, there are a number of 'threshold concepts' (Meyer & Land, 2006) to which students need to be exposed to enable them to apply research methods appropriately and effectively. Without a basic understanding of principles such as the fallibility of knowledge, the fundamental role of criticism, and the value of creativity, for example, students have little chance of becoming anything but 'normal scientists'. As we pointed out in Chap. 4, an appreciation of, say, the problem of induction and its solution may transform (and arguably enhance) how one actually goes about conducting a grounded theory study.

Another example is Popper's demarcation criterion between science and pseudoscience (i.e. that *scientific* theories have to be testable, and *scientists* willing to test them and give them up), which is an extremely useful concept to help students think critically about knowledge (Was a theory presented in a testable form? How confident should we be in the research findings? Have the authors claimed too much for their research?). Although these concepts can be difficult to grasp, our experience tells us that it is both possible and valuable to introduce them even to very inexperienced students. By way of example, Box 10.2 describes a simple practical task that can help early undergraduate students engage with the question of: what is science? It requires them to compare knowledge claims and make judgements about the value of different kinds of knowledge—the kind of activity they do all the time when reading a newspaper or watching TV, but often without reflection.

Box 10.2 'Defining Science' Activity for Early Undergraduate Students

Scenario: You are the performance director for a national Olympic squad. You have some funding to appoint a new staff member who can support your athletes. The following people apply for the role and you must rank them in order of preference for interview.

1. Homeopathic doctor
2. Crystal healer
3. Holistic life coach
4. Psychiatrist
5. Catholic priest
6. Accredited sport psychologist

Follow-up questions:

1. Which do you consider scientists? How are you able to make this judgement?
2. Did you put the scientists at the top of the list? If so, why?
3. What is different about scientific knowledge compared to other kinds of knowledge?

Alongside the teaching of important philosophical threshold concepts, Popper's four-stage schema is useful in addressing the balance of a research curriculum. As we noted earlier, many 'research methods' courses are dominated by detailed data collection and analysis classes, with a heavy bias for statistics (this may also be a reason why many students are turned-off research education classes). The crucially important step of clearly articulating an appropriate research problem is often neglected; and the difficult process of inventing or adapting imaginative theories as appropriate solutions to problems is limited to a partial function of a literature review, if covered at all. A critical rationalist curriculum, by contrast, would allocate roughly equal weighting to each main step of the research process. Each of the four stages would represent a 'pillar' or 'strand' of a curriculum, to which students would return in a deeper and more complex form in following years. Table 10.1 sketches the outline of just such a balanced, critical rationalist research curriculum. The suggested learning outcomes provide a general sense of what students would know and be able to do at the end of each stage, with the final row in the table effectively describing an early career researcher.

The student journey through such a programme would ideally be based on Jerome Bruner's proposal for a 'spiral curriculum': where fundamental ideas are simplified to a level appropriate to the students' level of understanding, before being carefully extended and repeated in an upward spiral of appreciation (see Harden & Stamper, 1999, for an applied example in medical education). As Bruner explains:

> If the understanding of number, measure and probability is judged critical in the pursuit of science, then instruction in these subjects should begin... as early as possible in a manner consistent with the child's forms of thought. Let the topics be developed and redeveloped in later grades... Many curricula are originally planned with a guiding idea much like the one set forth here. But as curricula are actually executed, as they grow and change, they often lose their original form and suffer relapse into a certain shapelessness. (1960: p. 54)

Table 10.1 A critical rationalist curriculum for research education

Attitude	Fallibilism (e.g. all theories, no matter how well supported, are likely to be wrong)		Critical attitude (e.g. no evidence can prove you right, but any evidence can prove you wrong)	
Method	P₁	TS	EE	P₂
Basic (early undergrad)	Identify the variables in a problem of personal interest (e.g. independent and dependent variables)	Identify a relevant theory to help solve the problem	Select and apply an appropriate 'test' of the theory Collect appropriate data and describe the findings	Comment on the status of the initial problem and make applied recommendations
Intermediate (late undergrad)	Justify the selection of a problem based on recommendations from existing research	Derive a testable hypothesis from an appropriate theory	Design a 'test' of the theory (or adapt an existing 'test') Collect valid/reliable/trustworthy/ authentic data and select appropriate analysis method	Make informed recommendations for future research
Advanced (postgrad)	Formulate a 'problem situation' based on historical analysis and justify its novelty	Determine the extent to which competing theories have been corroborated (evaluate the severity of the tests to which they have been subjected)	Justify an ethical and rigorous research design (inc.data collection and analysis process) Define appropriate criteria for judging quality of study	Evaluate strengths and weakness in own approach Comment on the extent of corroboration of theory

Clearly, there is still much flesh to add to these bones; we do not aim to be too prescriptive. The main point, rather, is that content of programmes is balanced, progressive and cumulative, containing threshold concepts concerning the attitude of a good researcher (e.g. see Box 9.2 in Chap. 9 on a professional ethics for sport and exercise psychology) *and* the more specific knowledge and skills associated with the execution of the critical rationalist method (problem setting and so on). Note that the method is also generic in nature, and may therefore be applicable to qualitative and quantitative, nomothetic and idiographic research approaches (e.g. 'error elimination' may involve a randomised controlled trial, or a series of life-history interviews, depending on the nature of the problem).

Turning briefly now to the question of *how* such a curriculum might best be delivered, we argue that it is best integrated within a wider sport and exercise psychology course (note: this is likely to be practically very difficult outside of single honours courses). Research education modules are typically delivered as 'appendages' to core substantive modules, leaving students to try make the connections and applications between research and, say, applied practice (see Model 1 in Fig. 10.1). In such circumstances, it is only highly engaged and dedicated students who will see, for example, that applied practitioners need to be wary of the fallibility of the theories they use to support interventions with athletes (cf. Keegan, 2015).

Model 1-The hopeful appendage approach

Semester	1			2		
Module	Sport psychology	Cognitive psychology	Social psychology	Exercise psychology	Applied practice	Research methods

Model 2-The deliberate integrated approach

Semester	1			2	
Module	Sport psychology	Cognitive psychology	Social psychology	Exercise psychology	Applied practice
	Research attitude and method				

Fig. 10.1 Two models for the delivery of research education

Following a more deliberate integrated approach to teaching and research would demand that research education is taught specifically, but also developed (and even assessed) across an entire course (Healey, 2005). Research attitudes and skills are arguably central to any higher education (Neary, 2012) and are therefore ideal material of synoptic teaching and assessment. In the example offered above (Model 2), students may undertake 'research-based' (Griffiths, 2004) assessment tasks in substantive modules—such as a mini research project in 'Social psychology' or some data collection and analysis in 'Exercise psychology'—in order to embed important attitudes and skills introduced through a parallel year-long research module. In short, it becomes the responsibility of *every* module and staff member in a course to develop and assess research education, since it is only through consistent and progressive *application* that research education effective.

Following the articulation of Popper's critical rationalism in Chap. 9, we argued that 'the primary goal of research education should be developing ingenuity in creating and criticising theories' (see Box 9.1 in Chap. 9). In order to achieve this goal, students need to be given the time and repeated opportunity to create and criticise theories in safe, supportive, low-risk environments. Formative assessment may therefore be more appropriate than summative assessment. Or, where summative assessment is used, students can be evaluated on process and understanding, rather than the production of error-free data and findings. Ingenuity also implies novel thinking, so educators should introduce students to theories, research designs and methods from outside of the discipline. By continuing to fill their heads with the well-worn theories (e.g. SDT), data collection tools and methods (e.g. psychometric questionnaires and correlation), we can hardly expect the next generation of sport and exercise psychologists to do anything 'revolutionary' in the future.

Conclusion

Sport and exercise psychology has come a long way from its humble beginnings; the recently young field has quickly gained considerable momentum, with many 'powerhouse' theories, methods and—of course—'big names'. Moreover, sport and exercise psychology has quickly reached the point where it is capable of contributing to the wider literature, rather than tending to 'borrow' ideas from its parent discipline (i.e. mainstream psychology). Growth, alone, however, is not necessarily a good indicator of success—some things that grow quickly, or aggressively, can be highly undesirable. As such, just as we recommend that practitioners engage in thorough and ongoing reflective practice and professional development, the overall discipline—especially its researchers—must review, reflect and adapt if we are to stay effective (and ethical). Strong candidates for the focus of this reflection include our philosophies of science, schools of thought, research traditions, paradigms and worldviews: all of which contribute to both our capabilities and limitations/boundaries: personal and collective. The analysis in this book has suggested that such limitations are common throughout science and that our discipline is no exception—and as such a rethink (or even revolution) may be needed in sport and exercise psychology. As noted elsewhere in the text, we hope that our efforts in researching, analysing and presenting this 'case' helps others from falling into a 'dogmatic slumber' (Kant, 1783/1985), or from learning important lessons the 'hard way'. In fact, the strategies and information presented in this chapter—and this book—should assist researchers in producing more meaningful and impactful work: work that really could change the world of sport and exercise psychology.

This final chapter has mapped out a number of paths forward: roads that may help us navigate round, through or over the metaphorical constraints and boundaries that can limit what (and how) we research. If we—as a field—are daring enough to start each new journey by rethinking how research is performed, communicated and educated, then this book (and the history of science) suggests that better outcomes would eventuate. Rethinking, however, is not enough. Without the courage to act, rethinking is merely an exhausting and futile exercise. We therefore hope that the concrete suggestions offered in this chapter will lead to change in the discipline. Change that is evident in how research is performed, manuscripts evaluated, conferences organised and education structured. It is up to each individual researcher, supervisor, editor, reviewer and director/leader. It is up to us.

References

Acierno, R., Hersen, M., & Van Hasselt, V. B. (1996). Accountability in psychological treatment. In *Sourcebook of psychological treatment manuals for adult disorders* (pp. 3–20). Boston: Springer US.

Adie, J. W., Duda, J. L., & Ntoumanis, N. (2012). Perceived coach-autonomy support, basic need satisfaction and the well-and ill-being of elite youth soccer players: A longitudinal investigation. *Psychology of Sport and Exercise, 13*, 51–59.

Agassi, J. (2008). *A philosopher's apprentice: In Karl Popper's workshop.* Amsterdam, The Netherlands: Rodopi.

Agassi, J. (2014). *Popper and his popular critics: Thomas Kuhn, Paul Feyerabend and Imre Lakatos.* London: Springer.

Albee, G. W. (2000). The Boulder model's fatal flaw. *American Psychologist, 55*(2), 247.

Alesina, A., & Ferrara, E. L. (2005). Ethnic diversity and economic performance. *Journal of Economic Literature, 43*, 762–800.

Allport, G. W. (1937). The functional autonomy of motives. *American Journal of Psychology, 50*, 141–156.

Allwood, C. M. (2012). The distinction between qualitative and quantitative research methods is problematic. *Quality and Quantity, 46*, 1417–1429.

Ames, C. (1992). Classrooms: Goals, structures, and student motivation. *Journal of Educational Psychology, 84*, 261–271.

© The Author(s) 2016
P. Hassmén et al., *Rethinking Sport and Exercise Psychology Research*,
DOI 10.1057/978-1-137-48338-6

Amiot, C. E., Sansfaçon, S., & Louis, W. R. (2014). How normative and social identification processes predict self-determination to engage in derogatory behaviours against outgroup hockey fans. *European Journal of Social Psychology, 44*(3), 216–230.

Andersen, M. B., McCullagh, P., & Wilson, G. J. (2007). But what do the numbers really tell us? Arbitrary metrics and effect size reporting in sport psychology research. *Journal of Sport and Exercise Psychology, 29*, 664.

Andreski, S. (1972). *Social sciences as sorcery*. London: André Deutsch Limited.

Bailey, R., & Collins, D. (2013). The standard model of talent development and its discontents. *Kinesiology Review, 2*(4), 248–259.

Balmer, A. (2012). For a sociology of sport. *Sociology of Sport Journal, 29*, 102–117.

Bakan, D. (1966). The test of significance in psychological research. *Psychological Bulletin, 66*, 423–437.

Barrett, S. (2003). *Environment and statecraft: The strategy of environmental treaty-making: The strategy of environmental treaty-making*. Oxford, UK: Oxford University Press.

Bartley, W. W., III. (1962). *The retreat to commitment*. La Salle, IL: Open Court.

Bartley, W. W., III. (1990). *Unfathomed knowledge, unmeasured wealth: On universities and the wealth of nations*. La Salle, IL: Open Court.

Bauerlein, M., Gad-el-Hak, M., Grody, W., McKelvey, B., and Trimble, S.W. (2010). We must stop the avalanche of low-quality research. *The Chronicle of Higher Education LVI, issue 38, back page Point of View, p. 80*, 10 June 2010.

Behar-Horenstein, L. S., & Niu, L. (2011). Teaching critical thinking skills in higher education: A review of the literature. *Journal of College Teaching & Learning, 8*, 25–42.

Belar, C. D. (2000). Revealing data on education and training. *Clinical Psychology: Science and Practice, 7*(4), 368–369.

Belar, C. D., & Perry, N. W. (1992). The national conference on scientist-practitioner education and training for the professional practice of psychology. *American Psychologist, 47*(1), 71.

Benjamin, L. T., Jr., & Baker, D. B. (2000). Boulder at 50: Introduction to the section. *American Psychologist, 55*(2), 233.

Biddle, S., Wang, C. J., Kavussanu, M., & Spray, C. (2003). Correlates of achievement goal orientations in physical activity: A systematic review of research. *European Journal of Sport Science, 3*(5), 1–20.

Biddle, S. J., Duda, J. L., Papaioannou, A., & Harwood, C. (2001). Physical education, positivism, and optimistic claims from achievement goal theorists: A response to Pringle (2000). *Quest, 53*(4), 457–470.

Blaug, M. (1991). Second thoughts on the Keynesian revolution. *History of Political Economy, 23*(2), 171–192.

Blodgett, A. T., Schinke, R. J., McGannon, K. R., & Fisher, L. A. (2015). Cultural sport psychology research: Conceptions, evolutions, and forecasts. *International Review of Sport and Exercise Psychology, 8*(1), 24–43.

Blumer, H. (1969). *Symbolic interactionism: Perspective and method.* Englewood Cliffs, NJ: Prentice Hall.

Boone, C., & Hendriks, W. (2008). Top management team diversity and firm performance: Moderators of functional-background and locus-of-control diversity. *Management Science, 55*(2), 165–180.

Borg, G. (1962). *Physical performance and perceived exertion* (Studia Psychologica et Paedagogica. Series altera, Investigationes XI). Lund, Sweden: Gleerup.

Borg, G. (1970). Perceived exertion as an indicator of somatic stress. *Scandinavian Journal of Rehabilitation Medicine, 2,* 92–98.

Borg, G. (1978). Subjective effort in relation to physical performance and working capacity. In H. L. Pick et al. (Eds.), *Psychology from research to practice* (pp. 333–361). New York: Plenum Publishing Corp.

Borg, G. (1998). *Borg's perceived exertion and pain scales.* Champaign, IL: Human Kinetics.

Boring, E. G. (1929). *A history of experimental psychology.* New York: Appleton.

Borsboom, D., & Mellenbergh, G. J. (2004). Why psychometrics is not pathological: A comment on Michell. *Theory & Psychology, 14,* 105–120.

Bortoli, L., Bertollo, M., & Robazza, C. (2009). Dispositional goal orientations, motivational climate, and psychobiosocial states in youth sport. *Personality and Individual Differences, 47*(1), 18–24.

Boudry, M., Blancke, S., & Pigliucci, M. (2015). What makes weird beliefs thrive? The epidemiology of pseudoscience. *Philosophical Psychology, 28,* 1177–1198.

Bourdieu, P. (1975). The specificity of the scientific field and the social conditions of the progress of reason. *Social Science Information, 14,* 19–47.

Bourdieu, P. (1991). The peculiar history of scientific reason. *Sociological Forum, 6*(1), 3–26.

Bourdieu, P. (2001). *Masculine domination.* Stanford, CA: Stanford University Press.

Bradley, J. V. (1981). Pernicious publication practices. *Bulletin of the Psychonomic Society, 18,* 31–34.

Bredemeier, B. J., Desertrain, G. S., Fisher, L. A., Getty, D., Slocum, N. E., Stephens, D. E., et al. (1991). Epistemological perspectives among women who participate in physical activity. *Journal of Applied Sport Psychology, 3,* 87–107.

Breen, L., & Darlaston-Jones, D. (2008). *Moving beyond the enduring dominance of positivism in psychological research: An Australian perspective.* Paper presented at the 43rd Australian Psychological Society Annual Conference.

Brembs, B., & Munafò, M. (2013). Deep impact: Unintended consequences of journal rank. *arXiv preprint arXiv:1301.3748.*

Brentano, F. (1874). *Psychology from an empirical standpoint.* Leipzig, Germany: Duncker & Humblot.

Bruner, J. S. (1960). *The process of education.* Cambridge, MA: Harvard University Press.

Brunet, J., & Sabiston, C. M. (2011). Exploring motivation for physical activity across the adult lifespan. *Psychology of Sport and Exercise, 12*, 99–105.

Bryant, A., & Charmaz, K. (Eds.). (2007). *The Sage handbook of grounded theory.* London: Sage.

Bryant, R. A. (2003). Early predictors of posttraumatic stress disorder. *Biological Psychiatry, 53*, 789–795.

Bryman, A. (2006). Integrating quantitative and qualitative research: How is it done? *Qualitative Research, 6*, 97–113.

Callaway, E. (2016). Publishing elite turns against impact factor. *Nature, 535*, 210–211.

Carter, D. A., D'Souza, F., Simkins, B. J., & Simpson, W. G. (2010). The gender and ethnic diversity of US boards and board committees and firm financial performance. *Corporate Governance: An International Review, 18*(5), 396–414.

Caspersen, C. J. (1989). Physical activity epidemiology: Concepts, methods, and applications to exercise science. *Exercise and Sport Sciences Reviews, 17*, 423–474.

Centre for Reviews & Dissemination (CRD). (2009). *Systematic reviews: CRD's guidance for undertaking reviews in health care.* Centre for Reviews and Dissemination.

Chamberlain, K. (2000). Methodolatry and qualitative health research. *Journal of Health Psychology, 5*, 285–296.

Chambless, D. L. (1999). Empirically validated treatments – What now? *Applied and Preventive Psychology, 8*(4), 281–284.

Chambless, D. L. (2006). Psychotherapy research and practice: Friends or foes? *PsycCRITIQUES, 52*(1), article 5.

Chambless, D. L., & Ollendick, T. H. (2001). Empirically supported psychological interventions. Controversies and evidence. *Annual Review of Psychology, 52*, 685–716.

Charmaz, K. (2000). Constructivist and objectivist grounded theory. *Handbook of Qualitative Research, 2,* 509–535.

Charmaz, K. (2006). *Constructing grounded theory* London: Sage.

Chin, N. S., Khoo, S., & Low, W. Y. (2012). Self-determination and goal orientation in track and field. *Journal of Human Kinetics, 33,* 151–161.

Church, M. A., Elliot, A. J., & Gable, S. L. (2001). Perceptions of classroom environment, achievement goals, and achievement outcomes. *Journal of Educational Psychology, 93*(1), 43.

Chwalisz, K. (2003). Evidence-based practice: A framework for twenty-first-century scientist-practitioner training. *The Counseling Psychologist, 31*(5), 497–528.

Corrie, S., & Callahan, M. M. (2000). A review of the scientist-practitioner model: Reflections on its potential contribution to counselling psychology within the context of current healthcare trends. *Psychology and Psychotherapy, 73,* 413.

Courtney, A., & Courtney, M. (2008). Comments regarding "on the nature of science". *Physics in Canada, 64,* 7–8.

Crits-Christoph, P., Chambless, D. L., & Markell, H. M. (2014). Moving evidence-based practice forward successfully: Commentary on Laska, Gurman, and Wampold. *Psychotherapy, 51,* 491–495.

Cronin, C., & Armour, K. M. (2015). Lived experience and community sport coaching: A phenomenological investigation. *Sport, Education and Society, 20,* 959–975.

Crowe, S. F., & Samartgis, J. (2015). ERA 2012 versus ERA 2010: Like the curate's egg … good in parts. *Australian Psychologist, 50,* 186–193.

Cruickshank, J. (2012). Positioning positivism, critical realism and social constructionism in the health sciences: A philosophical orientation. *Nursing Inquiry, 19,* 71–82.

Csikszentmihalyi, M. (2002). *Flow: The classic work on how to achieve happiness.* New York: Random House.

Culver, D., Gilbert, W., & Trudel, P. (2003). A decade of qualitative research published in sport psychology journals: 1990–1999. *The Sport Psychologist, 17,* 1–15.

Culver, D. M., Gilbert, W., & Sparkes, A. (2012). Qualitative research in sport psychology journals: The next decade 2000–2009 and beyond. *Sport Psychologist, 26,* 261–281.

Cunningham, G. B. (2008). Creating and sustaining gender diversity in sport organizations. *Sex Roles, 58*(1–2), 136–145.

Danziger, K. (1990). Generative metaphor and the history of psychological discourse. In *Metaphors in the history of psychology* (pp. 331–356). Cambridge, UK: Cambridge University Press.

Darbyshire, P. (2008). 'Never mind the quality, feel the width': The nonsense of 'quality', 'excellence', and 'audit' in education, health and research. *Collegian, 15*, 35–41.

Daud, N. M., & Husin, Z. (2004). Developing critical thinking skills in computer aided extended reading classes. *British Journal of Educational Technology, 35*(4), 477–487.

Deci, E. L., & Ryan, R. M. (2002). *Handbook of self-determination research.* Rochester, NY: University Rochester Press.

Demerouti, E., Bakker, A. B., Vardakou, I., & Kantas, A. (2003). The convergent validity of two burnout instruments: A multitrait-multimethod analysis. *European Journal of Psychological Assessment, 19*(1), 12–23.

Dennett, D. (1995). *Darwin's dangerous idea.* New York: Simon & Schuster.

Denzin, N. K. (2009). The elephant in the living room: Or extending the conversation about the politics of evidence. *Qualitative Research, 9*(2), 139–160.

Denzin, N. K. (2010). Moments, mixed methods, and paradigm dialogs. *Qualitative Inquiry, 16*(6), 419–427.

Denzin, N. K., & Lincoln, Y. S. (2005). *The Sage handbook of qualitative research.* London: Sage.

Dewar, A., & Horn, T. S. (1992). A critical analysis of knowledge construction in sport psychology. In *Advances in sport psychology* (pp. 13–22). Champaign, IL: Human Kinetics.

Dowling, G. R. (2014). Playing the citations game: From publish or perish to be cited or sidelined. *Australasian Marketing Journal, 22*, 280–287.

Downs, D. S., Savage, J. S., & Di Nallo, J. M. (2013). Self-determined to exercise? Leisure-time exercise behavior, exercise motivation, and exercise dependence in youth. *Journal of Physical Activity and Health, 10*(2), 176–184.

Doyle, J., & Cuthill, M. (2015). Does 'get visible or vanish' herald the end of 'publish or perish'? *Higher Education Research & Development, 34*(3), 671–674.

Drabick, D. A., & Goldfried, M. R. (2000). Training the scientist-practitioner for the 21st century: Putting the bloom back on the rose. *Journal of Clinical Psychology, 56*(3), 327–340.

Duda, J. L., & Allison, M. T. (1990). Cross-cultural analysis in exercise and sport psychology: A void in the field. *Journal of Sport & Exercise Psychology, 12*, 114–131.

Duda, J. L., & Hayashi, C. T. (1998). Measurement issues in cross-cultural research within sport and exercise psychology. *Advances in Sport and Exercise Psychology Measurement, 7*, 471–483.

Duda, J. L., & Nicholls, J. G. (1992). Dimensions of achievement motivation in schoolwork and sport. *Journal of Educational Psychology, 84*(3), 290–299.

Dunning, D. (2011). The Dunning-Kruger effect: On being ignorant of one's own ignorance. *Advances in Experimental Social Psychology, 44*, 247.

Dweck, C. S. (1986). Motivational processes affecting learning. *American Psychologist, 41*, 1040–1048.

Dweck, C. S., & Leggett, E. L. (1988). A social-cognitive approach to motivation and personality. *Psychological Review, 95*(2), 256–273.

Edmunds, J. A., Duda, J. L., & Ntoumanis, N. (2010). Psychological needs and the prediction of exercise-related cognitions and affect among an ethnically diverse cohort of adult women. *International Journal of Sport and Exercise Psychology, 8*(4), 446–463.

Elliot, A. J. (1999). Approach and avoidance motivation and achievement goals. *Educational Psychologist, 34*(3), 169–189.

Elliot, A. J., & Harackiewicz, J. M. (1996). Approach and avoidance achievement goals and intrinsic motivation: A mediational analysis. *Journal of Personality and Social Psychology, 70*, 461–475.

Elliot, A. J., & McGregor, H. A. (2001). A 2×2 achievement goal framework. *Journal of Personality and Social Psychology, 80*(3), 501–519.

Elliot, A. J., Murayama, K., & Pekrun, R. (2011). A 3×2 achievement goal model. *Journal of Educational Psychology, 103*(3), 632–648.

Eysenck, H. J. (1949). Training in clinical psychology: An English point of view. *American Psychologist, 4*(6), 173–176.

Farmanbar, R., Niknami, S., Lubans, D. R., & Hidarnia, A. (2013). Predicting exercise behaviour in Iranian college students: Utility of an integrated model of health behaviour based on the transtheoretical model and self-determination theory. *Health Education Journal, 72*(1), 56–69.

Farmer, J. D., & Foley, D. (2009). The economy needs agent-based modelling. *Nature, 460*(7256), 685–686.

Fechner, G. (1860/1966). *Elements of psychophysics.* New York: Holt, Rinehart and Winston (Original published in 1860).

Fechner, G. T. (1889). *Revision der Hauptpunkte der Psychophysik.* Wiesbaden, Germany: Breitkopf & Härtel.

Felde, K., Pensgaard, A. M., Lemyre, N., & Abrahamsen, F. E. (2010). Theory based Olympic intervention – The Norwegian experiences after Vancouver. Abstract in the Conference Proceedings of the 21st Annual Conference of the Association for the Advancement of Applied Sport Psychology (Miami, September 2006).

Fernandez-Duque, D., Evans, J., Christian, C., & Hodges, S. D. (2015). Superfluous neuroscience information makes explanations of psychological phenomena more appealing. *Journal of Cognitive Neuroscience, 27*, 926–944.

Feyerabend, P. (1970). Consolations for the specialist. In I. Lakatos & A. Musgrave (Eds.), *Criticism and the growth of knowledge* (pp. 197–230). Cambridge, UK: Cambridge University Press.

Feyerabend, P. (1975). *Against method.* London: Verso.

Feyerabend, P. (1978). *Science in a free society.* London: Verso.

Field, A. (2002). Appendix A: Required Pre-knowledge : A Linear Regression. In *Discovering Statistics with R* (Vol. 1, pp. 531–574). London: SAGE.

Field, A. (2013). *Discovering statistics using IBM SPSS statistics* (pp. 297–321). London: Sage.

Fischman, M. G. (2014). The importance of peer review: Thoughts on Knudson, Morrow, and Thomas (2014). *Research Quarterly for Exercise and Sport, 85*(4), 449–450.

Fisher, L. A., Butryn, T. M., & Roper, E. A. (2003). Applied research. *Sport Psychologist, 17*, 391–405.

Fisher, L. A., & Roper, E. A. (2015). Swimming upstream: Former diversity committee chairs' perceptions of the Association for Applied Sport Psychology's commitment to organizational diversity. *Journal of Applied Sport Psychology, 27*(1), 1–19.

Fortier, M. S., Wiseman, E., Sweet, S. N., O'Sullivan, T. L., Blanchard, C. M., Sigal, R. J., et al. (2011). A moderated mediation of motivation on physical activity in the context of the physical activity counseling randomized control trial. *Psychology of Sport and Exercise, 12*(2), 71–78.

Foucault, M. (1978). *The history of sexuality.* New York: Pantheon.

Frankfurt, H. (2005). *On Bullshit.* Princeton, NJ: Princeton University Press.

Fuller, S. (2006). *Kuhn vs. Popper: The struggle for the soul of science.* New York: Columbia University Press.

Fuller, S. (2014, July 13). Six principles for organising conferences in the 21st century. *The Sociological Imagination.* Retrieved from: http://sociologicalimagination.org/archives/15663

Gage, N. L. (1989). The paradigm wars and their aftermath. A "historical" sketch of research on teaching since 1989. *Educational Researcher, 18*, 4–10.

Gamberale, F. (1985). The perception of exertion. *Ergonomics, 28*, 299–308.

Garcia, J. (1981). Tilting at the paper mills of academia. *American Psychologist, 36*, 149–158.

Gardner, F. L., & Moore, Z. E. (2005). Using a case formulation approach in sport psychology consulting. *Sport Psychologist*, *19*(4), 430–445.

Gaston, A., Wilson, P. M., Mack, D. E., Elliot, S., & Prapavessis, H. (2013). Understanding physical activity behavior and cognitions in pregnant women: An application of self-determination theory. *Psychology of Sport and Exercise*, *14*(3), 405–412.

Gauch, H. G. (2003). *Scientific method in practice*. New York: Cambridge University Press.

Gaudiano, B. A., & Statler, M. A. (2001). The scientist-practitioner gap and graduate education: Integrating perspectives and looking forward. *The Clinical Psychologist*, *54*(4), 12–18.

Gill, D. L. (1994). A feminist perspective on sport psychology practice. *Sport Psychologist*, *8*, 411–411.

Gill, D. L. (2001). In search of feminist sport psychology: Then, now, and always. *Sport Psychologist*, *15*(4), 363–449.

Gillies, P. (1998). Effectiveness of alliances and partnerships for health promotion. *Health Promotion International*, *13*(2), 99–120.

Glaser, B. G. (1978). *Theoretical sensitivity: Advances in the methodology of grounded theory*. Mill Valley, CA: Sociology Press.

Glaser, B. G. (1992). *Emergence vs forcing: Basics of grounded theory analysis*. Mill Valley, CA: Sociology Press.

Glaser, B. G. (2015). The cry for help. *The Grounded Theory Review*, *14*(1), 3–10.

Glaser, B. G., & Strauss, A. L. (1967). *The discovery of grounded theory: Strategies for qualitative research*. Chicago: Aldine.

Goedeke, S. (2007). Teaching psychology at undergraduate level: Rethinking what we teach and how we teach it. *New Zealand Journal of Teacher's Work*, *4*(1), 48–63.

Gould, D., & Pick, S. (1995). Sport psychology: The Griffith era, 1920–1940. *The Sport Psychologist*, *9*, 391–405.

Graziano, A. M., & Raulin, M. L. (2010). *Research methods: A process of inquiry* (7th ed.). Boston: Pearson Education.

Green, C. D. (2003). Psychology strikes out: Coleman R. Griffith and the Chicago Cubs. *History of Psychology*, *6*, 267–283.

Griffith, C. R. (1925). Psychology and its relation to athletic competition. *American Physical Education Review*, *30*, 193–199.

Griffith, C. R. (1926). *The psychology of coaching: A study of coaching methods from the point of psychology*. New York: Scribner's.

Griffith, C. R. (1928). *Psychology and athletics: A general survey for athletes and coaches.* New York: Scribner's.

Griffiths, P., & Norman, I. (2013). Qualitative or quantitative? Developing and evaluating complex interventions: Time to end the paradigm war. *International Journal of Nursing Studies, 50,* 583–584.

Griffiths, R. (2004). Knowledge production and the research-teaching nexus: The case of the built environment disciplines. *Studies in Higher Education, 29*(6), 709–726.

Guba, E. G., & Lincoln, Y. S. (1994). Competing paradigms in qualitative research. In N. K. Denzin & Y. S. Lincoln (Eds.), *Handbook of qualitative research* (pp. 105–117). Thousand Oaks, CA: Sage.

Guba, E. G., & Lincoln, Y. S. (2000). *Handbook of qualitative research.* Thousand Oaks, CA: Sage.

Guzmán, J. F., & Kingston, K. (2012). Prospective study of sport dropout: A motivational analysis as a function of age and gender. *European Journal of Sport Science, 12*(5), 431–442.

Guzmán, J. F., Kingston, K., & Grijalbo, C. (2015). Predicting coaches' adherence/dropout: A prospective study. *International Journal of Sports Science & Coaching, 10*(2–3), 353–363.

Hammersley, M. (1990). *The dilemma of qualitative method: Herbert Blumer and the Chicago tradition.* London: Routledge.

Hands, D. W. (1985). Second thoughts on Lakatos. *History of Political Economy, 17,* 1–16.

Hanrahan, S. (2014). Athletes with physical *disabilities.* In S. Hanrahan & M. Andersen (Eds.), *Routledge handbook of applied sport psychology* (pp. 432–440). London: Routledge.

Hansen, J. T. (2004). Thoughts on knowing: Epistemic implications of counseling practice. *Journal of Counseling & Development, 82,* 131–138.

Harden, R., & Stamper, N. (1999). What is a spiral curriculum? *Medical Teacher, 21*(2), 141–143.

Hardy, L. (1996). Testing the predictions of the cusp catastrophe model of anxiety and performance. *Sport Psychologist, 10,* 140–156.

Harwood, C. (2015). *Doing sport psychology? Critical reflections as a scientist-practitioner. Proceedings of the FEPSAC Conference.* Retrieved September 8, 2015, from http://www.fepsac2015.ch/keynote_lectures.html#chris

Harwood, C., & Hardy, L. (2001). Persistence and effort in moving achievement goal research forward: A response to treasure and colleagues. *Journal of Sport & Exercise Psychology, 23*(4), 330–345.

Harwood, C., Hardy, L., & Swain, A. (2000). Achievement goals in sport: A critique of conceptual and measurement issues. *Journal of Sport & Exercise Psychology, 22*, 235–255.

Harwood, C., Spray, C. M., & Keegan, R. (2008). Achievement goal theories in sport. In T.S. Horn (Ed.), *Advances in sport psychology* (3rd ed., pp. 157–185, 444–448). Champaign, IL: Human Kinetics.

Harwood, C. G., Keegan, R. J., Smith, J. M., & Raine, A. S. (2015). A systematic review of the intrapersonal correlates of motivational climate perceptions in sport and physical activity. *Psychology of Sport and Exercise, 18*, 9–25.

Haslam, N., & Koval, P. (2010). Possible research area bias in the Excellence in Research for Australia (ERA) draft journal rankings. *Australian Journal of Psychology, 62*(2), 112–114.

Hassard, J. (1988). Overcoming hermeticism in organization theory: An alternative to paradigm incommensurability. *Human Relations, 41*(3), 247–259.

Hassmén, P., & Koivula, N. (1997). Mood, physical working capacity and cognitive performance in the elderly as related to physical activity. *Aging: Clinical and Experimental Research, 9*, 136–142.

Hayes, S. C., Barlow, D. H., & Nelson-Gray, R. O. (1999). *The scientist practitioner: Research and accountability in the age of managed care* (2nd ed.). Boston: Allyn & Bacon.

Hawking, S. (1988). *A brief history of time. From the Big Bang to black holes.* London: Bantam Dell Publishing Group.

Healey, M. (2005). Linking research and teaching to benefit student learning. *Journal of Geography in Higher Education, 29*(2), 183–201.

Hearnshaw, L. S. (1987). *The shaping of modern psychology.* London: Routledge & Kegan Paul.

Heisenberg, W. (1958). *Physics and philosophy.* London: Penguin Books Ltd.

Herdman, A. O., & McMillan-Capehart, A. (2010). Establishing a diversity program is not enough: Exploring the determinants of diversity climate. *Journal of Business and Psychology, 25*(1), 39–53.

Hesse-Biber, S. N. (2010). *Mixed methods research: Merging theory with practice.* New York: Guilford Press.

Hollings, S. C., Mallett, C. J., & Hume, P. A. (2014). The World Junior Athletics Championships: New Zealand athletes' lived experiences. *International Journal of Sports Science & Coaching, 9*, 1357–1374.

Holt, N. L., & Tamminen, K. A. (2010a). Moving forward with grounded theory in sport and exercise psychology. *Psychology of Sport and Exercise, 11*(6), 419–422.

Holt, N. L., & Tamminen, K. A. (2010b). Improving grounded theory research in sport and exercise psychology: Further reflections as a response to Mike Weed. *Psychology of Sport and Exercise, 11*(6), 405–413.

Horrobin, D. F. (1990). The philosophical basis of peer review and the suppression of innovation. *JAMA, 263*(10), 1438–1441.

Howitt, S. M., & Wilson, A. N. (2014). Revisiting "is the scientific paper a fraud?". *EMBO Reports, 15*(5), 481–484.

Hull, D. L. (1990). *Science as a process: An evolutionary account of the social and conceptual development of science.* Chicago: University of Chicago Press.

Hulleman, C. S., Schrager, S. M., Bodmann, S. M., & Harackiewicz, J. M. (2010). A meta-analytic review of achievement goal measures: Different labels for the same constructs or different constructs with similar labels? *Psychological Bulletin, 136*(3), 422.

Hume, D. (1738/9). *A treatise of human nature.* London: Noon.

Inoue, Y., Wegner, C. E., Jordan, J. S., & Funk, D. C. (2015). Relationships between self-determined motivation and developmental outcomes in sport-based positive youth development. *Journal of Applied Sport Psychology, 27*(4), 371–383.

Jackson, M. R. (2015). Resistance to qual/quant parity: Why the "paradigm" discussion can't be avoided. *Qualitative Psychology, 2*, 181–198.

Jackson, S. A. (1996). Toward a conceptual understanding of the flow experience in elite athletes. *Research Quarterly for Exercise and Sport, 67*(1), 76–90.

Jackson, S. A., Martin, A. J., & Eklund, R. C. (2008). Long and short measures of flow: Examining construct validity of the FSS-2, DFS-2 and new brief counterparts. *Journal of Sport and Exercise Psychology, 30*, 561–587.

Jackson, S. A., & Roberts, G. C. (1992). Positive performance states of athletes: Toward a conceptual understanding of peak performance. *The Sport Psychologist, 6*(2), 156–171.

Johnson, R. B., Onwuegbuzie, A. J., & Turner, L. A. (2007). Toward a definition of mixed methods research. *Journal of Mixed Methods Research, 1*(2), 112–133.

Kahneman, D. (2011). *Thinking, fast and slow.* New York: Farrar, Straus, and Giroux..

Kahneman, D. (2012). A proposal to deal with questions about priming effects. Open letter, September 26, 2012. http://www.nature.com/polopoly_fs/7.6716.1349271308!/suppinfoFile/Kah neman%20Letter.pdf

Kamphoff, C. S., Gill, D. L., Araki, K., & Hammond, C. C. (2010). A content analysis of cultural diversity in the Association for Applied Sport Psychology's conference programs. *Journal of Applied Sport Psychology, 22*(2), 231–245.

Kanfer, R. (1990). Motivation theory and industrial and organizational psychology. In M. D. Dunnerre (Ed.), *Handbook of industrial and organizational psychology* (Vol. 1, 2nd ed., pp. 75–130). Palo Alto, CA: Consulting Psychologists Press.

Kant, I. (1783/1985). Prolegomena to any future metaphysics that will be able to come forward as science (original published in 1783: Prolegomena zu einer jeden künftigen Metaphysik, die als Wissenschaft wird auftreten können). *Ellington, Philosophy of Material Nature.*

Kaplan, A., & Maehr, M. L. (2007). The contributions and prospects of goal orientation theory. *Educational Psychology Review, 19*(2), 141–184.

Kass, R. E., Caffo, B. S., Davidian, M., Meng, X.-L., Yu, B., & Reid, N. (2016). Ten simple rules for effective statistical practice. *PLoS Computational Biology, 12,* e1004961.

Keatley, D., Clarke, D. D., & Hagger, M. S. (2012). Investigating the predictive validity of implicit and explicit measures of motivation on condom use, physical activity and healthy eating. *Psychology & Health, 27*(5), 550–569.

Keegan, R. (2015). *Being a sport psychologist.* Basingstoke, UK: Palgrave Macmillan.

Keegan, R. J., Harwood, C. G., Spray, C. M., & Lavallee, D. (2014). A qualitative investigation of the motivational climate in elite sport. *Psychology of Sport and Exercise, 15*(1), 97–107.

Keegan, R., Spray, C. M., Harwood, C., & Lavallee, D. (2010). The motivational atmosphere in youth sport: Coach, parent and peer influences on motivation in specializing sport participants. *Journal of Applied Sport Psychology, 22,* 87–105

Kenttä, G., & Hassmén, P. (2002). Underrecovery and overtraining: A conceptual model. In M. Kellmann (Ed.), *Enhancing recovery: Preventing underperformance in athletes* (pp. 57–79). Champaign, IL: Human Kinetics.

Kerr, J. H. (1997). *Motivation and emotion in sport: Reversal theory.* Hove, UK: Psychology Press.

Khalil, E. (1987). Kuhn, Lakatos, and the history of economic thought. *International Journal of Social Economics, 14*(3/4/5), 118–131.

Kim, S. (2003). Research paradigms in organizational learning and performance: Competing modes of inquiry. *Information Technology, Learning, and Performance Journal, 21*(1), 9.

Kirschner, S. R. (2011). Critical thinking and the end(s) of psychology. *Journal of Theoretical and Philosophical Psychology, 31,* 173–183.

Knudson, D. V., Morrow, J. R., Jr., & Thomas, J. R. (2014). Advancing kinesiology through improved peer review. *Research Quarterly for Exercise and Sport, 85*(2), 127–135.

Koch, S. (1981). The nature and limits of psychological knowledge: Lessons of a century "qua science". *American Psychologist, 36*(3), 257–269.

Kornspan, A. S. (2013). Alfred W. Hubbard and the Sport Psychology Laboratory at the University of Illinois, 1950–1970. *The Sport Psychologist, 27,* 244–257.

Krane, V. (1994). A feminist perspective on contemporary sport psychology research. *Sport Psychologist, 8,* 393–410.

Krauss, S. (2008). A tripartite model of idiographic research: Progressing past the concept of idiographic research as a singular entity. *Social Behavior and Personality, 36,* 1123–1140.

Kroll, W., & Lewis, G. (1969). The first academic degree in physical education. *Journal of Health, Physical Education, Recreation, 40*(6), 73–74.

Kruger, J., & Dunning, D. (1999). Unskilled and unaware of it: How difficulties in recognizing one's own incompetence lead to inflated self-assessments. *Journal of Personality and Social Psychology, 77*(6), 1121–34. doi:10.1037/0022-3514.77.6.1121.

Kuhn, T. S. (1962/1996). *The structure of scientific revolutions.* Chicago: University of Chicago Press.

Kuhn, T. S. (1970). Logic of discovery or psychology of research? In I. Lakatos & A. Musgrave (Eds.), *Criticism and the growth of knowledge* (pp. 1–24). Cambridge, UK: Cambridge University Press.

Kuhn, T. S. (1974). Second thoughts on paradigms. *The Structure of Scientific Theories, 2,* 459–482.

Kvale, S. (1996). *InterViews: An introduction to qualitative research interviewing.* San Diego, CA: Sage Publications.

Lakatos, I. (1970). Falsification and the methodology of scientific research programmes. In I. Lakatos & A. Musgrave (Eds.), *Criticism and the growth of knowledge* (pp. 91–196). Cambridge, UK: Cambridge University Press.

Lakatos, I., & Musgrave, A. (1970). *Criticism and the growth of knowledge.* Cambridge, UK: Cambridge University Press.

Lambdin, C. (2012). Significance tests as sorcery: Science is empirical-significance tests are not. *Theory & Psychology, 22,* 67–90.

Lamiell, J. T. (1981). Toward an idiothetic psychology of personality. *American Psychologist, 36,* 276–289.

Landers, D. M. (1983). Whatever happened to theory testing in sport psychology? *Journal of Sport Psychology, 5,* 135–151.

Landers, D. M. (1995). Sport psychology: The formative years, 1950–1980. *The Sport Psychologist, 9,* 406–417.

Landers, D. M., & Arent, S. M. (2010). Arousal performance relationships. In J. M. Williams (Ed.), *Applied sport psychology* (pp. 221–246). Mountainview, CA: Mayfield.

Landrum, B., & Garza, G. (2015). Mending fences: Defining the domains and approaches of quantitative and qualitative research. *Qualitative Psychology, 2*(2), 199–209.

Laudan, L. (1977). *Progress and its problems: Towards a theory of scientific growth.* Berkeley, CA/Los Angeles: The University of California Press.

Lee, M. S. Y. (2002). Divergent evolution, hierarchy and cladistics. *Zool. Scripta, 31*(2), 217–219.

Lee, P. H., Macfarlane, D. J., Lam, T. H., & Stewart, S. M. (2011). Validity of the international physical activity questionnaire short form (IPAQ-SF): A systematic review. *International Journal of Behavioral Nutrition and Physical Activity, 8*, 115.

Lee, R. T., & Ashforth, B. E. (1996). A meta-analytic examination of the correlates of the three dimensions of job burnout. *Journal of Applied Psychology, 81*(2), 123–133.

Leslie, L. M. (2014). A status-based multilevel model of ethnic diversity and work unit performance. *Journal of Management.* doi:10.1177/0149206314535436.

Leunes, A., & Burger, J. (2000). Profile of mood states research in sport and exercise psychology: Past, present, and future. *Journal of Applied Sport Psychology, 12*, 5–15.

Leung, W., Shaffer, C. D., Reed, L. K., Smith, S. T., Barshop, W., Dirkes, W., et al. (2015). Drosophila Muller F elements maintain a distinct set of genomic properties over 40 million years of evolution. Genes, 5, 719–740

Lewin, B. D. (1952). Phobic symptoms and dream interpretation. *The Psychoanalytic Quarterly, 21*(3), 295–322.

Lilienfeld, S. O., Ammirati, R., & David, M. (2012). Distinguishing science from pseudoscience in school psychology: Science and scientific thinking as safeguards against human error. *Journal of School Psychology, 50*, 7–36.

Lincoln, Y. S. (2010). "What a long, strange trip it's been…": Twenty-five years of qualitative and new paradigm research. *Qualitative Inquiry, 16*, 3–9.

Lincoln, Y. S., & Guba, E. G. (1985). *Naturalistic inquiry* (Vol. 75). Beverly Hills, CA: Sage.

Lindahl, J., Stenling, A., Lindwall, M., & Colliander, C. (2015). Trends and knowledge base in sport and exercise psychology research: A bibliometric review study. *International Review of Sport and Exercise Psychology, 8*, 71–94.

Lingard, L., Albert, M., & Levinson, W. (2008). Grounded theory, mixed methods, and action research. *British Medical Journal, 337*(a567), 459–461.

Loehle, C. (1990). A guide to increased creativity in research-inspiration or perspiration? *Bioscience, 40,* 123–128.

Lovie, A. D. (1997). Commentary on Michell, quantitative science and the definition of measurement in psychology. *British Journal of Psychology, 88,* 393–394.

Lukes, S. (2005). *Power: A radical view.* Hampshire, UK: Palgrave.

Lunde, Å., Heggen, K., & Strand, R. (2012). Knowledge and power: Exploring unproductive interplay between quantitative and qualitative researchers. *Journal of Mixed Methods Research, 7,* 197–210.

Lundkvist, E., Gustafsson, H., Hjälm, S., & Hassmén, P. (2012). An interpretative phenomenological analysis of burnout and recovery in elite soccer coaches. *Qualitative Research in Sport, Exercise and Health, 4,* 400–419.

Lundkvist, E., Stenling, A., Gustafsson, H., & Hassmén, P. (2014). How to measure coach burnout: An evaluation of three burnout measures. *Measurement in Physical Education and Exercise Science, 18,* 209–226.

Macal, C. M., & North, M. J. (2010). Tutorial on agent-based modelling and simulation. *Journal of Simulation, 4*(3), 151–162.

Madill, A. (2015). Qualitative research is not a paradigm: Commentary on Jackson (2015) and Landrum and Garza (2015). *Qualitative Psychology, 2,* 214–220.

Magee, B. (1973). *Popper.* London: Penguin.

Magee, B. (1998). *Confessions of a philosopher.* London: Phoenix.

Marin, L. M., & Halpern, D. F. (2011). Pedagogy for developing critical thinking in adolescents: Explicit instruction produces greatest gain. *Thinking Skills and Creativity, 6,* 1–13.

Markland, D., & Tobin, V. J. (2010). Need support and behavioural regulations for exercise among exercise referral scheme clients: The mediating role of psychological need satisfaction. *Psychology of Sport and Exercise, 11*(2), 91–99.

Martens, M. P., Mobley, M., & Zizzi, S. J. (2000). Multicultural training in applied sport psychology. *Sport Psychologist, 14*(1), 81–97.

Martens, R. (1979). About smocks and jocks. *Journal of Sport Psychology, 1*(2), 94–99.

Martens, R. (1987). Science, knowledge, and sport psychology. *The Sport Psychologist, 1*(1), 29–55.

Martin, A. J. (2006). Personal bests (PBs): A proposed multidimensional model and empirical analysis. *British Journal of Educational Psychology, 76,* 803–825.

Martinent, G., Decret, J. C., Guillet-Descas, E., & Isoard-Gautheur, S. (2014). A reciprocal effects model of the temporal ordering of motivation and burnout among youth table tennis players in intensive training settings. *Journal of Sports Sciences, 32*(17), 1648–1658.

Maslach, C., & Jackson, S. E. (1981). The measurement of experienced burnout. *Journal of Organizational Behavior, 2*(2), 99–113.

Masterman, M. (1970). The nature of a paradigm. In I. Lakotos & A. Musgrave (Eds.), *Criticism and the growth of knowledge* (pp. 59–91). Cambridge, UK: Cambridge University Press.

Matos, L., Lens, W., & Vansteenkiste, M. (2007). Achievement goals, learning strategies and language achievement among Peruvian high school students. *Psychologica Belgica, 47*(1), 51–70.

McCann, T. V., & Clark, E. (2003). A grounded theory study of the role that nurses play in increasing clients' willingness to access community mental health services. *International Journal of Mental Health Nursing, 12*(4), 279–287.

McGannon, K. R., & Schweinbenz, A. N. (2011). Traversing the qualitative-quantitative divide using mixed methods: Some reflections and reconciliations for sport and exercise psychology. *Qualitative Research in Sport, Exercise and Health, 3*(3), 370–384.

McIntyre, N., & Popper, K. (1983). The critical attitude in medicine: The need for a new ethics. *British Medical Journal (Clinical research ed.), 287*(6409), 1919–1923.

McNair, D. M., Lorr, M., & Droppleman, L. F. (1971/1992). *Revised manual for the profile of mood states*. San Diego, CA: Educational and Industrial Testing Services.

Medawar, P. (1969). *Induction and intuition in scientific thought*. Philadelphia: American Philosophical Society.

Medawar, P. B. (1963). Is the scientific paper a fraud? In P. B. Medawar (Ed.) (1990), *The threat and the glory: Reflections on science and scientists* (pp. 228–233). London: HarperCollins.

Merton, R. K. (1968). *Social theory and social structure*. New York: Simon and Schuster.

Merton, R. K. (1975). Insiders and outsiders: A chapter in the sociology of knowledge. *American Journal of Sociology, 78*(1), 9–47.

Meyer, J., & Land, R. (2006). *Overcoming barriers to student understanding: Threshold concepts and troublesome knowledge*. London: Routledge.

Michell, J. (1990). *An introduction to the logic of psychological measurement*. Hillsdale, NJ: Erlbaum.

Michell, J. (1996). S.S. Stevens' definition of measurement: The illogicality of an intellectual virus. In C. R. Latimer & J. Michell (Eds.), *At once scientific and philosophic: A Festschrift for John Philip Sutcliffe* (pp. 81–96). Brisbane, Australia: Boombana.

Michell, J. (1997a). Quantitative science and the definition of measurement in psychology. *British Journal of Psychology, 88*, 355–383.

Michell, J. (1997b). Reply to Kline, Laming, Lovie, Luce and Morgan. *British Journal of Psychology, 88*, 401–406.

Michell, J. (1999). *Measurement in psychology: Critical history of a methodological concept*. Cambridge, UK: Cambridge University Press.

Michell, J. (2000). Normal science, pathological science and psychometrics. *Theory & Psychology, 10*(5), 639–667.

Mill, J. S. (1843). *A system of logic: Ratiocinative and inductive: Vol. I*. London: John W. Parker, West Strand.

Milne, D., & Paxton, R. (1998). A psychological re-analysis of the scientist-practitioner model. *Clinical Psychology & Psychotherapy, 5*(4), 216–230.

Morgan, W. P. (1985). Affective beneficence of vigorous physical activity. *Medicine & Science in Sports & Exercise, 17*, 94–100.

Motterlini, M. (1999). *For and against method: including Lakatos's lectures on scientific method and the Lakatos-Feyerabend correspondence*. Chicago: University of Chicago Press.

Moustafa, K. (2014). Don't fall in common science pitfall! *Frontiers in Plant Science, 5*, 536.

Munro, G. D., & Munro, J. E. (2000). Using daily horoscopes to demonstrate expectancy confirmation. *Teaching of Psychology, 27*, 114–116.

Munz, P. (1985). *Our knowledge of the growth of knowledge: Popper or Wittgenstein?* London: Routledge.

Murayama, K., Elliot, A., & Friedman, R. (2012). Achievement goals. In *The Oxford handbook of human motivation* (pp. 191–207). New York: Oxford University Press.

Naoi, A., Watson, J., Deaner, H., & Sato, M. (2011). Multicultural issues in sport psychology and consultation. *International Journal of Sport and Exercise Psychology, 9*(2), 110–125.

Narens, L., & Luce, R. D. (1986). Measurement: The theory of numerical assignments. *Psychological Bulletin, 99*(2), 166–180.

National Science Education Standards (1996). Washington, DC: National Academy Press.

Nauman, E. A., Breedlove, K. M., Breedlove, E. L., Talavage, T. M., Robinson, M. E., & Leverenz, L. J. (2015). Post-season neurophysiological deficits assessed by imPACT and fMRI in athletes competing in American Football. *Developmental Neuropsychology, 40*, 85–91.

Neary, M. (2012). Teaching politically: Policy, pedagogy and the new European university. *Journal for Critical Education Policy Studies, 10*(2), 233–257.

Nicholls, J. G. (1984). Achievement motivation: Conceptions of ability, subjective experience, task choice, and performance. *Psychological Review, 91*(3), 328–346.

Nicholls, J. G. (1989). *The competitive ethos and democratic education.* Cambridge, MA: Harvard University Press.

Noble, B. J., & Noble, J. M. (1998). Perceived exertion: The measurement. In J. L. Duda (Ed.), *Advances in sport and exercise psychology measurement* (pp. 351–360). Morgantown, West Virginia: Fitness Information Technology.

Norman, G. (2010). Likert scales, levels of measurement and the "laws" of statistics. *Advances in Health Sciences Education, 15*(5), 625–632.

Ntoumanis, N., & Biddle, S. J. (1999). A review of motivational climate in physical activity. *Journal of Sports Sciences, 17*(8), 655–665.

Ntoumanis, N., & Myers, N. D. (2015). *An introduction to intermediate and advanced statistical analyses for sport and exercise scientists.* London: Wiley.

Nunnally, J. (1978). *Psychometric methods.* New York: McGraw-Hill.

O'Cathain, A., Murphy, E., & Nicholl, J. (2007). Why, and how, mixed methods research is undertaken in health services research in England: A mixed methods study. *BMC Health Services Research, 7*, 85.

O'Gorman, J. (2001). The scientist-practitioner model and its critics. *Australian Psychologist, 36*(2), 164–169.

Oglesby, C. A. (2001). To unearth the legacy. *Sport Psychologist, 15*(4), 373–385.

Onwuegbuzie, A. J., & Leech, N. L. (2005). On becoming a pragmatic researcher: The importance of combining quantitative and qualitative research methodologies. *International Journal of Social Research Methodology, 8*, 375–387.

Oreskes, N., Shrader-Frechette, K., & Belitz, K. (1994). Verification, validation, and confirmation of numerical models in the earth sciences. *Science, 263*(5147), 641–646.

Page, A. (1996). The scientist-practitioner model: More faces than Eve. *Australian Psychologist, 31*(2), 103–108.

Panayides, P. (2013). Coefficient alpha. *Europe's Journal of Psychology, 9*, 687–696.

Petrie, T. A., Cogan, K. D., Van Raalte, J. L., & Brewer, B. W. (1996). Gender and the evaluation of sport psychology consultants. *Sport Psychologist, 10*, 132–139.

Piggott, D. (2010a). Listening to young people in leisure research: The critical application of grounded theory. *Leisure Studies, 29*(4), 415–433.

Piggott, D. (2010b). The grounded theory debate in sport psychology: Essentialism, anarchism or critical rationalism? *Paper presented at the BPS DSPE conference*, London.

Pintrich, P. (2000). An achievement goal theory perspective on issues in motivation terminology, theory, and research. *Contemporary Educational Psychology, 25*(1), 92–104.

Pitts, D., & Jarry, E. (2007). Ethnic diversity and organizational performance: Assessing diversity effects at the managerial and street levels. *International Public Management Journal, 10*(2), 233–254.

Plateau, J., & des lettres et des beaux-arts de Belgique Académie royale des sciences. (1872). *Sur la mesure des sensations physiques, et sur la loi qui lie l'intensité de la cause excitante.*

Ploszay, A. (2003). *The experience of providing expert sport psychology consultation: An existential phenomenological investigation.* Unpublished doctoral dissertation, University of Tennessee, Knoxville.

Poczwardowski, A., Aoyagi, M. W., Shapiro, J. L., & Van Raalte, J. L. (2014). Developing professional philosophy for sport psychology consulting practice. In A. Papaioannou & D. Hackfort (Eds.), *Routledge companion to sport and exercise psychology: Global perspectives and fundamental concepts* (pp. 895–907). London: Routledge.

Popper, K. (1945). *The open society and its enemies: Vols. 1 & 2..* London: Routledge.

Popper, K. (1959). *The logic of scientific discovery.* London: Hutchinson.

Popper, K. (1963/1969). *Conjectures and refutations. The growth of scientific knowledge.* London: Routledge.

Popper, K. (1978). *Unended quest: An intellectual autobiography.* London: Routledge.

Popper, K. (1994). *The myth of the framework: In defense of science and rationality.* London: Routledge.

Popper, K. R. (1934). *Logik der forschung.* London: Hutchinson.

Popper, K. R. (1963). *Conjectures and refutations: The growth of scientific knowledge.* New York: Harper & Row.

Popper, K. R. (1970). Normal science and its dangers. In I. Lakotos & A. Musgrave (Eds.), *Criticism and the growth of knowledge* (pp. 52–58). Cambridge, UK: Cambridge University Press.

Popper, K. R. (1974). Scientific reduction and the essential incompleteness of all science. In *Studies in the philosophy of biology* (pp. 259–284). London: Macmillan Education UK.

Popper, K. R. (2001). *The world of parmenides: Essays on the pre-socratic enlightenment.* London: Routledge.

Preston, J. (2008). *Kuhn's 'the structure of scientific revolutions': A reader's' guide.* London: Continuum.

Pringle, R. (2000). Physical education, positivism, and optimistic claims from achievement goal theorists. *Quest, 52*(1), 18–31.

Proctor, R., & Schiebinger, L. L. (Eds.). (2008). *Agnotology: The making and unmaking of ignorance*. Stanford, CA: Stanford University Press.

Raedeke, T. D., & Smith, A. L. (2001). Development and preliminary validation of an athlete burnout measure. *Journal of Sport & Exercise Psychology, 23,* 281–306.

Raimy, V. (Ed.). (1950). *Training in clinical psychology*. New York: Prentice-Hall.

Ram, N., Starek, J., & Johnson, J. (2004). Race, ethnicity, and sexual orientation: Still a void in sport and exercise psychology? *Journal of Sport & Exercise Psychology, 26,* 250–268.

Razon, S., Hutchinson, J., & Tenenbaum, G. (2012). Effort perception. In G. Tenenbaum, R. C. Eklund, & A. Kamata (Eds.), *Measurement in sport and exercise psychology* (pp. 265–278). Champaign, IL: Human Kinetics.

Reeves, T. C. (2006). Design research from the technology perspective. In J. V. Akker, K. Gravemeijer, S. McKenney, & N. Nieveen (Eds.), *Educational design research* (pp. 86–109). London: Routledge.

Remler, D. (2014). Are 90% of academic papers really never cited? Reviewing the literature on academic citations. London School of Economics Impact Blog.   http://blogs.lse.ac.uk/impactofsocialsciences/2014/04/23/academic-papers-citation-rates-remler/

Roberts, G. C. (2001). Understanding the dynamics of motivation in physical activity: The influence of achievement goals on motivational processes. In G. C. Roberts (Ed.), *Advances in motivation in sport and exercise* (pp. 1–50). Champaign, IL: Human Kinetics.

Roberts, G. C. (2012). Motivation in sport and exercise from an achievement goal theory perspective: After 30 years, where are we? In G. C. Roberts & D. C. Treasure (Eds.), *Advances in motivation in sport and exercise* (pp. 5–58). Champaign, IL: Human Kinetics.

Roberts, G. C., & Balagué, G. (1989, August). The development of a social-cognitive scale in motivation. In *Seventh World Congress of Sport Psychology, Singapore*.

Roberts, G. C., & Treasure, D. C. (2012). *Advances in motivation in sport and exercise* (3rd ed.). Champaign, IL: Human Kinetics.

Roberts, G. C., Treasure, D. C., & Balague, G. (1998). Achievement goals in sport: The development and validation of the perception of success questionnaire. *Journal of Sports Sciences, 16,* 337–347.

Romanyshyn, R. D. (1971). Method and meaning in psychology: The method has been the message. *Journal of Phenomenological Psychology, 2,* 93–114.

Roper, E. A., Fisher, L. A., & Wrisberg, C. A. (2005). Professional women's career experiences in sport psychology: A feminist standpoint approach. *The Sport Psychologist, 19*, 32–50.

Ross, L., & Ward, A. (1996). Naive realism in everyday life: Implications for social conflict and misunderstanding. In T. Brown, E. S. Reed, & E. Turiel (Eds.), *Values and knowledge* (pp. 103–135). Hillsdale, NJ: Erlbaum.

Rottensteiner, C., Tolvanen, A., Laakso, L., & Konttinen, N. (2015). Youth athletes' motivation, perceived competence, and persistence in organized team sports. *Journal of Sport Behavior, 38*(4), 432.

Rouse, P. C., Ntoumanis, N., Duda, J. L., Jolly, K., & Williams, G. C. (2011). In the beginning: Role of autonomy support on the motivation, mental health and intentions of participants entering an exercise referral scheme. *Psychology & Health, 26*(6), 729–749.

Rowbottom, D. P. (2011). Kuhn vs. Popper on criticism and dogmatism in science: A resolution at the group level. *Studies in History and Philosophy of Science, 42*(1), 117–124.

Rowley, A. J., Landers, D. M., Kyllo, L. B., & Etnier, J. F. (1995). Does the iceberg profile discriminate between successful and less successful athletes? A meta-analysis. *Journal of Sport and Exercise Psychology, 17*, 185–199.

Ryan, R. M., & Deci, E. L. (2000). Self-determination theory and the facilitation of intrinsic motivation, social development, and well-being. *American Psychologist, 55*(1), 68, 227–268.

Ryba, T. V., Schinke, R. J., & Tenenbaum, G. (2010). *The cultural turn in sport psychology*. Morgantown, WV: Fitness Information Technology.

Ryba, T. V., Stambulova, N. B., & Wrisberg, C. A. (2005). The Russian origins of sport psychology: A translation of an early work of A. C. Puni. *Journal of Applied Sport Psychology, 17*, 157–169.

Sagan, C. (1995). *Wonder and skepticism*. Skeptical Inquirer, 19, 1.

Sagan, C. (1996). *The demon-haunted world: Science as a candle in the dark* (pp. 304–306). New York: Balantine Books.

Sassower, R. (2006). *Popper's legacy: Rethinking politics, economics and science*. Stocksfield, UK: Acumen.

Sayer, A. (2010). *Method in social science*. London: Routledge.

Schaufeli, W. B., Leiter, M. P., Maslach, C., & Jackson, S. E. (1996). Maslach Burnout Inventory-General Survey. In C. Maslach, S. E. Jackson, & M. P. Leiter (Eds.), *The Maslach Burnout Inventory: Test manual* (3rd ed., pp. 22–26). Palo Alto, CA: Consulting Psychologists Press.

Schinke, R., & Hanrahan, S. J. (2009). *Cultural sport psychology*. Champaign, IL: Human Kinetics.

Schinke, R. J., McGannon, K. R., Parham, W. D., & Lane, A. M. (2012). Toward cultural praxis and cultural sensitivity: Strategies for self-reflexive sport psychology practice. *Quest, 64*(1), 34–46.

Schlösser, T., Dunning, D., Johnson, K. L., & Kruger, J. (2013). How unaware are the unskilled? Empirical tests of the "signal extraction" counterexplanation for the Dunning-Kruger effect in self-evaluation of performance. *Journal of Economic Psychology, 39*, 85–100.

Schmaltz, R., & Lilienfeld, S. O. (2014). Hauntings, homeopathy, and the Hopkinsville Goblins: Using pseudoscience to teach scientific thinking. *Frontiers in Psychology, 5*, 1–5.

Schneider, M. L., & Kwan, B. M. (2013). Psychological need satisfaction, intrinsic motivation and affective response to exercise in adolescents. *Psychology of Sport and Exercise, 14*(5), 776–785.

Schuklenk, U. (2015). On peer-review. *Bioethics, 29*, ii–iii.

Schwandt, T. A. (1996). Farewell to criteriology. *Qualitative Inquiry, 2*(1), 58–72.

Schwartz, M. A. (2008). The importance of stupidity in scientific research. *Journal of Cell Science, 121*(11), 1771.

Science and Engineering Indicators. (2016). https://www.nsf.gov/statistics/2016/nsb20161/uploads/1/nsb20161.pdf

Scripture, E. W. (1894). Tests of mental ability as exhibited in fencing. *Studies From the Yale psychological laboratory, 2*, 122–124.

Shapiro, D. (2002). Renewing the scientist practitioner model. *The Psychologist, 15*, 232–234.

Shapiro, M. B. (1955). Training of clinical psychologists at the Institute of Psychiatry. *Bulletin of the British Psychological Association, 8*, 1–6.

Shephard, R. J., & Aoyagi, Y. (2012). Measurement of human energy expenditure, with particular reference to field studies: An historical perspective. *European Journal of Applied Physiology, 112*, 2785–2815.

Shirom, A. (2005). Reflections on the study of burnout. *Work & Stress, 19*(3), 263–270.

Simons, J. P., & Andersen, M. B. (1995). The development of consulting practice in applied sport psychology: Some personal perspectives. *The Sport Psychologist, 9*, 449–468.

Skaalvik, E. M. (1997). Self-enhancing and self-defeating ego orientation: Relations with task and avoidance orientation, achievement, self-perceptions, and anxiety. *Journal of Educational Psychology, 89*(1), 71–81.

Smith, B., & Sparkes, A. (2012). Making sense of words and stories in qualitative research: Some strategies for consideration. In G. Tenenbaum, R. Eklund,

& A. Kamata (Eds.), *Handbook of measurement in sport and exercise psychology* (pp. 119–130). Champaign, IL: Human Kinetics.

Smith, B., & Sparkes, A. (2016). *Routledge handbook of qualitative research in sport and exercise.* London: Routledge.

Smith, B., & Sparkes, A. C. (2009). Narrative inquiry in sport and exercise psychology: What can it mean, and why might we do it? *Psychology of Sport and Exercise, 10*, 1–11.

Smith, D., & Bar-Eli, M. (2007). *Essential readings in sport and exercise psychology.* Darby, PA: DIANE Publishing Inc.

Smith, D. M. (2016). Neurophysiology of action anticipation in athletes: A systematic review. *Neuroscience and Biobehavioral Reviews, 60*, 115–120.

Smith, R. (2006). *The trouble with medical journals.* London: Royal Society of Medicine.

Sober, E. (1990). *Let's Razor Ockham's Razor. Royal Institute of Philosophy Supplement, 27*, 73–93. Retrieved from http://journals.cambridge.org/production/action/cjoGetFulltext?fulltextid=6217508

Sober, E. (1996). Parsimony and predictive equivalence. *Erkenntnis, 44*(1973), 167–197.

Sparkes, A. (2002). *Telling tales in sport and physical activity: A qualitative journey.* Champaign, IL: Human Kinetics.

Sparkes, A. C. (2013). Qualitative research in sport, exercise and health in the era of neoliberalism, audit and New Public Management: Understanding the conditions for the (im)possibilities of a new paradigm dialogue. *Qualitative Research in Sport, Exercise and Health, 5*, 440–459.

Sparkes, A. C. (2015). Developing mixed methods research in sport and exercise psychology: Critical reflections on five points of controversy. *Psychology of Sport and Exercise, 16*, 49–59.

Sparkes, A. C., & Smith, B. (2009). Judging the quality of qualitative inquiry: Criteriology and relativism in action. *Psychology of Sport and Exercise, 10*, 491–497.

Sparkes, A. C., & Smith, B. (2013). *Qualitative research methods in sport, exercise and health: From process to product.* London: Routledge.

Sproule, J., Martindale, R., Wang, J., Allison, P., Nash, C., & Gray, S. (2013). Investigating the experience of outdoor and adventurous project work in an educational setting using a self-determination framework. *European Physical Education Review, 19*(3), 315–328.

Standards for Educational and Psychological Testing (2014). Washington, DC: American Educational Research Association.

Statler, T. (2003). The art of applied sport psychology: Interviews with North America's outstanding consultants. In *20th AAASP Conference, Philadelphia, USA*.

Steel, P., & König, C. J. (2006). Integrating theories of motivation. *Academy of Management Review, 31*(4), 889–913.

Stellino, M., & Sinclair, C. D. (2013). Psychological predictors of children's recess physical activity motivation and behavior. *Research Quarterly for Exercise and Sport, 84*(2), 167–176.

Stevens, S. S. (1946). On the theory of scales of measurement. *Science, 103*, 677–680.

Stevens, S. S. (1951). Mathematics, measurement, and psychophysics. In *Handbook of experimental psychology* (pp. 1–49). Oxford, UK: Wiley.

Stevens, S. S. (1958). Problems and methods of psychophysics. *Psychological Bulletin, 55*, 177–196.

Stevens, S. S. (1961). To honor Fechner and repeal his law. *Science, 133*, 80–86.

Stevens, S. S. (1975). *Psychophysics: Introduction to its perceptual, neural, and social prospects*. New York: Wiley.

Stevens, S. S., & Davis, H. (1938). *Hearing: Its psychology and physiology*. New York: Wiley.

Stevens, S. S., Newman, E. B., & Volkmann, J. (1937). On the method of bisection and its relation to a loudness scale. *American Journal of Psychology, 49*, 134–137.

Stokes, D. E. (1997). *Pasteur's quadrant: Basic science and technological innovation*. Washington, DC: Brookings Institution Press.

Stoltenberg, C. D., Pace, T. M., Kashubeck-West, S., Biever, J. L., Patterson, T., & Welch, I. D. (2000). Training models in counseling psychology scientist-practitioner versus practitioner-scholar. *The Counseling Psychologist, 28*, 622–640.

Stoner, G., & Green, S. K. (1992). Reconsidering the scientist-practitioner model for school psychology practice. *School Psychology Review, 21*, 155–166.

Stove, D. C. (1982). *Popper and after: Four modern irrationalists*. Oxford, UK: Pergamon Press.

Straub, W. F., & Hinman, D. A. (1992). Profiles and professional perspectives of 10 leading sport psychologists. *Sport Psychologist, 6*, 297–312.

Strauss, A., & Corbin, J. (1994). Grounded theory methodology: an overview. In: N. Denzin & Y. Lincoln. (Eds), *Handbook of qualitative research*. (pp. 273-285). London: Sage.

Strauss, A., & Corbin, J. (1998). *Basics of qualitative research: Techniques and procedures for developing grounded theory*. Thousand Oaks, CA: Sage.

Strauss, B. (2002). Social facilitation in motor tasks: A review of research and theory. *Psychology of Sport and Exercise, 3*, 237-256.

Stricker, G. (1997). Are science and practice commensurable? *American Psychologist, 52*(4), 442–448.

Stricker, G. (2000). The scientist-practitioner model: Gandhi was right again. *American Psychologist, 55*(2), 253–254.

Suls, J., & Martin, R. (2009). The air we breathe: A critical look at practices and alternatives in the peer-review process. *Perspectives on Psychological Science, 4*(1), 40–50.

Swann, C., Crust, L., Keegan, R., Piggott, D., & Hemmings, B. (2015). An inductive exploration into the flow experiences of European tour golfers. *Qualitative Research in Sport, Exercise and Health, 7*, 210–234.

Swann, C., Keegan, R., Piggott, D., Crust, L., & Smith, M. F. (2012). Exploring flow occurrence in elite golf. *Athletic Insight, 4*, 171–186.

Taleb, N. N. (2007). *The black swan: The impact of the highly improbable.* New York: Random House.

Tapscott, D., & Williams, A. (2006). *Wikinomics: How mass communication changes everything.* New York: Portfolio.

Teddlie, C., & Tashakkori, A. (2011). Mixed methods research. In N. K. Denzin & Y. S. Lincoln (Eds.), *The Sage handbook of qualitative research* (pp. 285–300). London: Sage.

Teo, T. (2011). Radical philosophical critique and critical thinking in psychology. *Journal of Theoretical and Philosophical Psychology, 31*, 193–199.

Thomas, G., & James, D. (2006). Reinventing grounded theory: Some questions about theory, ground and discovery. *British Educational Research Journal, 32*(6), 767–795.

Thurber, J. (1939, February 18). The Scotty who knew too much. *New Yorker.*

Tourish, D. (2011). Leading questions: Journal rankings, academic freedom and performativity: What is, or should be, the future of *Leadership? Leadership, 7*, 367–381.

Trafimow, D., & Rice, S. (2009). Potential performance theory (PPT): Describing a methodology for analyzing task performance. *Behavior Research Methods, 41*, 359–371.

Treasure, D. C., & Robert, G. C. (2001). Students' perceptions of the motivational climate, achievement beliefs, and satisfaction in physical education. *Research Quarterly for Exercise and Sport, 72*, 165–175.

Tukey, J. W. (1962). The future of data analysis. *The Annals of Mathematical Statistics, 33*, 1–67.

Tversky, A., & Kahneman, D. (1974). Judgment under uncertainty: Heuristics and biases. *Science, 185*, 1124–1131.

Umans, T., Collin, S. O., & Tagesson, T. (2008). Ethnic and gender diversity, process and performance in groups of business students in Sweden. *Intercultural Education, 19*(3), 243–254.

Van den Berghe, L., Soenens, B., Vansteenkiste, M., Aelterman, N., Cardon, G., Tallir, I. B., et al. (2013). Observed need-supportive and need-thwarting teaching behavior in physical education: Do teachers' motivational orientations matter? *Psychology of Sport and Exercise, 14*(5), 650–661.

van Wesel, M. (2016). Evaluation by citation: Trends in publication behavior, evaluation criteria, and the strive for high impact publications. *Science and Engineering Ethics, 22*(1), 199–225.

Van Yperen, N. W. (2006). A novel approach to assessing achievement goals in the context of the 2×2 framework: Identifying distinct profiles of individuals with different dominant achievement goals. *Personality and Social Psychology Bulletin, 32*(11), 1432–1445.

Van Yperen, N. W., Blaga, M., & Postmes, T. (2014). A meta-analysis of self-reported achievement goals and nonself-report performance across three achievement domains (work, sports, and education). *PloS one, 9*(4), e93594.

Vansteenkiste, M., Lens, W., Elliot, A. J., Soenens, B., & Mouratidis, A. (2014). Moving the achievement goal approach one step forward: Toward a systematic examination of the autonomous and controlled reasons underlying achievement goals. *Educational Psychologist, 49*(3), 153–174.

Vaughn, B. K., & Daniel, S. R. (2012). Conceptualizing validity. In G. Tenenbaum, R. C. Eklund, & A. Kamata (Eds.), *Measurement in sport and exercise psychology* (pp. 33–39). Champaign, IL: Human Kinetics.

Vealey, R. S. (2006). Smocks and jocks outside the box: The paradigmatic evolution of sport and exercise psychology. *Quest, 58*, 128–159.

Vlachopoulos, S. P., Kaperoni, M., & Moustaka, F. C. (2011). The relationship of self-determination theory variables to exercise identity. *Psychology of Sport and Exercise, 12*(3), 265–272.

Waite, B. T., & Pettit, M. (1993). Work experiences of graduates from doctoral programs in sport psychology. *Journal of Applied Sport Psychology, 5*(2), 234–250.

Watson, J. D., & Crick, F. H. (1953). Molecular structure of nucleic acids. *Nature, 171*, 737–738.

Weed, M. (2009). Research quality considerations for grounded theory research in sport & exercise psychology. *Psychology of Sport and Exercise, 10*(5), 502–510.

Weed, M. (2010). A quality debate on grounded theory in sport and exercise psychology? A commentary on future areas for potential debate. *Psychology of Sport and Exercise*, 11, 414-418.

Weinberg, R. S. (1989). Applied sport psychology: Issues and challenges. *Journal of Applied Sport Psychology*, 1, 181–195.

Weinberg, R. S., & Gould, D. (1995). *Foundations of sport and exercise psychology* (1st ed.). Champaign, IL: Human Kinetics.

Weinberg, R. S., & Gould, D. (2015). *Foundations of sport and exercise psychology* (6th ed.). Champaign, IL: Human Kinetics.

Welk, G. (2002). *Physical activity assessments for health-related research.* Champaign, IL: Human Kinetics.

Williams, J. M. (2001). *Applied sport psychology: Personal growth to peak performance* (4th ed.). Palo Alto, CA: Mayfield Publishing.

Wundt, W. M. (1873–1874). *Grundzüge der physiologischen psychologie*, (2 volumes): *Principles of physiological psychology*. Leipzig, Germany: Engelmann.

Yambor, J., & Connelly, D. (1991). Issues confronting female sport psychology consultants working with male student-athletes. *The Sport Psychologist*, 5, 304–312.

Zahar, E. G. (1982). Feyerabend on observation and empirical content. *British Journal of the Philosophy of Science*, 33, 397–433.

Zajonc, R. B. (1965). *Social facilitation.* Research Center for Group Dynamics, Institute for Social Research, University of Michigan.

Zarrett, N., Sorensen, C., & Cook, B. S. (2015). Physical and social-motivational contextual correlates of youth physical activity in underresourced afterschool programs. *Health Education & Behavior*, 42, 518–529.

Zhu, W. (2012). Sadly, the earth is still round (p < 0.05). *Journal of Sport and Health Science*, 1, 9–11.

Zollman, C., & Vickers, A. (1999). ABC of complementary medicine: What is complementary medicine? *British Medical Journal*, 319(7211), 693.

Zuckerman, H. (1977). *Scientific elite: Nobel laureates in the United States.* London: Transaction Publishers.

Index

Note: Page numbers with "n" denote endnotes.

© The Author(s) 2016

P. Hassmén et al., *Rethinking Sport and Exercise Psychology Research*,
DOI 10.1057/978-1-137-48338-6